The Maudsley

The South London and Maudsley NHS Trust
&
Oxleas NHS Trust

2005–2006
PRESCRIBING
GUIDELINES

8th Edition

David Taylor
Carol Paton
Robert Kerwin

D0234100

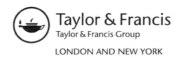

Taylor & Francis
Taylor & Francis Group

LONDON AND NEW YORK

© Taylor, Paton, Kerwin 2005

First published in the United Kingdom in 2005 by Taylor & Francis, an imprint of the Taylor & Francis Group, 2 Park Square, Milton Park, Abingdon, Oxon OX14 4RN

Tel.:   +44 (0)20 7017 6000
Fax.:   +44 (0)20 7017 6699
E-mail: info@dunitz.co.uk
Website: http://www.dunitz.co.uk

Although every effort has been made to ensure that all owners of copyright material have been acknowledged in this publication, we would be glad to acknowledge in subsequent reprints or editions any omissions brought to our attention.

Although every effort has been made to ensure that drug doses and other information are presented accurately in this publication, the ultimate responsibility rests with the prescribing physician. Neither the publishers nor the authors can be held responsible for errors or for any consequences arising from the use of information contained herein. For detailed prescribing information or instructions on the use of any product or procedure discussed herein, please consult the prescribing information or instructional material issued by the manufacturer.

A CIP record for this book is available from the British Library.

Library of Congress Cataloging-in-Publication Data

Data available on application

ISBN 1 84184 500 0

Distributed in North and South America by
Taylor & Francis
2000 NW Corporate Blvd
Boca Raton, FL 33431, USA

Within Continental USA
Tel: 800 272 7737; Fax: 800 374 3401
Outside Continental USA
Tel: 561 994 0555; Fax: 561 361 6018
E-mail: orders@crcpress.com

Distributed in the rest of the world by
Thomson Publishing Services
Cheriton House
North Way
Andover, Hampshire SP10 5BE, UK
Tel.: +44 (0)1264 332424
E-mail: salesorder.tandf@thomsonpublishingservices.co.uk

Composition by 𝕋 Tek-Art, Croydon, Surrey

Printed and bound in Great Britain by The Cromwell Press Ltd, Trowbridge, Wilts

Contents

Authors and editors

David Taylor, Senior Editor and Lead Author
Chief Pharmacist, South London and Maudsley NHS Trust
Honorary Senior Lecturer, Institute of Psychiatry

Carol Paton, Editor and Author
Chief Pharmacist, Oxleas NHS Trust

Robert Kerwin, Founding Editor
Professor of Clinical Neuropharmacology, Institute of Psychiatry
Consultant Psychiatrist, South London and Maudsley NHS Trust

Preface

The Maudsley Prescribing Guidelines have grown substantially in popularity in the last ten years, with over 100,000 copies sold of the first seven editions. *The Guidelines* are now widely used in the UK, Australia, New Zealand, Ireland and the Netherlands and have been translated into Italian, Japanese and Polish.

In this 8th edition we have expanded the scope of *The Guidelines* and included over twenty new sections. We have also revised and updated existing sections so as to include all data available to us at the end of January 2005.

We have also retained the standardised method in the construction of guidance and have studied literature reports identified from searches of EMBASE, Medline and PsychLIT performed during the last quarter of 2004 and January 2005. In addition, we have collected posters and abstracts from major conferences taking place throughout the world in 2003 and 2004. Retrieved reports have then been ranked according to their scientific validity in the usual way (meta-analyses first, then individual, randomised controlled trials, and so on) and guidance constructed where possible according to the ranking. We have again made use of the excellent Cochrane reviews of medication used in psychiatry. The number of references cited (over 1500 in this issue) continues to increase and to take-up a good deal of valuable space. In the next edition our intention is to place reference lists on the Internet (as is becoming customary) and therefore release space for practical guidance and discussion.

As with previous editions we are deeply indebted to a number of colleagues who have provided expert review of various sections. Particular thanks are due to Penny Maxwell, Specialist Clinical Pharmacist in Newcastle, Australia who, with colleagues, contributed the new section on prescribing in children. All of those who contributed to this edition are listed in the following acknowledgements section.

We hope that this 8th edition of *The Prescribing Guidelines* continues the tradition of providing practical and, where possible, evidence-based advice to mental health professionals. Remember that this is guidance, not instruction – the longer one works in mental health the more one is aware, to paraphrase Voltaire, that although doubt is uncomfortable, certainty is absurd.

David Taylor
February 2005

Acknowledgements

The Maudsley Prescribing Guidelines are a product of the authors' knowledge and expertise and the helpful contributions of a large number of specialists and experts. The input from these experts not only allows a greater range of subjects to be covered but also provides crucial, if informal, peer review of many sections. We are, therefore, deeply indebted to previous contributors and to the following contributors to the present edition of *The Guidelines*.

Caroline Ashley
David Ball
Thomas Barnes
David Burton
Anthony Cleare
Anne Connolly
Vivienne Curtis
Petrina Douglas-Hall
Sarah Elliot
Emily Finch
Bob Flanagan
Russel Foster
Maria Isaac
Mike Isaac
Cheryl Kipping
Julia Kuczynska
Nick Lintzeris
Shubhra Mace
Jane Marshall
Penelope Maxwell
Soraya Meyet
Kenneth Nunn
Banke Olofinjana
Maria O'Hagan
Veronica O'Keane
Suzanne Stewart
Karen Taylor
Arwel Thomas
Anne Uttley
Eromona Whiskey
Allan Young

Special thanks to

Jo Taylor

Notes on using *The Maudsley Prescribing Guidelines*

The main aim of *The Guidelines* is to provide clinicians with practically useful advice on the prescribing of psychotropic agents in commonly encountered clinical situations. The advice contained in this handbook is based on a combination of literature review, clinical experience and expert contribution. We do not claim that this advice is necessarily 'correct' or that it deserves greater prominence than guidance provided by other professional bodies or special interest groups. We hope, however, to have provided guidance that helps to assure the safe, effective and economic use of medicines in mental health. We hope also to have made clear the sources of information used to inform the guidance given.

Please note that many of the recommendations provided here go beyond the licensed or labelled indications of many drugs, both in the UK and elsewhere. Note also that, while we have endeavoured to make sure all quoted doses are correct, clinicians should always consult statutory texts before prescribing. Users of *The Guidelines* should also bear in mind that the contents of this handbook are based on information available to us up to January 2005. Much of the advice contained here will become outdated as more research is conducted and published.

No liability is accepted for any injury, loss or damage, however caused.

Notes on inclusion of drugs

The Guidelines are used in many other countries outside the UK. With this in mind, we have included in this edition those drugs in widespread use throughout the western world in January 2005. Thus, we have included, for example, ziprasidone, even though the drug is not marketed in the UK at this time. Its inclusion gives *The Guidelines* relevance in those countries where ziprasidone is marketed and may also be of benefit to UK readers, since many unlicensed drugs can be obtained through formal pharmaceutical importers. Many older drugs (methotrimeprazine, pericyazine, maprotiline, etc.) are either only briefly mentioned or not included on the basis that these drugs are not in widespread use at the time of writing.

Notes on commonly used abbreviations

Throughout this text we have abbreviated *British National Formulary* to *BNF* and extrapyramidal side-effects to EPSEs. All other abbreviations are explained in the text itself.

Notes on nomenclature

We have attempted to maintain uniformity in the naming of drug groups. However we are aware that new names emerge as time goes by. In particular, there is a clear trend to move away from terms such as 'typical' and 'atypical' in relation to antipsychotics. Many clinicians prefer the terms first- and second-generation antipsychotics since these terms perhaps imply no special properties for either group but simply indicate their time of arrival on the market. Nonetheless, these latter terms suffer some of the classification difficulties associated with the former. Is sulpiride typical or atypical? First or second generation? Is clozapine first or second generation or both? Is aripirazole third generation? Perhaps more importantly, the terms typical and atypical are common parlance and benefit from their relative brevity compared with the new nomenclature. Accordingly, we have persevered with using typical/atypical, at least for the time being.

chapter 1

Plasma level monitoring of psychotropics and anticonvulsants

Introduction

Plasma drug concentration or 'plasma level' monitoring is a process subject to considerable confusion and misunderstanding. Drug level monitoring, when appropriately used, is of considerable help in optimising treatment and assuring adherence. In psychiatry, as in other areas of medicine, plasma level determinations are frequently undertaken without good cause and results acted upon inappropriately. In other instances, plasma levels are underused.

Before taking a blood sample for plasma level assay, make sure that the following criteria are satisfied:

- **Is there a clinically useful assay method available?**
  Only a minority of drugs have available assays. The assay must be clinically validated and results available within a practical timescale.

- **Is the drug at 'steady state'?**
  Plasma levels are usually meaningful only when samples are taken after steady-state levels have been achieved. This takes 4–5 drug half-lives.

- **Is the timing of the sample correct?**
  Sampling time is vitally important for many but not all drugs. If the recommended sampling time is 12 hours post-dose, then the sample should be taken 11–13 hours post-dose if possible; 10–14 hours post-dose, if absolutely necessary. For trough or 'pre-dose' samples, take the blood sample immediately before the next dose is due. Do not, under any circumstances, withhold the next dose for more than 1 or (possibly) 2 hours until a sample is taken. Withholding for longer than this will inevitably give a misleading result (it will give a lower result than that ever seen in the usual, regular dosing), and this may lead to an inappropriate dose increase. Sampling time is less critical with drugs with a long half-life (e.g. olanzapine) but, as an absolute minimum, prescribers should always record the time of sampling and time of last dose.
  If a sample is not taken within 1–2 hours of the required time, it has the potential to mislead rather than inform. The only exception is if toxicity is suspected – sampling at the time of suspected toxicity is appropriate.

- **Will the level have any inherent meaning?**
  Is there a target range of plasma levels? If so, then plasma levels (from samples taken at the right time) will usefully guide dosing. If there is not an accepted target range, plasma levels can only indicate

adherence or toxicity. However, if the sample is being used to check compliance, then bear in mind that a plasma level of zero indicates only that the drug has not been taken in the past several days. Plasma levels above zero may indicate erratic compliance, full compliance or even long-standing non-compliance disguised by recent taking of prescribed doses. Note also that target ranges have their limitations: patients may respond to lower levels than the quoted range and tolerate levels above the range; also, ranges quoted by different laboratories vary sometimes widely without explanation.

- **Is there a clear reason for plasma level determination?**
  Only the following reasons are valid:
  – to confirm compliance (but see above)
  – if toxicity is suspected
  – if drug interaction is suspected
  – if clinical response is difficult to assess directly (and where a target range of plasma levels has been established)
  – if the drug has a narrow therapeutic index and toxicity concerns are considerable.

Interpreting sample results

The basic rule for sample level interpretation is to act upon assay results in conjunction with reliable clinical observation (*'treat the patient, not the level'*). For example, if a patient is responding adequately to a drug but has a plasma level below the accepted target range, then the dose should not normally be increased. If a patient has intolerable adverse effects but a plasma level within the target range, then a dose decrease may be appropriate.

Where a plasma level result is substantially different from previous results, a repeat sample is usually advised. Check dose, timing of dose and recent compliance but ensure, in particular, the correct timing of the sample. Many anomalous results are the consequence of changes in sample timing.

References for table opposite

1. Taylor D, Duncan D. Doses of carbamazepine and valproate in bipolar affective disorder. *Psychiatr Bull* 1997; **21**: 221–223.
2. Eadie MJ. Anticonvulsant drugs. *Drugs* 1984; **27**: 328–363.
3. Cohen AF, Land GS, Breimer DD *et al.* Lamotrigine, a new anticonvulsant: pharmacokinetics in normal humans. *Clin Pharmacol Ther* 1987; **42**: 535–541.
4. Kilpatrick ES, Forrest G, Brodie MJ. Concentration-effect and concentration-toxicity relations with lamotrigine: a prospective study. *Epilepsia* 1996; **37**: 534–538.
5. Johannessen SI, Battino D, Berry DJ *et al.* Therapeutic drug monitoring of the newer antiepileptic drugs. *Ther Drug Monit* 2003; **25**: 347–363.
6. Lardizabal DV, Morris HH, Hovinga CA *et al.* Tolerability and pharmacokinetics of oral loading with lamotrigine in epilepsy monitoring units. *Epilepsia* 2003; **44**: 536–539.
7. Taylor D, Duncan D. Plasma levels of tricyclics and related antidepressants: are they necessary or useful? *Psychiatr Bull* 1995; **19**: 548–550.
8. Davis R, Peters DH, McTavish D. Valproic acid – a reappraisal of its pharmacological properties and clinical efficacy in epilepsy. *Drugs* 1994; **47**: 332–372.
9. Perucca E. Pharmacological and therapeutic properties of valproate. *CNS Drugs* 2002; **16**: 695–714.

Further reading

Burke MJ, Preskorn SH. Therapeutic drug monitoring of antidepressants: cost implications and relevance to clinical practice. *Clin Pharmacokinet* 1999; **37**: 147–165.
Citrome L, Volavka J. Optimal dosing of atypical antipsychotics in adults: a review of the current evidence. *Harv Rev Psychiatry* 2002; **10**: 280–291.
Hiemke C, Dragicevic A, Grunder G *et al.* Therapeutic monitoring of new antipsychotic drugs. *Ther Drug Monit* 2004; **26**: 156–160.
Perry PJ. Therapeutic drug monitoring of antipsychotics. *Psychopharmacol Bull* 2001; **35**: 19–29.

Table Interpreting sample results

Drug	Target range	Sample timing	Time to steady state	Comments	References*
Carbamazepine	>7 mg/l bipolar disorder	Trough	2 weeks	Carbamazepine induces its own metabolism. Time to steady state dependent on autoinduction	1, 2
Clozapine	350–500 µg/l Upper limit of target range is ill-defined. See page 4	Trough	2–3 days	See page 4	See page 4
Lamotrigine	Not established but suggest 2.5–15 mg/l	Trough	5 days Auto-induction is thought to occur, so time to steady state may be longer	Some debate over utility of lamotrigine levels, especially in bipolar disorder. Toxicity may be increased above 15 mg/l	3–6
Lithium	0.6–1.0 mmol/l (may be >1.0 mmol/l in mania)	12 hours post-dose	5 days	Well-established target range	
Olanzapine	20–40 µg/l	12 hours post-dose	1 week	See page 6	See page 6
Phenytoin	10–20 mg/l	Trough	Variable	Follows zero-order kinetics. Free levels may be useful	2
Tricyclics	Nortriptyline 50–150 µg/l Amitriptyline 100–200 µg/l	Trough	2–3 days	Rarely used and of dubious benefit. Use ECG to assess toxicity	7
Valproate	50–100 mg/l Epilepsy and bipolar disorder	Trough	2–3 days	Some doubt over value of levels in epilepsy and bipolar disorder. Dosing should therefore be governed by clinical response and tolerability. Target range is a useful guide in the absence of clinical indicators	1, 2, 8, 9

Note: Plasma level monitoring of other drugs is not recommended (unless to confirm compliance or assess possible toxicity).
* For references see foot of page 2 opposite.

Clozapine plasma levels

Clozapine plasma levels are broadly related to daily dose[1], but there is sufficient variation to make impossible any precise prediction of plasma level. Plasma levels are generally lower in younger patients, males[2] and smokers[3]. A series of algorithms has been developed for the approximate prediction of clozapine levels according to patient factors and is recommended[4]. Algorithms cannot, however, account for other influences on clozapine plasma levels such as changes in adherence, inflammation[5] and infection[6].

The plasma level threshold for response to clozapine has been suggested to be 200 µg/l[7], 350 µg/l[8–10], 370 µg/l[11], 420 µg/l[12] and 504 µg/l[13].

Despite these varied estimates of response threshold, plasma levels can be useful in optimising treatment. In those not responding to clozapine, dose should be adjusted to give plasma levels in the range **350–500 µg/l**. Those not tolerating clozapine may benefit from a reduction to a dose giving plasma levels in this range. An upper limit to the clozapine target range has not been defined. Seizures occur more frequently in patients with levels above 1000 µg/l[14], so levels should probably be kept well below this. Note also that clozapine metabolism may become saturated at higher doses: the ratio of clozapine to norclozapine increases with increasing plasma levels, suggesting saturation[15–17]. The effect of fluvoxamine also suggests that metabolism via CYP1A2 to norclozapine can be overwhelmed[18].

A further consideration is that placing an upper limit on the target range for clozapine levels may discourage potentially worthwhile dose increases within the licensed dose range. Before plasma levels were widely used, clozapine was fairly often dosed to 900 mg/day, with valproate being added when the dose reached 600 mg/day. It remains unclear whether using these high doses can benefit patients with plasma levels already above the accepted threshold. Nonetheless, it is prudent to use valproate as prophylaxis against seizures and myoclonus when plasma levels are above 500–600 µg/l and certainly when levels approach 1000 µg/l.

References

1. Haring C, Fleischhacker WW, Schett P et al. Influence of patient-related variables on clozapine levels. Am J Psychiatry 1990; 147: 1471–1475.
2. Haring C, Meise M, Humpel C et al. Dose-related plasma levels of clozapine: influence of smoking behaviour, sex and age. Psychopharmacology 1989; 99: S38–S40.
3. Taylor D. Pharmacokinetic interactions involving clozapine. Br J Psychiatry 1997; 171: 109–112.
4. Rostami-Hodjegan A, Amin AM, Spencer EP et al. Influence of dose, cigarette smoking, age, sex and metabolic activity on plasma clozapine concentrations: a predictive model and nomograms to aid clozapine dose adjustment and to assess compliance in individual patients. J Clin Psychopharm 2004; 24: 70–78.
5. Haack MJ, Bak MLFJ, Beurskens R et al. Toxic rise of clozapine plasma concentrations in relation to inflammation. Eur Neuropsychopharm 2003; 13: 381–385.
6. De Leon J, Diaz FJ. Serious respiratory infections can increase clozapine levels and contribute to side effects: a case report. Prog Neuro-Psychoph 2003; 27: 1059–1063.
7. Vanderzwaag C, McGee M, McEvoy JP et al. Response of patients with treatment-refractory schizophrenia to clozapine within three serum level ranges. Am J Psychiatry 1996; 153: 1579–1583.
8. Perry PJ, Miller DD, Arndt SV, Cadoret RJ. Clozapine and norclozapine plasma concentrations and clinical response of treatment refractory schizophrenic patients. Am J Psychiatry 1991; 148: 231–235.
9. Miller DD. Effect of phenytoin on plasma clozapine concentrations in two patients. J Clin Psychiatry 1991; 52: 23–25.
10. Spina E, Avenoso A, Facciola G et al. Relationship between plasma concentrations of clozapine and norclozapine and therapeutic response in patients with schizophrenia resistant to conventional neuroleptics. Psychopharmacology 2000; 148: 83–89.
11. Hasegawa M, Gutierrez-Esteinou R, Way L et al. Relationship between clinical efficacy and clozapine concentrations in plasma in schizophrenia: effect of smoking. J Clin Psychopharm 1993; 13: 383–390.

12. Potkin SG, Bera R, Gulasekaram B *et al.* Plasma clozapine concentrations predict clinical response in treatment-resistant schizophrenia. *J Clin Psychiatry* 1994; **55**(Suppl. B): 133–136.
13. Perry PJ. Therapeutic drug monitoring of atypical antipsychotics. *CNS Drugs* 2000; **13**: 167–171.
14. Greenwood-Smith C, Lubman DI, Castle DJ. Serum clozapine levels: a review of their clinical utility. *J Psychopharmacol* 2003; **17**: 234–238.
15. Volpicelli SA, Centorrino F, Puopolo PR *et al.* Determination of clozapine, norclozapine, and clozapine-*N*-oxide in serum by liquid chromatography. *Clin Chem* 1993; **39**: 1656–1659.
16. Guitton C, Kinowski JM, Abbar M, *et al.* Clozapine and metabolite concentrations during treatment of patients with chronic schizophrenia. *J Clin Pharmacol* 1999; **39**: 721–728.
17. Palego L, Biondi L, Giannaccini G *et al.* Clozapine, norclozapine plasma levels, their sum and ratio in 50 psychotic patients: influence of patient-related variables. *Prog Neuro-Psychoph* 2002; **26**: 473–480.
18. Wang CY, Zhang ZJ, Li WB *et al.* The differential effects of steady-state fluvoxamine on the pharmacokinetics of olanzapine and clozapine in healthy volunteers. *J Clin Pharmacol* 2004; **44**: 785–792.

Olanzapine plasma levels

Plasma levels of olanzapine are linearly related to daily dose, but there is substantial variation[1], with higher levels seen in women[2], non-smokers[3] and those on enzyme inhibiting drugs[3,4]. With once-daily dosing, the threshold level for response has been suggested to be 9.3 µg/l (trough sample)[5], 23.2 µg/l (12-hour post-dose sample)[2] and 23 µg/l at a mean of 13.5 hours postdose[6]. Severe toxicity is uncommon but may be associated with levels above 100 µg/l, and death is occasionally seen at levels above 160 µg/l[7] (albeit when other drugs or physical factors are relevant). A target range for therapeutic use of **20–40 µg/l** (12-hour post-dose sample) has been proposed[8].

In practice, the dose of olanzapine should be governed by response and tolerability. Plasma level determinations should be reserved for those suspected of non-adherence or those not responding to the maximum licensed dose. In the latter case, dose may then be adjusted to give 12-hour plasma levels of 20–40 µg/l.

References

1. Aravagiri M, Ames D, Wirshing WC *et al.* Plasma level monitoring of olanzapine in patients with schizophrenia: determination by high-performance liquid chromatography with electrochemical detection. *Ther Drug Monit* 1997; **19**: 307–313.
2. Perry PJ. Therapeutic drug monitoring of atypical antipsychotics. *CNS Drugs* 2000; **13**: 167–171.
3. Gex-Fabry M, Balant-Gorgia AE, Balant LP. Therapeutic drug monitoring of olanzapine: the combined effect of age, gender, smoking, and comedication. *Ther Drug Monit* 2003; **25**: 46–53.
4. Bergemann N, Frick A, Parzer P, Kopitz J. Olanzapine plasma concentration, average daily dose, and interaction with co-medication in schizophrenic patients. *Pharmacopsychiatry* 2004; **37**: 63–68.
5. Perry PJ, Sanger T, Beasley C. Olanzapine plasma concentrations and clinical response in acutely ill schizophrenic patients. *J Clin Psychopharm* 1997; **6**: 472–477.
6. Fellows L, Ahmad F, Castle DJ *et al.* Investigation of target plasma concentration–effect relationships for olanzapine in schizophrenia. *Ther Drug Monit* 2003; **25**: 682–689.
7. Rao ML, Hiemke C, Grasma der K, Bauman P. Olanzapine: pharmacology, pharmacokinetics and therapeutic drug monitoring. *Fortschr Neurol Psych* 2001; **69**: 510–570.
8. Robertson MD, McMullin MM. Olanzapine concentrations in clinical serum and postmortem blood specimens – when does therapeutic become toxic? *J Forensic Sci* 2000; **42**: 418–421.

chapter 2

Schizophrenia

General introduction to antipsychotics*

The class of drugs used to treat schizophrenia and other psychotic illnesses is known as 'antipsychotics' (the terms 'neuroleptics' and 'major tranquillisers' are also sometimes used although neither is strictly correct).

The antipsychotic potency of most antipsychotics is directly proportional to their ability to block dopamine receptors in the brain, although the exact mechanism by which they exert their antipsychotic effect is probably more complicated than this. They vary greatly in their selectivity for dopamine receptors, many also having significant effects on acetylcholine, noradrenaline, histamine and serotonin pathways. A wide range of side-effects is therefore to be expected, the most common of which are listed below.

Extra-pyramidal side-effects

- **Dystonic reactions** (such as oculogyric spasm and torticollis) may be treated with oral, im or iv anticholinergics, depending on their severity. Approximately 10% of patients exposed to the older typical drugs develop an acute dystonic reaction[1]. This is more likely in the early stages of treatment or after an increase in dose and can be both painful and very frightening. Adverse early experiences are likely to reduce long-term willingness to take medication. Dystonia may also occur on drug withdrawal.
- **Pseudoparkinsonism** (characterised by tremor, bradykinesia and rigidity) is seen in approximately 20% of patients prescribed typical drugs[2]. It can be treated with anticholinergic drugs, but *not* dopamine agonists, as these would obviously diminish the dopamine antagonistic action of the antipsychotics. Anticholinergics should not be prescribed prophylactically with antipsychotics. The majority of patients appear to cope without them in the long term. It is also worth noting that anticholinergics have their own side-effects (dry mouth, blurred vision, constipation, cognitive impairment, etc.) and are thought to exacerbate tardive dyskinesia. They can also be misused for their euphoric effects and have a 'street value'.
- **Akathisia** (a subjectively unpleasant state of motor restlessness) responds poorly to anticholinergics. It is decidedly unpleasant and contributes to anxiety and dysphoria. Approximately 20–25% of patients prescribed the older drugs are affected[3]. If this is severe, it is often best to try

* This section contains a brief overview of antipsychotic properties. Many issues are covered in greater depth in later sections.

a drug with evidence of a lower liability for akathisia – usually an atypical (see page 16). Alternatively a non-selective beta-blocker such as propranolol (10–20 mg t.d.s.)[4] is well supported, and the antihistamine cyproheptadine (4–8 mg b.d.)[5,6] may be worth a try. These approaches are probably equally effective[7]. It is important that akathisia is distinguished from agitation secondary to psychosis, as it may have serious consequences if left untreated (akathisia has been linked to violence and suicide)[8]. For further guidance see page 76.

- **Tardive dyskinesia** (TD) has traditionally been thought to be caused by super-sensitivity of dopamine receptors, which develops because of prolonged therapy with dopamine-blocking drugs. This denervation supersensitivity theory has been supported by the observation that TD is temporarily improved by increasing the dose of the offending drug (this is the wrong approach clinically, as it can only perpetuate the problem). Undoubtedly, the aetiology of TD is more complex, probably involving GABA pathways to a significant extent. In the present state of our knowledge, TD is best dealt with by:
  - reducing and discontinuing anticholinergics
  - reducing the antipsychotic dose to the minimum that is effective
  - substituting older drugs with atypical antipsychotics[9]
  - trying clozapine if appropriate (may actually treat TD as well as psychosis)[10].

If the above fail to control the abnormal movements, various other options (tetrabenazine, sodium valproate, etc.) may be worth pursuing depending on the circumstances of each individual case[11]. See page 78 for further guidance.

It is worth noting that dyskinesia indistinguishable from TD was seen in psychiatric patients long before the introduction of antipsychotic drugs[12,13] (and indeed occurs independently of psychiatric illness in around 2% of the normal elderly population)[14]. There was a recorded prevalence of 5% in patients with schizophrenia before the introduction of antipsychotics, rising to up to 20% thereafter[14]. Recent studies of older patients with schizophrenia who have never been treated with antipsychotic drugs show a prevalence rate similar to populations treated with antipsychotics. All patients treated with antipsychotics are at risk of developing TD, although patients with affective illness, diabetes and learning disabilities; females; and the elderly seem to be more likely to be affected[14]. Those with mood disorders may also be more at risk of developing tardive dystonia. The presence of EPSEs during treatment with antipsychotics is associated with a threefold increase in risk of TD, and it is likely that the newer atypical antipsychotics (which produce less frequent EPSEs) will be associated with a lower incidence of TD[9].

Hyperprolactinaemia

This is an expected phenomenon as prolactin is under the inhibitory control of dopamine. Hyperprolactinaemia can lead to galactorrhoea, amenorrhoea, gynaecomastia, hypogonadism, sexual dysfunction and an increased risk of osteoporosis[15–17]. Long-stay psychiatric female inpatients have been noted to have a ninefold increase in the risk of breast cancer when compared to the normal population[18]. Although other risk factors are undoubtedly important in this group of patients, prolonged hyperprolactinaemia is likely to be a contributing factor.

A measurement of serum prolactin can be a useful indicator that the (older, typical) antipsychotic drug is being taken and is reaching CNS dopamine receptors. Prolactin levels of several thousand micrograms/litre may be seen when very high doses of antipsychotics are prescribed.

Of the newer, atypical antipsychotics, sertindole, quetiapine, ziprasidone, aripiprazole and clozapine have no important effect on prolactin. Olanzapine has a transient minimal effect. Risperidone, amisulpride and zotepine have potent prolactin-elevating effects, similar to conventional drugs. For further guidance on hyperprolactinaemia, see page 74.

Reduced seizure threshold

Grand mal seizures are a recognised side-effect of antipsychotic therapy (the higher the dose, the greater the risk). As a very general rule of thumb, the more sedative and less potent drugs carry a higher risk than the more potent, less sedative drugs. Clozapine carries the greatest risk[19]. Some antipsychotics have little or no effect on seizure threshold. See page 259 for further information on treating patients with pre-existing epilepsy.

Postural hypotension

Postural hypotension is mediated through adrenergic α_1-blockade, and so can usually be predicted for any drug with significant antagonist activity at this receptor. It is a particular risk when phenothiazines are prescribed for the elderly, but can also occur with higher doses of other antipsychotics in much younger patients. The atypical antipsychotics clozapine, risperidone, quetiapine and sertindole all have important affinity for α_1-receptors, making dosage titration necessary.

Anticholinergic side-effects

Anticholinergic side-effects include dry mouth (which may contribute to dental decay, ill-fitting dentures), blurred vision (which can contribute to falls in the elderly) and constipation (impaction can occur). Clozapine in particular has been associated with severe constipation resulting in gastrointestinal obstruction[20]. Anticholinergic effects may also have a detrimental impact on cognitive functioning

Antipsychotics with potent anticholinergic effects (notably chlorpromazine and clozapine) should never be given to patients who have closed-angle glaucoma. Drugs with less potent anticholinergic side-effects (e.g. haloperidol) can be used with caution in open-angle glaucoma that is being treated and monitored, as long as the dosage used does not produce mydriasis. Drugs such as haloperidol, trifluoperazine and sulpiride may be used in prostatic hypertrophy.

Neuroleptic malignant syndrome (NMS)[21-23]

NMS may occur in as many as 0.5% of newly treated patients and is thought to be greatly underdiagnosed. It is a potentially life-threatening complication of neuroleptic treatment, with the mortality rate estimated as being up to 20%. The main symptoms of NMS are mild hyperthermia, fluctuating consciousness, muscular rigidity, autonomic instability and severe EPSEs (primarily rigidity). Serum CPK is always raised. Leucocytosis (with a left shift) and abnormal LFTs are common. The enormous load of muscle breakdown products can lead to severe renal damage. The syndrome is believed to be caused by the rapid blockade of hypothalamic and striatal dopamine receptors, leading to a 'resetting' of the thermoregulatory systems and severe skeletal muscle spasm, which contributes to a considerable heat load that cannot be dissipated. The risk is greater the higher the starting dose of the antipsychotic and the more rapidly it is increased. All antipsychotics and other psychotropics, lithium and SSRIs have been implicated in NMS, with the majority of cases attributable to haloperidol. It is difficult to know if this is an inherent characteristic of haloperidol or if it is better explained by the fact that haloperidol is very widely prescribed in situations where initial high-dose antipsychotic therapy may be indicated.

Although it is primarily associated with antipsychotics, other drugs that interfere with dopaminergic neurotransmission have also been implicated in NMS[21] (e.g. MAOIs, TCAs, metoclopramide and tetrabenazine). Levodopa withdrawal has also been implicated.

Weight gain

In comparison with the general population, people with schizophrenia are more likely to be overweight and have increased quantities of visceral fat[24,25]. They are also at greater risk of developing hypertension, cardiovascular disease, type 2 diabetes and dyslipidaemia. In addition, antipsychotic-induced weight gain, particularly with atypicals, can be significant.

A substantial proportion of patients will gain 7% of their baseline body weight, which increases the risk of obesity-related morbidity (type 2 diabetes, heart disease, some cancers, etc.). Relative weight gain is difficult to determine, as there is no standard way of measuring it (5% gain, 7% gain, BMI, etc.). In general, clozapine has the greatest potential to cause weight gain, followed by

9

olanzapine, then quetiapine and risperidone, and then amisulpride. Ziprasidone[26,27] and aripiprazole may be relatively weight neutral[28]. See page 83 for further information. Several case reports/case series associate clozapine and olanzapine with the development of hyperglycaemia, diabetes mellitus and ketoacidosis. Being male, non-Caucasian and aged around 40 years, and possibly being obese/having recent weight gain, would appear to be risk factors. The maximum period of risk may be the first 6 months of treatment. The likely mechanism is insulin resistance and this does not seem to be clearly dose-related. In approximately one-third of cases, ongoing treatment with oral hypoglycaemics or insulin is required, despite treatment with clozapine or olanzapine being discontinued[29]. See page 92 for further guidance on weight gain and diabetes.

Others

Some antipsychotic drugs are sedative, some are cardio-toxic and many are associated with idiosyncratic side-effects. Further information can be found under the individual drug headings. Antipsychotic treatment is a risk factor for venous thromboembolism[30].

References

1. American Psychiatric Association. Practice guideline for the treatment of patients with schizophrenia. *Am J Psychiatry* 1997; 154(Suppl. 1): 1–63.
2. Bollini P, Pampallona S, Orza MJ *et al*. Antipsychotic drugs: is more worse? A meta-analysis of the published randomised controlled trials. *Psychol Med* 1994; 24: 307–316.
3. Halstead SM, Barnes TRE, Speller JC. Akathisia: prevalence and associated dysphoria in an in-patient population with chronic schizophrenia. *Br J Psychiatry* 1994; 164: 177–183.
4. Miller CH, Fleischhaker WW. Managing antipsychotic-induced acute and chronic akathisia. *Drug Safety* 2000; 22: 73–81.
5. Weiss D, Aizenberg D, Hermesh H *et al*. Cyproheptadine treatment in neuroleptic-induced akathisia. *Br J Psychiatry* 1995; 167: 483–486.
6. Poyurovsky M, Weizman A. Serotonin-based pharmacotherapy for acute neuroleptic-induced akathisia: a new approach to an old problem. *Br J Psychiatry* 2001; 179: 4–8.
7. Tsvi F, Haggai H, Aizenberg D *et al*. Cyproheptadine versus propranolol for the treatment of acute neuroleptic-induced akathisia: a comparative double-blind study. *J Clin Psychopharm* 2001; 21: 612–615.
8. Van Putten T, Marder SR. Behavioral toxicity of antipsychotic drugs. *J Clin Psychiatry* 1987; 48(Suppl. 9): 13–19.
9. Glazer W. Expected incidence of tardive dyskinesia associated with atypical antipsychotics. *J Clin Psychiatry* 2000; 61(Suppl. 4): 21–26.
10. Simpson GM. The treatment of tardive dyskinesia and tardive dystonia. *J Clin Psychiatry* 2000; 61(Suppl. 4): 39–44.
11. Duncan D, McConnell H, Taylor D. Tardive dyskinesia: how is it prevented and treated? *Psychiatr Bull* 1997; 21: 422–425.
12. Fenton WS. Prevalence of spontaneous dyskinesia in schizophrenia. *J Clin Psychiatry* 2000; 61(Suppl. 4): 10–14.
13. McCreadie RG, Padmavali R, Thara R *et al*. Spontaneous dyskinesia and parkinsonism in never-medicated, chronically ill patients with schizophrenia: 18-month follow-up. *Br J Psychiatry* 2002; 181:135–137.
14. American Psychiatric Association. *Tardive Dyskinesia: A Task Force Report of the American Psychiatric Association.* Washington, DC: American Psychiatric Association, 1992.
15. Dickson RA, Seeman MV, Corenblum B. Hormonal side effects in women: typical versus atypical antipsychotic treatment. *J Clin Psychiatry* 2000; 61(Suppl. 3): 10–15.
16. Halbreich U, Paller S. Accelerated osteoporosis in psychiatric patients: possible pathophysiological processes. *Schizophr Bull* 1996; 22: 447–454.
17. Smith SM, O'Keane V, Murray R. Sexual dysfunction in patients taking conventional antipsychotic medication. *Br J Psychiatry* 2002; 181: 49–55.
18. Halbreich U, Shen J, Panorov V. Are chronic psychiatric patients at increased risk for developing breast cancer? *Am J Psychiatry* 1996; 153: 559–560.
19. Devinsky O, Honigfeld G, Patin J. Clozapine-related seizures. *Neurology* 1991; 41: 369–371.
20. Anon. Clozapine (Clozaril) and gastrointestinal obstruction. *Current Problems in Pharmacovigilance* 1999; 25: 5.
21. Velamoor VR. Neuroleptic malignant syndrome: recognition, prevention and management. *Drug Safety* 1998; 19: 73–82.
22. Pelonero AL, Levenson JL, Pandurangi AK. Neuroleptic malignant syndrome: a review. *Psychiatr Serv* 1999; 49: 1163–1172.
23. Adityanjee A, Aderibigbe YA, Mathews T. Epidemiology of neuroleptic malignant syndrome. *Clin Neuropharmacol* 1999; 22: 151–158.
24. Mayer JM. Effects of atypical antipsychotics on weight and serum lipid levels. *J Clin Psychiatry* 2001; 62: 27–34.
25. Thakore JH, Mann JN, Vlahos I *et al*. Increased visceral fat distribution in drug-naive and drug-free patients with schizophrenia. *Int J Obes Relat Metab Disord* 2002; 26: 137–141.
26. Taylor DM, McAskill R. Atypical antipsychotics and weight gain – a systematic review. *Acta Psychiatr Scand* 2000; 101: 416–432.
27. Allison DB, Mentore JL, Moonseong H *et al*. Antipsychotic induced weight gain: a comprehensive research synthesis. *Am J Psychiatry* 1999; 156: 1686–1696.
28. Jody D, Saha AR, Iwamoto T *et al*. Meta-analysis of weight effects with aripiprazole. Poster presented at the American Psychiatric Association 155th Annual Meeting, May 2002, Philadelphia.
29. Mir S, Taylor D. Atypical antipsychotics and hyperglycaemia. *Int Clin Psychopharmacol* 2001; 16: 63–74.
30. Zornberg GL, Jick H. Antipsychotic drug use and risk of first-time idiopathic venous thromboembolism: a case control study. *Lancet* 2000; 356: 1219–1223.

Antipsychotics – equivalent doses

Antipsychotic drugs vary greatly in potency and this is usually expressed as differences in 'neuroleptic equivalents'. Most of the data relating to neuroleptic equivalents originate from early central dopamine binding studies (antipsychotic efficacy is, of course, undoubtedly far more complex than simple D_2 blockade), and atypical antipsychotics such as clozapine fare poorly in such comparative studies. *BNF* maximum doses for antipsychotic drugs bear little relationship to their 'neuroleptic equivalents'. If we bear these major limitations in mind and use the comparisons as a rough guide for the purpose of transferring a patient from one typical drug to another, followed by an early review, the table below represents the best guide from the information presently available[1,2].

Table Equivalent doses		
Drug	**Equivalent dose (consensus) (mg/day)**	**Range of values in literature (mg/day)**
Chlorpromazine	100	–
Thioridazine	100	75–100
Fluphenazine	2	2–5
Trifluoperazine	5	2.5–5
Flupentixol	3	2–3
Zuclopenthixol	25	25–60
Haloperidol	3	1.5–5
Sulpiride	200	200–270
Pimozide	2	2
Loxapine	10	10–25
Fluphenazine *depot*	5/week	1–12.5/week
Pipotiazine *depot*	10/week	10–12.5/week
Flupentixol *depot*	10/week	10–20/week
Zuclopenthixol *depot*	100/week	40–100/week
Haloperidol *depot*	15/week	5–25/week

It is illogical to convert atypical antipsychotics into 'equivalents' and dosage guidelines are discussed under each individual drug. See pages 15–19 for further discussion.

References

1. Foster P. Neuroleptic equivalence. *Pharm J* 1989; **243**: 431–432.
2. Atkins M, Burgess A, Bottomley C *et al*. Chlorpromazine equivalents: a consensus of opinion for both clinical and research applications. *Psychiatr Bull* 1997; **21**: 224–226.

Antipsychotics – minimum effective doses

The table below suggests the minimum dose of antipsychotic likely to be effective in schizophrenia (first episode or relapse). At least some patients will respond to the dose suggested, although others may require higher doses. Given the variation in individual response, all doses should be considered approximate. Primary references are provided where available, but consensus opinion has also been used (as have standard texts such as the *BNF* and *Summaries of Product Characteristics*). Only oral treatment with commonly used drugs is covered.

Table Minimum effective dose/day – antipsychotics

Drug	1st episode	Relapse	References
Chlorpromazine	200 mg*	300 mg	–
Haloperidol	2 mg	>4 mg	1–3
Sulpiride	400 mg*	800 mg	4
Trifluoperazine	10 mg*	15 mg	–
Amisulpride	400 mg*	800 mg	5–7
Aripiprazole	15 mg*	15 mg	8
Olanzapine	5 mg	10 mg	9–10
Quetiapine	150 mg*	300 mg	11–13
Risperidone	2 mg	4 mg	14, 15
Ziprasidone	80 mg*	80 mg	16, 17
Zotepine	75 mg*	150 mg	18, 19

*Estimate – too few data available.

References

1. Oosthuizen P, Emsley R, Turner J *et al.* Determining the optimal dose of haloperidol in first-episode psychosis. *J Psychopharmacol* 2001; **15**: 251–255.
2. McGorry P. Recommended haloperidol and risperidone doses in first-episode psychosis. *J Clin Psychiatry* 1999; **60**: 794–795.
3. Waraich P, Adams C, Roque M *et al.* Haloperidol dose for the acute phase of schizophrenia (Cochrane Review). In: The Cochrane Library, Issue 4, 2002. Oxford: Update Software.
4. Soares BGO, Fenton M, Chue P. Sulpiride for schizophrenia (Cochrane Review). In: The Cochrane Library, Issue 4, 2002. Oxford: Update Software.
5. Mota Neto JIS, Lima MS, Soares BGO. Amisulpride for schizophrenia (Cochrane Review). In: The Cochrane Library, Issue 4, 2002. Oxford: Update Software.
6. Puech A, Fleurot O, Rein W. Amisulpride, an atypical antipsychotic, in the treatment of acute episodes of schizophrenia: a dose-ranging study vs. haloperidol. *Acta Psychiatr Scand* 1998; **98**: 65–72.
7. Moller H, Boyer P, Fleurot O *et al.* Improvement of acute exacerbations of schizophrenia with amisulpride: a comparison with haloperidol. *Psychopharmacology* 1997; **132**: 396–401.
8. Taylor D. Aripiprazole: a review of its pharmacology and clinical utility. *Int J Clin Pract* 2003; **57**: 49–54.
9. Sanger T, Lieberman J, Tohen M *et al.* Olanzapine versus haloperidol treatment in first-episode psychosis. *Am J Psychiatry* 1999; **156**: 79–87.
10. Kasper S. Risperidone and olanzapine: optimal dosing for efficacy and tolerability in patients with schizophrenia. *Int Clin Psychopharmacol* 1998; **13**: 253–262.
11. Small J, Hirsch S, Arvanitis L. Quetiapine in patients with schizophrenia. *Arch Gen Psychiatry* 1997; **54**: 549–557.
12. Peuskens J, Link C. A comparison of quetiapine and chlorpromazine in the treatment of schizophrenia. *Acta Psychiatr Scand* 1997; **96**: 265–273.

13. Arvantis LA, Miller BG. Multiple fixed doses of 'Seroquel' (quetiapine) in patients with acute exacerbation of schizophrenia: a comparison with haloperidol and placebo. The Seroquel Trial 13 Study Group. *Biol Psychiatry* 1997; **42**: 233–246.
14. Lane H-Y, Chiu W-C, Chou J *et al.* Risperidone in acutely exacerbated schizophrenia: dosing strategies and plasma levels. *J Clin Psychiatry* 2000; **61**: 209–214.
15. Williams R. Optimal dosing with risperidone: updated recommendations. *J Clin Psychiatry* 2001; **62**: 282–289.
16. Bagnall A-M, Lewis R, Leitner M. Ziprasidone for schizophrenia and severe mental illness (Cochrane Review). In: The Cochrane Library, Issue 4, 2002. Oxford: Update Software.
17. Taylor D. Ziprasidone – an atypical antipsychotic. *Pharm J* 2001; **266**: 396–401.
18. Petit M, Raniwalla J, Tweed J. A comparison of an atypical and typical antipsychotic, zotepine versus haloperidol, in patients with acute exacerbation of schizophrenia: a parallel-group double-blind trial. *Psychopharmacol Bull* 1996; **32**: 81–87.
19. Palmgren K, Wighton A, Reynolds C *et al.* The safety and efficacy of zotepine in the treatment of schizophrenia: results of a one-year naturalistic clinical trial. *Int J Psychiatry Clin Pract* 2000; **4**: 299–306.

Antipsychotics – licensed maximum doses

The table below lists the UK licensed maximum doses of antipsychotics.

Drug	Maximum dose (mg/day)
Chlorpromazine	1000
Thioridazine	600 (see *BNF*)
Fluphenazine	20
Trifluoperazine	None (suggest 50)
Flupentixol	18
Zuclopenthixol	150
Haloperidol	30 (see *BNF*)
Sulpiride	2400
Pimozide	20
Loxapine	250
Amisulpride	1200
Aripiprazole	30
Clozapine	900
Risperidone	16 (see *BNF*)
Olanzapine	20
Quetiapine	750/800 (see *BNF*)
Ziprasidone*	160
Zotepine	300
Fluphenazine depot	50/week
Pipotiazine depot	50/week
Haloperidol depot	300 every 4 weeks
Flupentixol depot	400/week
Zuclopenthixol depot	600/week

Note: Doses above these maxima should only be used in extreme circumstances: there is no evidence for improved efficacy.

* Not available in the UK at time of publication. US labelling used.

New antipsychotics – costs

Newer antipsychotics are relatively costly medicines, although their benefits may make them cost-effective in practice. Cost minimisation is a practical option that reduces drug expenditure without compromising patient care or patient quality of life. It involves using the right drug for the most appropriate condition (see Protocols) and using the minimum effective dose in each patient. The table below gives the cost (£/patient per 30 days) as of January 2005 of atypicals at their estimated lowest effective dose, their approximate average clinical dose and their licensed maximum dose. The table allows comparison of different doses of the same drug and of different drugs at any of the three doses. It is hoped that the table will encourage the use of lower doses of less expensive drugs, given equality in other respects and allowing for clinical requirements.

Table Monthly costs of new antipsychotics

Drug	Minimum effective dose cost (see page 12)	Approximate average clinical dose cost	Maximum dose cost
Amisulpride*	400 mg/day (depends on indication – see *BNF*) £66.00	800 mg/day £132.00	1200 mg/day £198.00
Aripiprazole	15 mg/day £108.89	20 mg/day £217.78	30 mg/day £217.78
Olanzapine	10 mg/day £85.12	15 mg/day £127.69**	20 mg/day £170.25**
Risperidone (oral)	4 mg/day £68.69	6 mg/day £101.01	16 mg/day £200.01
Risperidone (injection)	25 mg/2 weeks £165.86	37.5 mg/2 weeks £231.68	50 mg/2 weeks £297.10
Quetiapine	300 mg/day £85.00	500 mg/day £141.55	750 mg/day £226.55
Zotepine	150 mg/day £50.62	300 mg/day £94.55	300 mg/day £94.55

*Generic version expected – check latest price.
**Using 10 mg tablets.

Notes:
- costs for UK adults (30 days), MIMS, January 2005
- average clinical doses for inpatients receiving maintenance therapy
- clozapine costs not included because it has different indications.

Choice of antipsychotic

The *BNF* states that 'the various antipsychotic drugs differ somewhat in predominant actions and side-effects. Selection is influenced by the degree of sedation required and the patient's susceptibility to EPSEs. However, the differences between antipsychotic drugs are less important than the greater variability in patient response.'

Phenothiazines

These are often divided into a further three subgroups, depending on their basic chemistry and, coincidentally, the degree of sedation they produce.

Chlorpromazine and **promazine** are the most sedative, and chlorpromazine the most widely pre-scribed phenothiazine. The pharmacology of chlorpromazine is complex but well documented. As well as the side-effects common to all antipsychotics, chlorpromazine causes photosensitivity reac-tions (hence the need for liberal amounts of high-factor sunscreen and straw hats in the summer), and occasionally a hypersensitivity reaction resembling obstructive jaundice (the block being bio-chemical and not mechanical). Chlorpromazine is epileptogenic in a dose-dependent fashion and can cause significant weight gain. Promazine has a relatively good side-effect profile and so is suit-able for the elderly, if it is sufficient to control symptoms. It is not effective in schizophrenia.

Thioridazine, **pericyazine** and **pipotiazine** are relatively less likely to produce EPSEs. Because of concerns over QTc prolongation[1], the product licence for thioridazine has been restricted to the second line treatment of schizophrenia in patients who are under the direct care of a consultant psychiatrist[2]. There are further restrictions on its use in patients with cardiovascular disease or those receiving a wide range of other drugs[1]. It is essentially impossible to prescribe thioridazine within its product licence. Long-term therapy with high doses of thioridazine is not recommended because of its ability to cause pigmentary retinopathy. Thioridazine will be withdrawn from the UK market in 2005. Pericyazine has achieved some success in curbing acts of spontaneous aggression/antisocial behaviour in younger people, most probably because of its potent sedative effect.

Fluphenazine and **trifluoperazine** are the least sedative phenothiazines but are more likely to cause EPSEs. Trifluoperazine is available as tablets, liquid and controlled-release capsules. There is little rationale in prescribing the more expensive controlled-release preparation, as, sedation aside, most antipsychotics can be administered once daily in their conventional form.

Butyrophenones

Haloperidol is the most widely prescribed drug in this group. It is a very potent D_2 blocker. It has been suggested that plasma levels of 5–12 µg/l are associated with optimal response and that such levels are achievable with daily doses of no more than 20 mg. Studies have shown that optimal response is achieved from daily doses of no more than 10 mg although much higher doses are com-monly seen (and are associated with a high prevalence of EPSEs)[3]. Some studies suggest a non-linear relationship between dose and response, with a paradoxical response being possible when high doses are used. It has been suggested that the observed paradoxical response may be due to an increased incidence of EPSEs, akathisia and akinesia being interpreted as increased agitation and an increase in negative symptoms, respectively. The *BNF* maximum dose for oral haloperidol has decreased from 120 to 15 mg/day (or 30 mg in treatment-resistant schizophrenia: September 2004 edition). **Droperidol** is no longer available in the UK (because of an association with QTc prolongation).

Thioxanthines

Flupentixol is the most widely prescribed member of this group and is used mostly in depot form. Low doses of flupentixol are claimed to have an antidepressant effect and, although there is a small hint (by no means proven) in some very old literature that this may be the case in psychosis, it is not a suitable treatment for depression.

Diphenylbutylpiperidines

Pimozide is the only member of this group that is still prescribed. It is relatively specific for dopamine receptors and therefore has a narrower side-effect profile. It is claimed to be particularly useful in the treatment of monosymptomatic hypochondriacal psychoses (marketing hype originating from a small open case series – a very poor evidence base). In August 1990, the Committee on Safety of Medicines (CSM) reported that 13 reports of sudden, unexpected death associated with the use of pimozide had been received, which led them to recommend a maximum daily dose of 20 mg, and also that anyone receiving more than 16 mg daily should have periodic ECGs carried out. The Committee went on to request reports of ventricular arrhythmia and sudden, unexpected death associated with any antipsychotic[4].

Atypical antipsychotics

The term 'atypical' was originally associated with the inability of a compound to produce catalepsy in laboratory animals (a screening model thought to have good predictive validity in identifying potential antipsychotic agents). Atypical antipsychotics were also defined as having no effect on serum prolactin. More recently, the term has been used to describe antipsychotics that are highly selective D_2 blockers, those that are relatively selective for D_2 receptors in mesolimbic areas, those that have a high $5HT_2:D_2$ receptor blocking ratio and those that are claimed to have an effect on negative symptomatology. The definition of this term is likely to become even more confused in the future, should any of the more novel compounds presently being developed reach the market (dopamine autoreceptor agonists, NMDA agonists, $5HT_3$ antagonists, sigma antagonists, etc.). Atypical antipsychotics do cause fewer EPSEs than most of the older drugs, but are not devoid of other side-effects. These effects are discussed for individual drugs below.

Clozapine

Clozapine is the archetypal atypical antipsychotic. Clozapine has been around since the 1960s and was withdrawn from use after an association with neutropenia (incidence 3%) and agranulocytosis (0.8%) was made. The pivotal study by Kane et al.[5] in the late 1980s proved that clozapine was more effective than conventional antipsychotics, and it was reintroduced in the UK with compulsory haematological monitoring. Patients must be registered with an approved clozapine monitoring services (CPMS, ZTAS, etc.) and have a full blood count performed weekly for the first 18 weeks (when the risk of neutropenia/agranulocytosis is greatest)[6], fortnightly until 52 weeks of treatment, and then monthly thereafter if haematologically stable (the incidence of agranulocytosis after 1 year is similar to that associated with the phenothiazines[6]). Studies have shown that 30% of patients who have previously been refractory to treatment improve significantly after 6 weeks' treatment with clozapine, and up to 60% respond after 1 year. Local experience has shown that even patients who have not been identified as 'responders' by staff feel subjectively better on clozapine and that levels of aggression and violence in this population have fallen[7]. Clozapine is perhaps most useful in patients who are actively and floridly psychotic. Although claims are made for its efficacy in negative symptomatology, clinical gains in this area are much less marked[8,9]. Clozapine treatment has been linked to a reduction in suicidality[10] and the data are sufficient[11] for specific labelling for this indication in the USA. (See page 58.)

The pharmacology of clozapine is unusual compared with other antipsychotics in that it only binds weakly to D_1 and D_2 receptors, while having an affinity for D_4, $5HT_2$, $5HT_3$, α_1 and α_2 adrenergic, and ACh M_1 and H_1 receptors. Which one/combination of any of these effects is responsible for the superior clinical profile of clozapine is a subject of extensive speculation, but as of yet, no firm conclusion.

Clozapine also has a unique side-effect profile in that it has been associated with an extremely low incidence of EPSEs, and is thought not to cause/precipitate TD (it has even been suggested that clozapine can be an effective treatment for existing TD – see page 78. Clozapine does not raise prolactin levels and so is not associated with amenorrhoea. Menstruation will return and effective contraception is essential in sexually active females.

Clozapine is associated with a greater incidence of seizures than other antipsychotics and this is probably related to high plasma levels in susceptible individuals. The incidence of seizures increases markedly at doses of 600 mg/day or above and is probably related to plasma level. Grand mal seizures may be prevented with sodium valproate.

Clozapine also has other troublesome side-effects in that sialorrhoea can be a significant problem. The mechanism of this effect is not completely understood – it has been suggested that it is mediated through cholinergic, adrenergic and 5HT pathways. It is best dealt with practically (by encouraging patients to sleep with their head propped up on several pillows or with a towel over their pillow). Several pharmacological strategies have been tried such as anticholinergics (procyclidine, hyoscine, pirenzepine, atropine), amitriptyline, propranolol, clonidine and desmopressin[12]. All of these approaches are associated with their own side-effects, both physical and psychiatric, and should be tried with caution. See page 63 for further details.

Raised body temperature can also be a problem during initiation of clozapine treatment. Although this problem is described in the literature as benign hyperthermia, temperatures of over 40 °C have been described. Unless the temperature becomes very elevated (above 38.5 °C with paracetamol cover), there is no reason for stopping clozapine, as this effect is transient (it must, of course, be differentiated from fever secondary to neutropenia). Fever may also be associated with myocarditis (see page 81).

Clozapine has also been linked to the development of hypersensitivity myocarditis[13] (risk estimated to be increased 1000-fold in the first month of treatment) and cardiomyopathy[13] (risk estimated to be increased five-fold). It is unclear at present whether this risk is higher than that associated with other antipsychotics. See page 54 et seq for further information about the side-effects of clozapine and how to manage them.

A therapeutic range may exist for clozapine where serum concentrations of >350 µg/l are required for efficacy. There are many limitations to these data and serum levels should be interpreted with caution[14]. See page 4 for further discussion and guidelines.

A 'withdrawal syndrome' has been described when clozapine treatment is withdrawn abruptly[15] (as it must be when the blood profile dictates). Whether this represents rapid return of the original psychopathology, super-sensitivity psychosis, a true withdrawal syndrome, or a mixture of all three is unclear.

Other atypical antipsychotics[16]

The other 'atypical antipsychotics', sulpiride, amisulpride, risperidone, sertindole, olanzapine, quetiapine, ziprasidone and zotepine have not been proven to be effective in treating resistant illness. They are advocated as better tolerated first-line treatments[17].

Sulpiride was arguably the first member of this group to be marketed and is often termed typical or at least grouped with them. Conventional antipsychotics are all effective in treating positive symptoms (i.e. formal thought disorder, passivity feelings, delusions and hallucinations) and, given prophylactically, they substantially reduce the relapse rate for many patients (see page 44). None of these compounds, however, directly or significantly, improve the manifestations of negative symptomatology (i.e. anergia, apathy, flattening of affect and poverty of speech), all of which are a major cause of long-term deterioration, withdrawal and isolation amongst patients with schizophrenia.

Sulpiride was the first antipsychotic for which claims were made regarding its effect upon negative symptomatology (although it must be noted that this effect is not striking). It has a dose-related selectivity for pre-synaptic D_4 and post-synaptic D_2 receptors. In low doses (less than 800 mg/day) the main affinity is for D_4 receptors, which are auto-inhibitory. The inhibitory control of dopamine release is therefore decreased and more dopamine is available in the synaptic cleft. Above 800 mg/day the affinity for D_2 receptors dominates, resulting in the post-synaptic blockade of D_2 receptors. Sulpiride is associated with fewer EPSEs than the older drugs and, as such, may also be associated with less potential for causing TD.

Amisulpride is similar to sulpiride in that lower doses (300 mg/day or less) selectively block pre-synaptic dopamine receptors, leading to an increase in dopamine transmission in the prefrontal cortex (the site supposedly responsible for the genesis of negative symptoms). At higher doses, it blocks post-synaptic dopamine receptors and is relatively selective for limbic rather than striatal areas, which translates clinically into a low potential for EPSEs. Amisulpride is relatively free from sedation, anticholinergic side-effects and postural hypotension, but, like sulpiride, is a particularly potent elevator of serum prolactin. The difference clinically between amisulpride and sulpiride is unclear. Amisulpride is significantly more expensive at the time of writing, but a cheaper generic form is expected.

Risperidone is a potent $5HT_2$:D_2 antagonist. It was developed in line with the observation that ritanserin (a potent $5HT_2$ receptor antagonist), when given in combination with conventional antipsychotics, was effective in treating the negative and affective symptoms of schizophrenia[18]. In doses of 6 mg or less per day, risperidone is associated with a low incidence of EPSEs and sedation. It is associated with hyperprolactinaemia. Risperidone has a first-dose hypotensive effect (due to α_1 blockade), and in order to minimise this, an increasing-dosage regime is used over the first few days. There have been reports of nausea, dyspepsia, abdominal pain, dyspnoea and chest pain associated with its use.

Prescribing surveys have shown that risperidone is frequently prescribed in both doses greater than 8 mg/day (so that EPSEs are produced), and in combination with other antipsychotics (where treatment resistance is the real issue)[19]. This is illogical.

Sertindole is also associated with significant α_1 blockade and therefore dosage titration is required. Its major advantages are that it produces virtually no EPSEs within the licensed dosage range and has no effect on prolactin. Its major disadvantage is that it is associated with QTc prolongation, and it is recommended that an ECG is obtained before initiating therapy. (A survey of junior doctors in psychiatry demonstrated that less than 20% were able to identify a prolonged QTc interval on an ECG[20].) Sertindole has been tentatively linked with a number of cases of 'antipsychotic-associated sudden death'[21], and in November 1998 its licence was suspended by several European countries. Sertindole was subsequently voluntarily withdrawn from general use by the manufacturers, but has now been reintroduced, following studies demonstrating its apparent safety.

Olanzapine is also a $5HT_2$:D_2 blocker. It is sedative, produces some postural hypotension and has anticholinergic side-effects. Although chemically and pharmacologically very similar to clozapine, olanzapine has been licensed as a first-line antipsychotic, and there is currently no compelling evidence to support its efficacy in treatment-resistant illness. Olanzapine has minimal effects on serum prolactin and may be associated with a lower incidence of sexual dysfunction than other antipsychotics. Clinical trials have shown that 10–20 mg olanzapine/day is the most effective dose. Because it is well tolerated (notwithstanding its longer-term effects, see pages 83, 92), prescribers may feel tempted to increase the dose above 20 mg (the licensed maximum) in partial or non-responders. Such patients would be more appropriately treated with clozapine. Olanzapine serum levels can be measured and this may be useful when non-compliance is suspected. See page 6 for further guidance on plasma level monitoring.

Quetiapine has a low affinity for D_1, D_2 and $5HT_2$ receptors and moderate affinity for adrenergic α_1 and α_2 receptors. It is relatively mesolimbic-specific and does not raise serum prolactin; however, it does require dosage titration (like risperidone and sertindole). Quetiapine is considered to be an effective and well-tolerated antipsychotic. There are very few data to suggest that it may be effective in treatment-resistant illness. The early published efficacy data for quetiapine have been said to be less compelling compared with the other atypicals. This mainly relates to the high dropout rates reported in short-term trials[22] and is highly controversial (quetiapine trials included some low doses and all antipsychotics have high dropout rates in trials). Quetiapine has rarely been associated with the development of cataracts in laboratory animals. There are also some reports in humans[23] but a direct causal relationship has not been firmly established. Quetiapine has also been associated with raised plasma lipids (this is true for clozapine and olanzapine as well – there are fewer data for the other atypical antipsychotics).

Zotepine is an antagonist at $5HT_{2a}$, $5HT_{2c}$, D_1, D_2, D_3 and D_4 receptors, a potent inhibitor of noradrenaline reuptake, and a potent H_1 antagonist (sedative), with some α_1 adrenergic blocking activity (postural hypotension) and possibly some activity at NMDA receptors. It raises serum prolactin and is associated with a high incidence of seizures. Doses above 300 mg/day (frequently used according to the available literature) and antipsychotic polypharmacy increase this risk. There are very few trial data comparing zotepine with other atypical antipsychotics. There is no study of any quality in refractory illness reported in the English language literature.

References

1. Reilly JG, Ayis SA, Ferrier IN et al. QTc interval abnormalities and psychotropic drug therapy in psychiatric patients. Lancet 2000; 355: 1048–1052.
2. Melleril SPC. Datasheet compendium, 2002.
3. Hilton T, Taylor D, Abel K. Which dose of haloperidol? Psychiatr Bull 1996; 20: 359–362.
4. Committee on Safety of Medicines. Cardiotoxic effects of pimozide. Current Problems 1990; 29: 1.
5. Kane J, Honifeld G, Singer J et al. Clozapine for the treatment resistant schizophrenic. Arch Gen Psychiatry 1988; 45: 789–796.
6. Atkin F, Kendall F, Gould D et al. Neutropenia and angranulocytosis in patients receiving clozapine in the UK and Ireland. Br J Psychiatry 1996; 169: 483–488.
7. Wolfson PM, Paton C. Clozapine audit: what do patients and relatives think? J Ment Health 1996; 5: 267–273.
8. Rosenheck R, Dunn L, Peszke M et al. Impact of clozapine on negative symptoms and on the deficit syndrome in refractory schizophrenia. Am J Psychiatry 1999; 156: 88–93.
9. Breier AF, Malhotra AK, Su T et al. Clozapine and risperidone in chronic schizophrenia: effects on symptoms, parkinsonian side effects and neuroendocrine response. Am J Psychiatry 1999; 156: 294–298.
10. Meltzer HY, Okayli G. Reduction of suicidality during clozapine treatment of neuroleptic resistant schizophrenia: impact on risk-benefit assessment. Am J Psychiatry 1995; 152: 183–190.
11. Meltzer HY, Alphs L, Green AI et al. Clozapine treatment for suicidality in schizophrenia. International Suicide Prevention Trial (InterSePT). Arch Gen Psychiatry 2003; 60: 82–91.
12. Cree A, Mir S, Fahy T. A review of the treatment options for clozapine-induced hypersalivation. Psychiatr Bull 2001; 25: 114–116.
13. Killan JG, Kerr K, Lawrence C et al. Myocarditis and cardiomyopathy associated with clozapine. Lancet 1999; 354: 1841–1845.
14. Taylor D, Duncan D. The use of clozapine plasma levels in optimising therapy. Psychiatr Bull 1995; 19: 753–755.
15. Ekblom B, Eriksson K, Lindstrom LH. Supersensitivity psychosis in schizophrenic patients after sudden clozapine withdrawal. Psychopharmacology 1984; 83: 293–294.
16. Leysen JE, Janssen PMF, Heylen L et al. Receptor interactions of new antipsychotics: relation to pharmacodynamic and clinical effects. Int J Psychiatry Clin Pract 1998; 2(Suppl. 1): 3–17.
17. Taylor DM, Duncan-McConnell D. Refractory schizophrenia and atypical antipsychotics. J Psychopharmacol 2000; 14: 409–418.
18. Duinkerke SJ, Botter PA, Jansen AA. Ritanserin, a selective 5HT2/1C antagonist, and negative symptoms in schizophrenia. Br J Psychiatry 1993; 164: 451–455.
19. Taylor D, Holmes R, Hilton T et al. Evaluating and improving the quality of risperidone prescribing. Psychiatr Bull 1997; 21: 680–683.
20. Warner JP, Gledhill JA, Connell F et al. How well do psychiatric trainees interpret electrocardiographs? Psychiatr Bull 1996; 20: 651–652.
21. Pritze J, Bandelow B. The QT interval and the atypical antipsychotic sertindole. Int J Psychiatry Clin Prac 1998; 2: 265–273.
22. Srisurapsanont M, Disayavanish C, Taimkaewk K. Quetiapine for schizophrenia (Cochrane review). In: The Cochrane Library, Issue 3. Oxford: Update Software, 2000.
23. Valibhai F, Phan NB, Still DJ. Cataracts and quetiapine. Am J Psychiatry 2001; 158: 966.

Newer antipsychotics

Ziprasidone

Ziprasidone has been available in the USA and some European countries for several years. It is a D_2:$5HT_2$ antagonist with significant agonist activity at $5HT_{1A}$ receptors and moderately potent inhibition of monoamine reuptake[1,2]. Efficacy is similar to haloperidol[3] and olanzapine[4] and tolerability is good; most adverse effects occur at the same frequency as placebo and EPSEs, hyperprolactinaemia and weight gain are uncommon[5,6]. More recent studies suggest that ziprasidone is more effective in the treatment of negative symptoms than haloperidol[7] and as effective as amisulpride[8]. Ziprasidone has a moderate effect on the QT interval, which may, at least in theory, make it relatively more likely than other antipsychotics to cause ventricular arrhythmia (see page 87)[9]. This potential problem should be set against the clear advantages of ziprasidone in relation to weight gain[10] and impaired glucose tolerance[11]. Switching to ziprasidone because of the adverse effects of other antipsychotics seems to be safe and effective[12].

References

1. Taylor D. Ziprasidone – an atypical antipsychotic. *Pharm J* 2001; **266**: 396–401.
2. Davis R, Markham A. Ziprasidone. *CNS Drugs* 1997; **8**: 153–159.
3. Goff DC, Posever T, Herz L *et al.* An exploratory haloperidol-controlled dose-finding study of ziprasidone in hospitalized patients with schizophrenia or schizoaffective disorder. *J Clin Psychopharm* 1998; **18**: 296–304.
4. Simpson GM, Glick ID, Weiden P *et al.* Randomized, controlled, double-blind multicenter comparison of the efficacy and tolerability of ziprasidone and olanzapine in acutely ill inpatients with schizophrenia or schizoaffective disorder. *Am J Psychiatry* 2004; **161**: 1837–1847.
5. Keck P, Buffenstein A, Ferguson J *et al.* Ziprasidone 40 and 120 mg/day in the acute exacerbation of schizophrenia and schizoaffective disorder: a 4-week placebo-controlled trial. *Psychopharmacology* 1998; **140**: 173–184.
6. Keck P, Reeves K, Harrigan E. Ziprasidone in the short-term treatment of patients with schizoaffective disorder: results from two double-blind, placebo-controlled, multicenter studies. *J Clin Psychopharm* 2001; **21**: 27–35.
7. Hirsch S, Werner K, Bauml J *et al.* A 28-week comparison of ziprasidone and haloperidol in outpatients with stable schizophrenia. *J Clin Psychiatry* 2002; **63**: 516–522.
8. Olie J-P, Spina E, Benattia I. Ziprasidone vs amisulpride for negative symptoms of schizophrenia. Poster presented at ECNP annual conference. Barcelona, Spain, October 2002.
9. Taylor D. Ziprasidone in the management of schizophrenia: the QT interval issue in context. *CNS Drugs* 2003; **17**: 423–430.
10. Taylor DM, McAskill R. Atypical antipsychotics and weight gain – a systematic review. *Acta Psychiatr Scand* 2000; **101**: 416–432.
11. Kingsbury SJ, Fayek M, Trufasiu D *et al.* The apparent effects of ziprasidone on plasma lipids and glucose. *J Clin Psychiatry* 2001; **62**: 347–349.
12. Weiden PJ, Simpson GM, Potkin SG *et al.* Effectiveness of switching to ziprasidone for stable but symptomatic outpatients with schizophrenia. *J Clin Psychiatry* 2003; **64**: 580–588.

Aripiprazole

Aripiprazole is a partial agonist at D_2 receptors: full binding to D_2 receptors reduces dopaminergic neuronal activity by about 30% (in the absence of dopamine, aripiprazole acts as a weak agonist)[1]. It is a potent antagonist at $5HT_{2A}$ receptors and a partial agonist at $5HT_{1A}$ receptors[2].

Aripiprazole appears to be at least as effective as haloperidol[3] and risperidone[4] and is well tolerated with a low incidence (placebo level) of extra-pyramidal symptoms[5]. It seems not to be associated with symptomatic hyperprolactinaemia, QTc prolongation, impaired glucose tolerance or substantial weight gain[6–8]. Switching to aripiprazole from other antipsychotics seems safe and effective by any method[9]. Despite these promising findings, Cochrane is lukewarm about aripiprazole[10], arguably without justification. Recent data not considered by Cochrane suggest that aripiprazole is antimanic[11] and has useful activity in depressive[12] and negative symptoms[13]. Early clinical experience suggests tolerability may be improved in some by starting at 10 mg daily.

References

1. Burris KD, Molski TF, Ryan E *et al.* Aripiprazole is a high affinity partial agonist at human D_2 dopamine receptors. *Int J Neuropsychopharm* 2000; 3(Suppl. 1): S129.
2. Jordan S, Koprivica V, Chen R *et al.* The antipsychotic aripiprazole is a potent, partial agonist at the human $5HT_{1A}$ receptor. *Eur J Pharmacol* 2002; 441: 137–140.
3. Kane JM, Carson WH, Saha AR *et al.* Efficacy and safety of aripiprazole and haloperidol versus placebo in patients with schizophrenia and schizoaffective disorder. *J Clin Psychiatry* 2002; 63: 763–771.
4. Potkin SG, Saha AR, Kujawa MJ *et al.* Aripiprazole, an antipsychotic with a novel mechanism of action, and risperidone vs placebo in patients with schizophrenia and schizoaffective disorder. *Arch Gen Psychiatry* 2003; 60: 681–690.
5. Petrie JL, Saha AR, McEvoy JP. Aripiprazole, a new atypical antipsychotic: phase 2 clinical trial results. *Eur Neuropsychopharm* 2002; 7(Suppl. 1): S157.
6. Pigott TA, Carson WH, Saha AR *et al.* Aripiprazole for the prevention of relapse in stabilized patients with chronic schizophrenia: a placebo-controlled 26-week study. *J Clin Psychiatry* 2003; 64: 1048–1056.
7. Stock F, Marder SR, Saha AR *et al.* Safety and tolerability meta-analysis of aripiprazole in schizophrenia. *Int J Neuropsychopharm* 2002; 5(Suppl. 1): S185.
8. Jody D, Saha AR, Iwamoto T *et al.* Meta-analysis of weight effects with aripiprazole. Poster presented at American Psychiatric Association 155th Annual Meeting, 18–23 May 2002, Philadelphia.
9. Casey DE, Carson WH, Saha AR *et al.* Switching patients to aripiprazole from other antipsychotic agents: a multicenter randomized study. *Psychopharmacology* 2003; 166: 391–399.
10. El-Sayeh HG, Morganti C. Aripiprazole for schizophrenia. Cochrane Database of Systematic Reviews 2004, Issue 2. Art No.: CD004578.pub2. DOI: 10.1002/14651858.CD004578.pub2.
11. Keck PE Jr, Marcus R, Tourkodimitis S *et al.* A placebo-controlled, double-blind study of the efficacy and safety of aripiprazole in patients with acute bipolar mania. *Am J Psychiatry* 2003; 160: 1651–1658.
12. Stock EG, Archibald DG, Tourkodimitris S *et al.* Long-term effects of aripiprazole and haloperidol on affective symptoms of schizophrenia. Twelfth Biennial Winter Workshop on Schizophrenia, Davos, Switzerland, 7–13 February 2004.
13. Kostic D, Manos G, Stock EG *et al.* Long-term effects of aripiprazole on the negative symptoms of schizophrenia. 16th Congress of the European College of Neuropsychopharmacology, 20–24 September 2003, Prague, Czech Republic.

Further reading

Taylor DM. Aripiprazole: a review of its pharmacology and clinical use. *Int J Clin Pract* 2003; 57: 49–53.

Antipsychotics – general principles of prescribing

- The **lowest possible dose** should be used. For each patient, the dose should be titrated to the lowest known to be effective; dose increases should then take place only after 2 weeks of assessment during which the patient is clearly showing poor or no response. With depot medication, plasma levels rise for 6–12 weeks after initiation, even without a change in dose. Dose increases during this time are therefore inappropriate (see page 35).

- For the large majority of patients, the use of a **single antipsychotic** (with or without additional mood stabiliser or sedatives) is recommended (see page 40).

- **Polypharmacy** of antipsychotics should be undertaken only where response to a single antipsychotic (including clozapine) has been clearly demonstrated to be inadequate. In such cases, the effect of polypharmacy should be carefully evaluated and documented. Where there is no clear benefit, treatment should revert to single antipsychotic therapy (see page 40).

- In general, **antipsychotics should not be used as 'PRN' sedatives**. Short courses of benzodiazepines or general sedatives (e.g. promethazine) are recommended.

- Responses to antipsychotic drug treatment should be **assessed by recognised rating scales** and be documented in patients' records.

Atypical antipsychotics – summary of NICE guidance[1]

- Choice of antipsychotic should be made jointly by the prescriber and the (properly informed) patient and/or carer.

- When consultation with the patient is not possible and where there is no advance directive, an atypical drug should be used. The patient's carer or advocate should be consulted whenever possible.

- Atypical drugs should be considered in the choice of first-line treatments.

- Atypical drugs should be considered for patients showing or reporting unacceptable adverse effects caused by typical agents (see page 27).

- Patients unresponsive to two different antipsychotics (one an atypical) should be given clozapine.

- Depot medication should be used where there are grounds to suspect that a patient may be unlikely to adhere to prescribed oral therapy.

- Where more than one atypical is appropriate, the drug with the lowest purchase cost should be prescribed.

- 'Advance directives' regarding patients' preference for treatment should be developed and documented.

- Drug treatment should be considered only part of a comprehensive package of care.

- Atypical and typical antipsychotics should not be prescribed together except during changeover of medication.

Reference

1. National Institute of Clinical Excellence. Health Technology Appraisal No. 43. NICE, London, 2002.

1st episode schizophrenia

Treatment algorithm

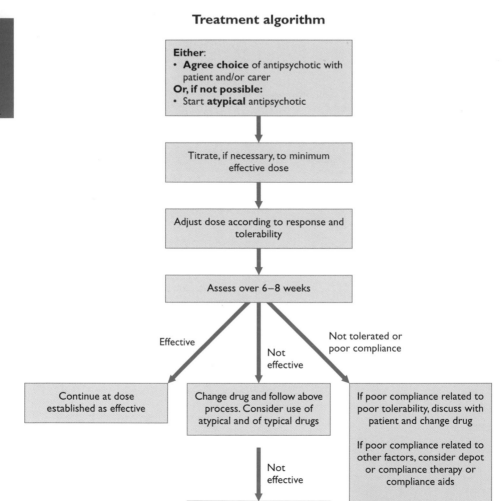

Either:
- **Agree choice** of antipsychotic with patient and/or carer
Or, if not possible:
- Start **atypical** antipsychotic

Titrate, if necessary, to minimum effective dose

Adjust dose according to response and tolerability

Assess over 6–8 weeks

Effective

Not effective

Not tolerated or poor compliance

Continue at dose established as effective

Change drug and follow above process. Consider use of atypical and of typical drugs

If poor compliance related to poor tolerability, discuss with patient and change drug

If poor compliance related to other factors, consider depot or compliance therapy or compliance aids

Repeat above process

Not effective

Clozapine

Relapse or acute exacerbation of schizophrenia

(full adherence to medication confirmed)

Treatment algorithm

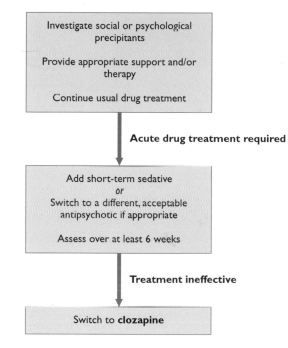

Investigate social or psychological precipitants

Provide appropriate support and/or therapy

Continue usual drug treatment

Acute drug treatment required

Add short-term sedative
or
Switch to a different, acceptable antipsychotic if appropriate

Assess over at least 6 weeks

Treatment ineffective

Switch to **clozapine**

Relapse or acute exacerbation of schizophrenia

(adherence doubtful or known to be poor)

Treatment algorithm

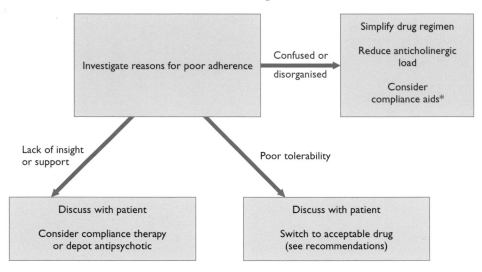

Investigate reasons for poor adherence	Confused or disorganised → Simplify drug regimen / Reduce anticholinergic load / Consider compliance aids*
Lack of insight or support → Discuss with patient / Consider compliance therapy or depot antipsychotic	Poor tolerability → Discuss with patient / Switch to acceptable drug (see recommendations)

* Compliance aids (e.g. Medidose system) are not a substitute for patient education. The ultimate aim should be to promote independent living, perhaps with patients filling their own compliance aid, having first been given support and training. Note that such compliance aids are of little use unless the patient is clearly motivated to adhere to prescribed treatment. Note also that some medicines are not suitable for storage in compliance aids.

Switching antipsychotics because of poor tolerability – recommendations

Schizophrenia

Adverse effect	Suggested drugs	Alternatives	References
Acute EPSEs	Quetiapine Olanzapine Aripiprazole	Risperidone (<6 mg/day) Clozapine Ziprasidone	1–5
Hyperprolactinaemia	Quetiapine Olanzapine (small, transient rise in prolactin[6], although symptoms rarely observed[7]) Aripiprazole	Ziprasidone Clozapine	8–11
Weight gain	Amisulpride Haloperidol Trifluoperazine Aripiprazole	Quetiapine Ziprasidone Risperidone	12–15
Tardive dyskinesia	Clozapine	Olanzapine Quetiapine Risperidone (<6 mg/day)	16–18
Impaired glucose tolerance	Amisulpride Ziprasidone Aripiprazole	Risperidone	19–22
QT prolongation	Amisulpride Aripiprazole	Olanzapine	23–25
Sedation	Amisulpride Risperidone Sulpiride Haloperidol Aripiprazole		–
Postural hypotension	Amisulpride Sulpiride Haloperidol Trifluoperazine Aripiprazole		–

References

1. Stanniland C, Taylor D. Tolerability of atypical antipsychotics. *Drug Safety* 2000; **22**: 195–214.
2. Daniel T, Baldessarini RJ, Tarazi FI. Effects of newer antipsychotics on extrapyramidal function. *CNS Drugs* 2002; **16**: 23–45.
3. Caroff SN, Mann SC, Campbell EC *et al.* Movement disorders associated with atypical antipsychotic drugs. *J Clin Psychiatry* 2002; **63**: 12–19.
4. Lemmens P, Brecher M, Van Baelen B. A combined analysis of double-blind studies with risperidone vs. placebo and other antipsychotic agents: factors associated with extrapyramidal symptoms. *Acta Psychiatr Scand* 1999; **99**: 160–170.
5. Taylor DM. Aripiprazole: a review of its pharmacology and clinical use. *Int J Clin Pract* 2003; **57**: 49–54.
6. Crawford AM, Beasley C, Tollefson GD. The acute and long-term effect of olanzapine compared with placebo and haloperidol on serum prolactin concentrations. *Schizophr Res* 1997; **26**: 41–54.
7. Licht R, Arngrim T, Christensen H. Olanzapine-induced galactorrhea. *Psychopharmacology* 2002; **162**: 94–95.

8. Turrone P, Kapur S, Seeman M *et al.* Elevation of prolactin levels by atypical antipsychotics. *Am J Psychiatry* 2002; **159**: 133–135.

9. David S, Taylor C, Kinon B *et al.* The effects of olanzapine, risperidone and haloperidol on plasma prolactin levels in patients with schizophrenia. *Clin Ther* 2000; **22**: 1085–1095.

10. Hammer MB, Arana GW. Hyperprolactinaemia in antipsychotic-treated patients: guidelines for avoidance and management. *CNS Drugs* 1998; **10**: 209–222.

11. Haddad PM, Wieck A. Antipsychotic-induced hyperprolactinaemia. Mechanisms, clinical features and management. *Drugs* 2004; **64**. 2291–2314.

12. Taylor DM, McAskill R. Atypical antipsychotics and weight gain – a systemic review. *Acta Psychiatr Scand* 2000; **101**: 416–432.

13. Allison D, Mentore J, Moonseong H *et al.* Antipsychotic-induced weight gain: a comprehensive research synthesis. *Am J Psychiatry* 1999; **156**: 1686–1696.

14. Brecher M, Rak I, Melvin R *et al.* The long-term effect of quetiapine (Seroquel) monotherapy on weight in patients with schizophrenia. *Int J Psychiatry Clin Pract* 2000; **4**: 287–291.

15. Casey DE, Carson WH, Saha AR *et al.* Switching patients to aripiprazole from other antipsychotic agents: a multicenter randomized study. *Psychopharmatology* 2003; **166**: 391–399.

16. Lieberman J, Johns C, Cooper T *et al.* Clozapine pharmacology and tardive dyskinesia. *Psychopharmacology* 1989; **99**: S54–S59.

17. O'Brien J, Barber R. Marked improvement in tardive dyskinesia following treatment with olanzapine in an elderly subject. *Br J Psychiatry* 1998; **172**: 186.

18. Sacchetti E, Valsecchi P. Quetiapine, clozapine and olanzapine in the treatment of tardive dyskinesia induced by first-generation antipsychotics: a 124 week case report. *Int Clin Psychopharmacol* 2003; **18**: 357–359.

19. Haddad PM. Antipsychotics and diabetes: a review of non-prospective data. *Br J Psychiatry* 2004; **184**(suppl 47): 580–586.

20. Berry S, Mahmoud R. Normalization of olanzapine-associated abnormalities of insulin resistance and insulin release after switch to risperidone: the risperidone rescue study. Poster presented at the European College of Neuropsychopharmacology 15th Annual Meeting, 5–9 October 2002, Barcelona, Spain.

21. Gianfrancesco F, Grogg A, Mahmoud R *et al.* Differential effects of risperidone, olanzapine, clozapine, and conventional antipsychotics on type 2 diabetes: findings from a large health plan database. *J Clin Psychiatry* 2002; **63**: 920–930.

22. Mir S, Taylor D. Atypical antipsychotics and hyperglycaemia. *Int Clin Psychopharmacol* 2001; **16**: 63–73.

23. Glassman A, Bigger J. Antipsychotic drugs: prolonged QTc interval, torsade de pointes, and sudden death. *Am J Psychiatry* 2001; **158**: 1774–1782.

24. Taylor D. Antipsychotics and QT prolongation. *Acta Psychiatr Scand* 2003; **107**: 85–95.

25. Titier K, Girodet P-O, Verdoux H. Atypical antipsychotics – from potassium channels to torsade de pointes and sudden death. *Drug Safety* 2005; **28**: 35–51.

Further reading

Devlin MJ, Yanovski SZ, Wilson GT. Obesity: what mental health professionals need to know. *Am J Psychiatry* 2000; **157**: 854–866.

National Institute of Clinical Excellence. Guidance on the use of newer (atypical) antipsychotic drugs for the treatment of schizophrenia. Health Technology Appraisal No. 43, NICE, London, 2002.

Slovenko R. Update on legal issues associated with tardive dyskinesia. *J Clin Psychiatry* 1999; **61**(Suppl. 4): 45–57.

Van Harten PN, Hoek HW, Kahn RS. Acute dystonia induced by drug treatment. *BMJ* 1999; **319**: 623–626.

Typical antipsychotics – clinical utility

Typical and atypical antipsychotics are not categorically delineated. Typical drugs are those which can be expected to give rise to acute EPSEs, hyperprolactinaemia and, in the longer term, tardive dyskinesia. Atypicals, by any sensible definition, might be expected not to be associated with these adverse effects. However, some atypicals show dose-related EPSEs, some induce hyperprolactinaemia and some may eventually give rise to tardive dyskinesia. To complicate matters further, it has been suggested that the therapeutic and adverse effects of typical drugs can be separated by careful dosing[1] – thus making typical drugs atypical (there is much evidence to the contrary, incidentally[2–4]).

Given these observations, it seems unwise to consider so-called typical and atypical drugs as distinct groups of drugs. The essential difference between the two is the therapeutic index in relation to acute EPSEs; for instance, haloperidol has an extremely narrow index (probably substantially less than 0.5 mg/day); olanzapine a wide index (20–40 mg/day).

Typical drugs still play an important role in schizophrenia and offer a valid alternative to atypicals where atypicals are poorly tolerated. Their main drawbacks are, of course, acute EPSEs (see page 71), hyperprolactinaemia and tardive dyskinesia. Hyperprolactinaemia is probably unavoidable in practice and, even when not symptomatic, may grossly affect hypothalamic function[5]. It is firmly associated with sexual dysfunction[6], but be aware that the autonomic effects of some atypicals may also cause sexual dysfunction[7].

Tardive dyskinesia probably occurs more frequently with typicals than atypicals[8–10] (notwithstanding difficulties in defining what is atypical), although this is far from certain[11]. Careful observation of patients and the prescribing of the lowest effective dose are essential to help reduce the risk of this serious adverse event[12,13].

References

1. Oosthuizen P, Emsley R, Turner J et al. Determining the optimal dose of haloperidol in first-episode psychosis. J Psychopharmacol 2001; 154: 251–255.
2. Zimbroff DL, Kane JM, Tamminga CA et al. Controlled, dose-response study of sertindole and haloperidol in the treatment of schizophrenia. Am J Psychiatry 1997; 154: 783–791.
3. Jeste DV, Lacro JP, Palmer B et al. Incidence of tardive dyskinesia in early stages of low-dose treatment with typical neuroleptics in older patients. Am J Psychiatry 1999; 156: 309–311.
4. Meltzer HY, Fang VS. The effect of neuroleptics on serum prolactin in schizophrenia patients. Arch Gen Psychiatry 1976; 33: 279–286.
5. Smith S, Wheeler M, Murray R et al. The effects of antipsychotic-induced hyperprolactinaemia on the hypothalamic-pituitary-gonadal axis. J Clin Psychopharm 2001; 22: 109–114.
6. Smith S, O'Keane V, Murray R. Sexual dysfunction in patients taking conventional antipsychotic medication. Br J Psychiatry 2002; 181: 49–55.
7. Aizenberg D, Modai I, Landa A et al. Comparison of sexual dysfunction in male schizophrenia patients maintained on treatment with classical antipsychotics versus clozapine. J Clin Psychiatry 2001; 62: 541–544.
8. Tollefson G, Beasley C, Tamura R et al. Double-blind, controlled, long-term study of the comparative incidence of treatment-emergent tardive dyskinesia with olanzapine or haloperidol. Am J Psychiatry 1997; 154: 1248–1254.
9. Beasley C, Dellva M, Tamura R et al. Randomised double-blind comparison of the incidence of tardive dyskinesia in patients with schizophrenia during long-term treatment with olanzapine or haloperidol. Br J Psychiatry 1999; 174: 23–30.
10. Correll CU, Leucht S, Kane JM. Lower risk for tardive dyskinesia associated with second-generation antipsychotics: a systematic review of 1-year studies. Am J Psychiatry 2004; 161: 414–425.
11. Halliday J, Farrington S, Macdonald S et al. Nithsdale schizophrenia surveys 23: movement disorders. Br J Psychiatry 2002; 181: 422–427.
12. Jeste D, Caligiuri M. Tardive dyskinesia. Schizophr Bull 1993; 19: 303–315.
13. Cavallaro R, Smeraldi E. Antipsychotic-induced tardive dyskinesia: recognition, prevention and management. CNS Drugs 1995; 4: 278–293.

New antipsychotics – recommended monitoring

Table

Drug	Obligatory monitoring		Suggested
	Baseline	Continuation	Baseline
Amisulpride	None	None	FPG/HbA$_{1C}$ Prolactin U&Es Weight Blood lipids
Clozapine	FBC Prescriber and pharmacist must register	FBC – weekly for 18 wks – at least every 2 wks for 1 year – monthly thereafter	FPG/HbA$_{1C}$[1,2] BP ECG (optional) LFTs U&Es Weight Blood lipids
Olanzapine	None	None	FPG/HbA$_{1C}$ BP FBC LFTs U&Es Prolactin Weight Blood lipids
Quetiapine	None	None	FPG/HbA$_{1C}$ BP LFTs TFTs U&Es Weight Blood lipids
Risperidone	None	None	FPG/HbA$_{1C}$ BP LFTs Prolactin U&Es Blood lipids Weight

additional monitoring		Actions
	Continuation	
FPG/HbA$_{IC}$	– 12 monthly	Perform FPG if HbA$_{IC}$ raised
Prolactin	– if symptoms occur	Stop if prolactin-related effects intolerable
U&Es	– 6 monthly	
Weight	– as needed	
Blood lipids	– after 3/12 then yearly	
CPK	– if NMS suspected	Stop if NMS suspected
FPG/HbA$_{IC}$	– at 1 month; 4–6 monthly	Perform FPG if HbA$_{IC}$ raised
BP	– 4 hourly during titration	Stop if neutrophils below 1.5×10^9/l
CPK	– if NMS suspected	Refer to specialist care if neutrophils below 0.5×10^9/l
ECG[3,4] (optional)	– when maintenance dose is reached	Stop if ECG shows important changes or if signs of heart failure noted
EEG[5,6]	– if myoclonus or seizures occur	Use valproate if EEG show epileptiform changes
LFTs[7]	– every 6 months for first year	Stop if LFTs indicate hepatitis or reduced hepatic function (PT or albumin)
U&Es[8]	– every 12 months	
Weight	– as needed	
Blood lipids	– 3 monthly then yearly	
FPG/HbA$_{IC}$[1,9,10]	– at 1 month; 4–6 monthly	Perform FPG if HbA$_{IC}$ raised
BP	– frequently during initiation	
CPK	– if NMS suspected	Stop if NMS suspected
FBC[11,12]	– 12 monthly	Stop if neutrophils below 1.5×10^9/l
LFTs	– at 3 and 6 months	Stop if PT or albumin change
U&Es	– 12 monthly	
Prolactin	– if symptoms occur (rare)	
Weight	– as needed	
Blood lipids	– 3 monthly then yearly	
FPG/HbA$_{IC}$[13]	– 12 monthly	Perform FPG if HbA$_{IC}$ raised
BP	– frequently during titration	
CPK	– if NMS suspected	Stop if NMS suspected
LFTs	– at 3 and 6 months	Stop if PT or bilirubin change
TFTs	– 12 monthly	
U&Es	– 12 monthly	
Weight	– as needed	
Blood lipids	– 3 monthly then yearly	
FPG/HbA$_{IC}$	– 12 monthly	Perform FPG if HbA$_{IC}$ raised
BP	– frequently during titration	
CPK	– if NMS suspected	Stop if NMS suspected
LFTs	– 12 monthly	Use with caution in hepatic/renal failure
Prolactin	– if symptoms occur	Stop if prolactin-related effects intolerable
U&Es	– 12 monthly	
Blood lipids	– after 3/12 then yearly	
Weight	– as needed	

New antipsychotics – recommended monitoring

| Drug | Obligatory monitoring | | Suggested |
	Baseline	Continuation	Baseline
Zotepine	None (ECG in some circumstances)	None (ECG in some circumstances)	FPG/HbA$_{1C}$ BP ECG LFTs Prolactin U&Es Weight Blood lipids
Ziprasidone	None (ECG in some circumstances)	None (ECG in some circumstances)	FPG/HbA$_{1C}$ BP FBC LFTs U&Es Weight Blood lipids
Aripiprazole	None	None	FPG/HbA$_{1C}$ BP FBC LFTs U&Es Weight Blood lipids

KEY: BP = blood pressure
CPK = creatinine phosphokinase
ECG = electrocardiograph
EEG = electroencephalograph
FBC = full blood count
FPG = fasting plasma glucose
HbA$_{1C}$= glycosylated haemoglobin
LFTs = liver function tests
PT = prothrombin time
TFTs = thyroid function tests
U&Es = urea and electrolytes

additional monitoring		Actions
	Continuation	

FPG/HbA$_{1C}$
BP
CPK
EEG[14]
ECG
 	
LFTs
Prolactin
U&Es
Weight
Blood lipids
	– 12 monthly
	– frequently during titration
	– if NMS suspected
	– if seizures occur
	– if necessary when
	   maintenance
	   dose is reached
	– 12 monthly
	– if symptoms occur
	– 12 monthly
	– as needed
	– after 3/12 then yearly
		Perform FPG if HbA$_{1C}$ raised
		
		Stop if NMS suspected
		Use valproate if EEG shows epileptiform
		changes
		
		Stop if ECG shows important changes
		
		Stop if renal function deteriorates

FPG/HbA$_{1C}$ BP FBC LFTs U&Es Weight Blood lipids	– 12 monthly – frequently during initiation – 6–12 monthly – 6 monthly – 6 monthly – as required – after 3/12 then yearly	Perform FPG if HbA$_{1C}$ raised Stop if FBC shows pathological changes Stop PT or bilirubin change
FPG/HbA$_{1C}$ BP FBC LFTs U&Es Weight Blood lipids	– 12 monthly – frequently during initiation – 12 monthly – 12 monthly – 12 monthly – as required – after 3/12 then yearly	Perform FPG if HbA$_{1C}$ raised Stop if FBC shows pathological changes Stop if PT or bilirubin change

Sources of information

Monitoring recommendations for new antipsychotics are derived from:
- normal clinical practice with new medicines (e.g. FBC, LFTs, U&Es)
- relevant summaries of product characteristics
- specific references (see below).

References

1. Wirshing DA, Spellberg BJ, Erhart SM *et al*. Novel antipsychotics and new onset diabetes. *Biol Psychiatry* 1998; 44: 778–783.
2. Hägg S, Joelsson L, Mjörndal T *et al*. Prevalence of diabetes and impaired glucose tolerance in patients treated with clozapine compared with patients treated with conventional depot neuroleptic medications. *J Clin Psychiatry* 1998; 59: 294–299.
3. Leo RJ, Kreeger JL, Kim KY. Cardiomyopathy associated with clozapine. *Ann Pharmacother* 1996; 30: 603–605.
4. Low RA, Fuller MA, Popli A. Clozapine induced atrial fibrillation (Letter). *ClinPsychopharmacol* 1998; 18: 170.
5. Silvestri RC, Bromfield EB, Khoshbin S. Clozapine-induced seizures and EEG abnormalities in ambulatory psychiatric patients. *Ann Pharmacother* 1998; 32: 1147–1151.
6. Taner E, Cosar B, Isik E. Clozapine-induced myoclonic seizures and valproic acid. *Int J Psychiatry Clin Pract* 1998; 2: 53–55.
7. Hummer M, Kurz M, Kurzthaler I *et al*. Hepatotoxicity of clozapine. *J Clin Psychopharm* 1997; 17: 314–317.
8. Elias TJ, Bannister KM, Clarkson AR *et al*. Clozapine: first report of acute interstitial nephritis: case report. *Lancet* 1999; 354: 1180–1181.
9. Ober SK, Hudak R, Rusterholtz A. Hyperglycemia and olanzapine. *Am J Psychiatry* 1999; 156: 970.
10. Lindenmayer JP, Patel R. Olanzapine-induced ketoacidosis with diabetes mellitus. *Am J Psychiatry* 1999; 156: 1471.
11. Naumann R, Felber W, Heilemann H *et al*. Olanzapine-induced agranulocytosis. *Lancet* 1999; 354: 566–567.
12. Duggal HS, Gates C, Pathak PC. Olanzapine-induced neutropenia: mechanism and treatment. *J Clin Psychopharm* 2004; 24: 234–235.
13. Sobel M, Jaggers ED, Franz MA. New-onset diabetes mellitus associated with the initiation of quetiapine treatment. *J Clin Psychiatry* 1999; 60: 556–557.
14. Prakash A, Lamb HM. Zotepine: a review of its pharmacodynamic and pharmacokinetic properties and therapeutic efficacy in the management of schizophrenia. *CNS Drugs* 1998; 9: 153–175.

Further reading

Marder SR, Essock SM, Miller AL *et al*. Physical health monitoring of patients with schizophrenia. *Am J Psychiatry* 2004; 161: 1334–1349.
Taylor D. Monitoring the new antipsychotic drugs. *Prog Neurolo Psychiatry* 1997; 1: 13–15.

See also sections on ECG monitoring (page 87), weight gain (page 83) and impaired glucose tolerance (page 92).

Depot antipsychotics

Advice on prescribing depot medication

- **Give a test dose.**
  Depots are long-acting. Any adverse effects that result from injection are likely to be long-lived. Thus a small test dose is essential to help avoid severe, prolonged adverse effects. See table below and manufacturer's information.

- **Begin with the lowest therapeutic dose.**
  There are few data showing clear dose–response effects for depot preparations. There is some information indicating that low doses are at least as effective as higher ones. Low doses are likely to be better tolerated and are certainly less expensive.

- **Administer at the longest possible licensed interval.**
  All depots can be safely administered at their licensed dosing intervals. There is no evidence to suggest that shortening the dose interval improves efficacy. Moreover, injections are painful, so less frequent administration is desirable. The 'observation' that some patients deteriorate in the days before the next depot is due is probably fallacious. For some hours (or even days with some preparations) plasma levels of antipsychotics continue to fall, albeit slowly, after the next injection. Thus patients are most at risk of deterioration immediately after a depot injection and not before it. Moreover, in trials, relapse seems only to occur 3–6 months after withdrawing depot therapy; roughly the time required to clear steady-state depot drug levels from the blood.

- **Adjust doses only after an adequate period of assessment.**
  Attainment of peak plasma levels, therapeutic effect and steady-state plasma levels are all delayed with depot injections. Doses may be *reduced* if adverse effects occur, but should only be *increased* after careful assessment over at least 1 month, and preferably longer. The use of adjunctive oral medication to assess depot requirements may be helpful, but it too is complicated by the slow emergence of antipsychotic effects. Note that at the start of therapy, plasma levels of antipsychotic released from a depot increase over several weeks without increasing the given dose. Dose increases during this time to steady-state plasma levels are thus illogical and impossible to evaluate properly.

Differences between depots

Zuclopenthixol is claimed to be more effective in aggressive patients, flupentixol decanoate in those who are depressed, haloperidol decanoate in the prophylaxis of manic illness and pipotiazine palmitate when EPSEs are problematic. Fluphenazine decanoate is said to be associated with depressed mood (which is common anyway in this patient group). The bulk of the literature in this area originates from the 1970s and 1980s, and the objective data contained therein do little to support the above 'folklore'. Many of these claimed differences are more the result of marketing strategies than of objective scientific evidence. The following *BNF* statement concerning 'choice of antipsychotic' should be borne in mind when considering depot as well as oral antipsychotics:

> *The various drugs differ somewhat in predominant actions and side-effects. Selection is influenced by the degree of sedation required and the patient's susceptibility to extrapyramidal side-effects. However, the differences between antipsychotic drugs are less important than the great variability in patient response; moreover, tolerance to these secondary effects usually develops.*

One very real difference that does exist is that flupentixol decanoate can be given in very much higher 'neuroleptic equivalent' doses than the other depot preparations and still remain 'within *BNF* limits'. It is doubtful that this confers any real therapeutic advantage.

Table Antipsychotic depot injections – suggested doses and frequencies[1]

Drug	Trade name	Test dose (mg)	Dose range (mg/week)	Dosing interval (weeks)	Comments
Flupentixol decanoate	Depixol	20	12.5–400	2–4	? Mood elevating; may worsen agitation
Fluphenazine decanoate	Modecate	12.5	6.25–50	2–5	? Avoid in depression High EPS
Haloperidol decanoate	Haldol	25*	12.5–75	4	High EPS, low incidence of sedation
Pipotiazine palmitate	Piportil	25	12.5–50	4	? Lower incidence of EPS (unproven)
Zuclopenthixol decanoate	Clopixol	100	100–600	2–4	? Useful in agitation and aggression

Notes:
- Give a quarter or half stated doses in elderly.
- After test dose, wait 4–10 days before starting titration to maintenance therapy (see product information for individual drugs).
- Dose range is given in mg/week for convenience only – avoid using shorter dose intervals than those recommended except in exceptional circumstances (e.g. long interval necessitates high volume (>3–4 ml) injection).

*Test dose not stated by manufacturer.

Intramuscular anticholinergics and depots

Depot antipsychotics do not produce acute EPSEs at the time of administration[2]: this may take hours to days. The administration of intramuscular procyclidine routinely with each depot is illogical, as the effects of the anticholinergic drug will have worn off before plasma antipsychotic levels peak.

References

1. Taylor D, Duncan D. Antipsychotic depot injections – suggested doses and frequencies. *Psychiatr Bull* 1995; **19**: 357.
2. Kane JM, Aguglia E, Altamura C *et al.* Guidelines for depot antipsychotic treatment in schizophrenia. *Eur Neuropsychopharm* 1998; **8**: 55–66.

Further reading

Adams CE, Fenton MKP, Quraishi S *et al.* Systematic meta-review of depot antipsychotic drugs for people with schizophrenia. *Br J Psych* 2001; **179**: 290–299.
Taylor D. Depot antipsychotics revisited. *Psychiatr Bull* 1999; **23**: 551–553.
Walbum J, Gray R, Gournay K *et al.* Systematic review of patient and nurse attitudes to depot antipsychotic medication. *Br J Psych* 2001; **179**: 300–307.

Risperidone long-acting injection

Risperidone is the only atypical drug available as a depot or long-acting, injectable formulation. Doses of 25–50 mg every 2 weeks appear to be as effective as oral doses of 2–6 mg/day[1]. The long-acting injection also seems to be well tolerated – less than 10% experience EPSEs and less than 6% withdrew from a long-term trial because of adverse effects[2]. Few data are available relating to effects on prolactin but problems might be predicted[3]. There is confusion over the dose–response relationship for RLAI. Studies randomising subjects to different doses of RLAI show no differences or trends towards differences in response according to dose[4]. Naturalistic studies indicate doses higher than 25 mg/week are frequently required[5,6]. One study suggests higher doses are associated with better outcome[7].

Risperidone long-acting injection differs importantly from other depots and the following should be noted:

- Risperidone depot is not an esterified form of the parent drug. It contains risperidone coated in polymer to form microspheres. These microspheres have to be suspended in an aqueous base immediately before use.

- The injection must be stored in a fridge (consider the practicalities for CPNs).

- It is available as doses of 25, 37.5 and 50 mg. The whole vial must be used (because of the nature of the suspension). This means that there is limited flexibility in dosing. In clinical studies 25 mg was as effective as 50 mg/2 weeks.

- A test dose is not required or sensible. (Testing tolerability with oral risperidone is desirable but not always practical.)

- It takes 3–4 weeks for the first injection to produce therapeutic plasma levels. Patients must be maintained on a full dose of their previous antipsychotic for at least 3 weeks after the administration of the first risperidone injection. Oral antipsychotic cover is sometimes required for longer (6–8 weeks). If the patient is not already receiving an oral antipsychotic, oral risperidone should be prescribed. (See table for advice on switching from depots.)

- Risperidone depot must be administered every 2 weeks. The pharmacokinetic profile does not allow longer intervals between doses. There is no flexibility to negotiate with patients about the frequency of administration.

For guidance on switching to risperidone long-acting injection see the table on page 38.

References

1. Chue P, Eerdekens M, Augustyns I et al. Efficacy and safety of long-acting risperidone microspheres and risperidone oral tablets. Poster presented at the 11th Biennial Winter Workshop on Schizophrenia, 24 February–1 March 2002, Davos, Switzerland.
2. Fleischhacker WW, Eerdekens M, Karcher K et al. Treatment of schizophrenia with long-acting injectable risperidone: a 12-month open-label trial of the first long-acting second-generation antipsychotic. J Clin Psychopharm 2003; 64: 1250–1257.
3. Kleinber DI, Davies JM, de Costa R et al. Prolactin levels and adverse events in patients treated with risperidone. J Clin Psychopharm 1999; 19: 57–61.
4. Kane JM, Eerdekens M, Lindenmayer JP et al. Long-acting injectable risperidone: efficacy and safety of the first long-acting atypical antipsychotic. Am J Psychiatry 2003; 160: 1125–1132.
5. Turner M, Eerdekens E, Jacko M et al. Long-acting injectable risperidone: safety and efficacy in stable patients switched from conventional depot antipsychotics. Int Clin Psychopharmacol 2004; 19: 241–249.
6. Taylor DM, Young CL, Mace S et al. Early clinical experience with risperidone long-acting injection: a prospective, 6-month follow-up of 100 patients. J Clin Psychiatry 2004; 65: 1076–1083.
7. Taylor D, Young C, Patel M. Six month follow-up of patients receiving risperidone long-acting injection – factors predicting clinical outcome. J Clin Psychiatry, submitted.

Switching to risperidone long-acting injection (RLAI)

Table		
Switching from	*Recommended method of switching*	*Comments*
No treatment (new patient or recently non-compliant)	Start risperidone oral at 2 mg/day and increase to 3 or 4 mg/day on day 2. If tolerated, give RLAI 25 mg on day 3. Continue with oral risperidone for at least 3 weeks then taper over 1–2 weeks. Be prepared to continue oral risperidone for longer	Use oral risperidone before giving injection to ensure good tolerability
Oral risperidone	Give RLAI 25 mg. Continue with oral risperidone for at least 3 weeks, then taper over 1–2 weeks	RLAI 25 mg and 50 mg appear to have the same efficacy. However, for patients maintained on more than 4 mg/day oral risperidone, higher doses of RLAI may, in theory, be required. Consider initiation with 37.5 mg/2 weeks in such patients
Oral antipsychotics (not risperidone)	*Either:* (a) Switch to oral risperidone and then, if tolerated give injection (25 mg) *or:* (b) Give RLAI 25 mg and then slowly discontinue oral antipsychotics after 3–4 weeks. Be prepared to continue oral treatment for longer	Dose of RLAI difficult to predict. Best practice is perhaps to start at 25 mg every 2 weeks and then adjust as necessary. May be worth initiating RLAI at 37.5 mg/2 weeks in those previously maintained on doses in the upper range of licensed doses
Depot antipsychotic	Give RLAI 25 mg one week *before* the last depot injection is given, or give RLAI in place of the last depot injection	Dose of RLAI difficult to predict. Best practice is perhaps to start at 25 mg every 2 weeks and then adjust as necessary. May be worth initiating RLAI at 37.5 mg/2 weeks in those previously maintained on doses in the upper range of licensed doses
Antipsychotic polypharmacy with depot	Give RLAI 25 mg one week before the last depot injection is given, or in place of the last depot injection. Slowly taper oral antipsychotics 3–4 weeks later. Be prepared to continue oral antipsychotics for longer	Aim to treat patient with RLAI as the sole antipsychotic. As before, 25 mg every 2 weeks is recommended initially for all patients, but consider starting at higher dose in those previously on high doses

Management of patients on long-term depots

Such patients should be seen by their consultant at least once a year (ideally more frequently) in order to review their progress and treatment. There is no simple formula for deciding when to reduce the dose; therefore, a risk/benefit analysis must be done for every patient, taking the following factors into consideration:

- Is the patient symptom-free and if so for how long? Long-standing, non-distressing symptoms which have not previously been responsive to medication may be excluded.

- What is the severity of the side-effects (EPSEs, TD, obesity, etc.)?

- What is the previous pattern of illness? Consider the speed of onset, duration and severity of episodes and any danger posed to self or others.

- Has dosage reduction been attempted before? If so, what was the outcome?

- What are the patient's current social circumstances? Is it a period of relative stability, or are stressful life events anticipated?

- What is the social cost of relapse (e.g. is the patient the sole breadwinner for a family)?

- Is the patient able to monitor his/her own symptoms? If so, will he/she seek help?

If after consideration of the above, the decision is taken to reduce medication, the patient's family should be involved and a clear explanation given of what should be done if symptoms return/worsen. It would then be reasonable to proceed in the following manner:

- If it has not already been done, oral antipsychotic medication should be discontinued first.

- The interval between injections should be increased to up to 4 weeks before decreasing the dose given each time. Note: *not* with risperidone.

- The dose should be reduced by no more than a third at any one time. Note: special considerations apply to risperidone.

- Decrements should, if possible, be made no more frequently than every 3 months.

- Discontinuation should be seen as the end point of the above process.

If the patient becomes symptomatic, this should be seen not as a failure, but rather as an important step in determining the minimum effective dose that the patient requires.

Antipsychotic polypharmacy

There is no good objective evidence that antipsychotic polypharmacy offers any efficacy advantage over the use of a single antipsychotic, but such prescriptions are commonly seen[1]. National surveys have repeatedly shown that up to 50% of patients prescribed atypical antipsychotics receive a typical drug as well[2,3]. Anticholinergic medication is then often required[3].

A UK audit of antipsychotic prescribing in hospitalised patients found that 20% of all patients prescribed antipsychotics were prescribed doses above the *BNF* maximum. Very few of these prescriptions were for single antipsychotics[1] (high doses were the result of antipsychotic polypharmacy). Monitoring of patients receiving high doses or combinations was very poor. Prescribers would seem not to be aware of the additive side-effects resulting from antipsychotic polypharmacy. Clinical factors such as age (young), gender (male) and diagnosis (schizophrenia) were associated with antipsychotic polypharmacy, albeit only a small proportion of the total[4]. One study has shown a past history of violence to be an important factor[5]. The majority of such prescribing, however, remains unexplained.

Another study which followed a cohort of patients with schizophrenia prospectively over a 10-year period found that receiving more than one antipsychotic concurrently was associated with increased mortality[6]. There was no association with the total number of antipsychotics given sequentially as monotherapy, the maximum daily antipsychotic dose, duration of exposure, lifetime intake, or any other measure of illness severity. Interestingly, the prescription of anticholinergics was associated with increased survival. Although these data should be interpreted with some important caveats in mind, they should serve to remind us that antipsychotic monotherapy is desirable and should be the norm. This is emphasised by a more recent study which demonstrated longer patient hospital stay and more frequent adverse effects in people receiving antipsychotic polypharmacy[7]. It follows that it should be standard practice to document the rationale for using antipsychotic polypharmacy in individual cases in clinical notes along with a clear account of any benefits and side-effects. Medicolegally, that would seem to be wise although in practice it is rarely done[8].

Note that the NICE explicitly demands that atypicals and typicals be not prescribed together except when switching[9]. Note also that clozapine augmentation strategies often involve polypharmacy and this is perhaps the sole therapeutic area where such practice is supportable.

References

1. Harrington M, Lelliott P, Paton C *et al.* The results of a multi-centre audit of the prescribing of antipsychotic drugs for in-patients in the UK. *Psychiatr Bull* 2002; **26**: 414–418.
2. Taylor D, Mace S, Mir S *et al.* A prescription survey of the use of atypical antipsychotics for hospital patients in the UK. *Int J Psychiatry Clin Pract* 2000; **4**: 41–46.
3. Paton C, Lelliott P, Harrington M *et al.* Patterns of antipsychotic and anticholinergic prescribing for hospital inpatients. *J Clin Psychopharm* 2003; **26**: 419–423.
4. Lelliott P, Paton C, Harrington M. The influence of patient variables on polypharmacy and combined high dose of antipsychotic drugs prescribed for in-patients. *Psychiatr Bull* 2002; **26**: 411–414.
5. Wilkie A, Preston N, Wesby R. High dose neuroleptics – who gives them and why? *Psychiatr Bull* 2001; **25**: 179–183.
6. Waddington JL, Youssef HA, Kinsella A. Mortality in schizophrenia: antipsychotic polypharmacy and absence of adjunctive anticholinergics over the course of a 10 year prospective study. *Br J Psychiatry* 1998; **173**: 325–329.
7. Centorrino F, Goren JL, Hennen J *et al.* Multiple versus single antipsychotic agents for hospitalized psychiatric patients: Case-control study of risks versus benefits. *Am J Psychiatry* 2004; **161**: 700–706.
8. Taylor D, Mir S, Mace S *et al.* Co-prescribing of atypical and typical antipsychotics – prescribing sequence and documented outcome. *Psychiatr Bull* 2002; **26**: 170–172.
9. National Institute for Clinical Excellence. *Guidance on the Use of Newer (Atypical) Antipsychotic Drugs for the Treatment of Schizophrenia.* London: NICE, June 2002.

High-dose antipsychotics: prescribing and monitoring

'High dose' can result from the prescription of either:

1. a single antipsychotic in a dose that is above the recommended maximum.
Or
2. two or more antipsychotics that, when expressed as a percentage of their respective maximum recommended doses and added together, result in a cumulative dose of >100%.

Efficacy

There is no firm evidence that high doses of antipsychotics are any more effective than standard doses. This holds true for the use of antipsychotics in rapid tranquillisation, the management of acute psychotic episodes, chronic aggression and relapse prevention[1].

There are a small number of RCTs that examine the efficacy of high versus standard doses in patients with treatment-resistant schizophrenia[2,3]. Some demonstrated benefit[4] but the majority of these studies are old, the number of patients randomised is small and study design is poor by current standards. Some studies used doses equivalent to more than 10 g chlorpromazine. A recent review of the dose–response effects of a variety of antipsychotics revealed no evidence whatever for increasing doses above accepted therapeutic ranges[5]. Effect appears to be optimal at low doses: 4 mg/day risperidone; 300 mg/day quetiapine, etc.

Adverse effects

The majority of side effects associated with antipsychotic treatment are dose related. These include EPSEs, sedation, postural hypotension, anticholinergic effects and QTc prolongation. High-dose antipsychotic treatment has insufficient support in the scientific literature and clearly worsens adverse effect incidence and severity[6,7]. Polypharmacy (with the exception of augmentation strategies for clozapine) also seems to be ineffective[8,9] and to produce more severe adverse effects[9,10].

References

1. Royal College of Psychiatrists. Revised Consensus Statement on High Dose Antipsychotic Medication. Expected 2005.
2. Hirsch SR, Barnes TRE. Clinical use of high dose neuroleptics. *Br J Psychiatry* 1994; **164**: 94–96.
3. Thompson C. The use of high-dose antipsychotic medication. *Br J Psychiatry* 1994; **164**: 448–458.
4. Aubree JC, Lader MH. High and very high dosage antipsychotics: a critical review. *J Clin Psychiatry* 1980; **41**: 341–350.
5. Davis JM, Chen N. Dose response and dose equivalence of antipsychotics. *J Clin Psychopharm* 2004; **24**: 192–208.
6. Bollini P, Pampallona S, Orza MJ *et al.* Antipsychotic drugs: is more worse? A meta-analysis of the published randomized control trials. *Psychol Med* 1994; **24**: 307–316.
7. Baldessarini RJ, Cohen BM, Teicher MH. Significance of neuroleptic dose and plasma level in the pharmacological treatment of psychoses. *Arch Gen Psychiatry* 1988; **45**: 79–91.
8. Taylor D, Mir S, Mace S *et al.* Co-prescribing of atypical and typical antipsychotics – prescribing sequence and documented outcome. *Psychiatr Bull* 2002; **26**: 170–172.
9. Centorrino F, Goren JL, Hennen J *et al.* Multiple versus single antipsychotic agents for hospitalized psychiatric patients: case-control study of risks versus benefits. *Am J Psychiatry* 2004; **161**: 700–706.
10. Waddington JL, Youssef HA, Kinsella A. Mortality in schizophrenia. *Br J Psychiatry* 1998; **173**: 325–329.

Prescribing high-dose antipsychotics

Before using high doses, ensure that:
- Sufficient time has been allowed for response (see page 24).
- At least two different antipsychotics have been tried (one atypical).
- Clozapine has failed or not been tolerated due to agranulocytosis. Most other side-effects can be managed: see page 54 et seq. A very small proportion of patients may also refuse clozapine outright.
- Compliance is not in doubt (use of blood tests, liquids/dispersible tablets, depot preparations, etc.).
- Adjunctive medications such as antidepressants or mood stabilisers are not indicated.
- Psychological approaches have failed or are not appropriate.

The decision to use high doses should:
- be made by a consultant psychiatrist
- involve the multidisciplinary team
- be done if possible, with the patient's informed consent.

Process:
- Exclude contraindications (ECG abnormalities, hepatic impairment).
- Document the decision to prescribe high doses in the clinical notes along with a description of target symptoms. The use of an appropriate rating scale is advised.
- Adequate time for response should be allowed after each dosage increment before a further increase is made.

Monitoring:
- Physical monitoring should be carried out as outlined on page 30.
- All patients on high doses should have regular ECGs (baseline, when steady-state serum levels have been reached after each dosage increment, and then every 6 to 12 months). Additional monitoring is advised if drugs that are known to cause electrolyte disturbances or QTc prolongation are subsequently coprescribed.
- Target symptoms should be assessed after 6 weeks and 3 months. If insufficient improvement in these symptoms has occurred, the dose should be decreased to the normal range.

Negative symptoms

A good deal of advertising material for new antipsychotics emphasises improved efficacy against negative symptoms when compared to older alternatives. Some points are worthy of consideration. The aetiology of negative symptoms is complex and it is important to determine the most likely cause in any individual case before embarking on a treatment regime. Negative symptoms can be either primary (transient or enduring) or secondary to positive symptoms (e.g. asociality secondary to paranoia), EPSEs (e.g. bradykinesia, lack of facial expression), depression (e.g. social withdrawal) or institutionalisation[1]. Secondary negative symptoms are obviously best dealt with by treating the relevant cause (EPSEs, depression, etc.). In general:

- The earlier a psychotic illness is effectively treated, the less likely is the development of negative symptoms over time[2].

- Older antipsychotics have only a small effect against primary negative symptoms and can cause secondary negative symptoms (EPSEs).

- Atypical antipsychotics cause few EPSEs but are not strikingly effective against primary negative symptoms. Many trials report statistically significant differences in favour of the atypical, but the clinical significance of the small mean changes observed is questionable. More robust data support the effectiveness of amisulpride in primary negative symptoms[3,4] but even this effect seems no better than haloperidol[5].

- Low serum folate concentrations have been found in patients with predominantly negative symptoms[6].

References

1. Carpenter WT. The treatment of negative symptoms: pharmacological and methodological issues. *Br J Psychiatry* 1996; **168**(Suppl. 29): 17–22.
2. Waddington JL, Youssef HA, Kinsella A. Sequential cross sectional and 10 year prospective study of severe negative symptoms in relation to duration of initially untreated psychosis in chronic schizophrenia *Psychol Med* 1995; **25**: 849–857.
3. Boyer P, Lecrubier Y, Puech AJ *et al.* Treatment of negative symptoms in schizophrenia with amisulpride. *Br J Psychiatry* 1995; **166**: 68–72.
4. Danion JM, Rein W, Fleurot O. Improvement of schizophrenia patients with primary negative symptoms treated with amisulpride. Amisulpride Study Group. *Am J Psychiatry* 1999; **156**: 610–616.
5. Speller JC, Barnes TR, Curson DA *et al.* One-year, low-dose neuroleptic study of in-patients with chronic schizophrenia characterised by persistent negative symptoms. Amisulpride v. haloperidol. *Br J Psychiatry* 1997; **171**: 564–568.
6. Goff DC, Bottiglieri T, Arning E *et al.* Folate, homocysteine and negative symptoms in schizophrenia. *Am J Psychiatry* 2004; **161**: 1705–1708.

Schizophrenia

Antipsychotic prophylaxis

First episode of psychosis

A placebo-controlled study has shown that when no prophylactic treatment is given, 57% of first-episode patients have relapsed at 1 year[1]. After 1–2 years of being well on antipsychotic medication, the risk of relapse remains high (figures of 10–15% per month have been quoted), but this area is less well researched[2,3]. Although the current consensus is that antipsychotics should be prescribed for 1–2 years after a first episode of schizophrenia[4,5], Gitlan *et al*.[6] found that withdrawing antipsychotic treatment in line with this consensus led to a relapse rate of almost 80% after 1 year medication-free and 98% after 2 years. In practice, a firm diagnosis of schizophrenia is rarely made after a first episode and the majority of prescribers and/or patients will have at least attempted to stop antipsychotic treatment within 1 year[7]. It is vital that patients, carers and keyworkers are aware of the early signs of relapse and how to access help. Antipsychotics should not be considered the only intervention. Psychosocial and psychological interventions are clearly also important.

Multi-episode schizophrenia

The majority of those who have one episode of schizophrenia will go on to have further episodes. With each subsequent episode, the baseline level of functioning deteriorates[8] and the majority of this decline is seen in the first decade of illness. Suicide risk (10%) is also concentrated in the first decade of illness. Those who receive targeted antipsychotics (i.e. only when symptoms re-emerge) have a worse outcome than those who receive prophylactic antipsychotics[9,10] and the risk of TD may also be higher. The figure below depicts the relapse rate in a large cohort of patients with psychotic illness, the majority of whom had already experienced multiple episodes[11]. All had originally received or were still receiving treatment with typical antipsychotics. Note that many of the studies included in this data set were old, and unstandardised diagnostic criteria were used. Variable definitions of relapse and short follow-up periods were the norm and other psychotropic drugs were not controlled for.

Figure Effect of prophylactic antipsychotics

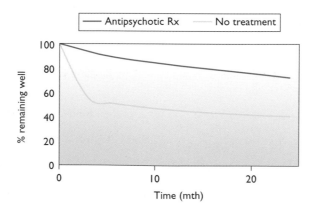

There is some evidence to support improved long-term outcomes with atypical antipsychotics. Csernansky *et al.*[12] found that relapse rates over 2 years were 34% for risperidone and 60% for haloperidol. A naturalistic study found that almost 70% of those discharged from hospital on risperidone or olanzapine were not readmitted over the next 2 years, compared with 52% of those who were treated with conventional antipsychotics[13]. Another naturalistic study found relapse rates and service costs to be significantly lower with risperidone than with conventional drugs[14].

Dose for prophylaxis

Many patients probably receive higher doses than necessary (particularly of the older drugs) when acutely psychotic[15,16]. In the longer term a balance needs to be made between effectiveness and side-effects. Lower doses of the older drugs (8 mg haloperidol/day or equivalent) are, when compared with higher doses, associated with less severe side-effects[17], better subjective state and better community adjustment[18]. Very low doses increase the risk of psychotic relapse[15,19]. There are no data to support the use of lower than standard doses of the newer drugs as prophylaxis.

How and when to stop[20]

The decision to stop antipsychotic drugs requires a risk benefit analysis for each patient. Withdrawal of antipsychotic drugs after long-term treatment should be gradual and closely monitored. The relapse rate in the first 6 months after abrupt withdrawal is double that seen after gradual withdrawal (defined as slow taper down over at least 3 weeks for oral antipsychotics or abrupt withdrawal of depot preparations)[21]. Abrupt withdrawal may also lead to discontinuation symptoms (e.g. headache, nausea, insomnia) in some patients[22].

The following factors should be considered[20]:

- Is the patient symptom-free, and if so, for how long? Long-standing, non-distressing symptoms which have not previously been responsive to medication may be excluded.

- What is the severity of side-effects (EPSEs, TD, obesity, etc.)?

- What was the previous pattern of illness? Consider the speed of onset, duration and severity of episodes and any danger posed to self and others.

- Has dosage reduction been attempted before, and, if so, what was the outcome?

- What are the patient's current social circumstances? Is it a period of relative stability, or are stressful life events anticipated?

- What is the social cost of relapse (e.g. is the patient the sole breadwinner for a family)?

- Is the patient/carer able to monitor symptoms, and, if so, will they seek help?

As with first-episode patients, patients, carers and keyworkers should be aware of the early signs of relapse and how to access help. Those with a history of aggressive behaviour or serious suicide attempts and those with residual psychotic symptoms should be considered for life-long treatment.

Key points that patients should know

- Antipsychotics do not 'cure' schizophrenia. They treat symptoms in the same way that insulin treats diabetes.

- Long-term treatment is required to prevent relapses.

- Many antipsychotic drugs are available. Different drugs suit different patients. Perceived side-effects should always be discussed, so that the best tolerated drug can be found.

- Antipsychotics should not be stopped suddenly.

References

1. Crow TJ, McMillan JP, Johnson AL et al. The Northwick Park study of first episodes of schizophrenia II. A randomised controlled trial of prophylactic neuroleptic treatment. Br J Psychiatry 1986; 148: 120–127.
2. Neuchterlein KH, Gitlin M, Subotnik KL. The early course of schizophrenia and long-term maintenance neuroleptic therapy. Arch Gen Psychiatry 1995; 52: 193–195.
3. Davis JM, Metalon L, Watanabe MD et al. Depot antipsychotic drugs: place in therapy. Drugs 1994; 47: 741–773.
4. Sheitman BB, Lee H, Strausi R et al. The evaluation and treatment of first-episode psychosis. Schizophr Bull 1997; 23: 653–661.
5. American Psychiatric Association. Practice guideline for the treatment of patients with schizophrenia. Am J Psychiatry 1997; 154(4 Suppl. 1): 1–63.
6. Gitlan M, Neuchterlein K, Subotnik KL. Clinical outcome following neuroleptic discontinuation in patients with remitted recent-onset psychosis. Am J Psychiatry 2001; 158: 1835–1842.
7. Johnson DAW, Rasmussen JGC. Professional attitudes in the UK towards neuroleptic maintenance therapy in schizophrenia: the problem of inadequate prophylaxis. Psychiatr Bull 1997; 21: 394–397.
8. Wyatt RJ. Neuroleptics and the natural course of schizophrenia. Schizophr Bull 1991; 17: 325–351.
9. Jolly AG, Hirsch SR, McRink A et al. Trial of brief intermittent neuroleptic prophylaxis for selected schizophrenic outpatients: clinical outcomes at one year. BMJ 1989; 298: 985–990.
10. Herz MI, Glazer WM, Mostert MA et al. Intermittent vs maintenance medication in schizophrenia: 2 year results. Arch Gen Psychiatry 1991; 48: 333–339.
11. Gilbert PL, Harris MJ, McAdams LA et al. Neuroleptic withdrawal in schizophrenic patients. Arch Gen Psychiatry 1995; 52: 173–188.
12. Csernansky JG, Mahmoud R, Brenner R. A comparison of risperidone and haloperidol for the prevention of relapse in patients with schizophrenia. New Engl J Med 2002; 346: 16–22.
13. Rabinowitz J, Lichtenberg P, Kaplan Z et al. Rehospitalisation rates of chronically ill schizophrenic patients discharged on a regimen of risperidone, olanzapine or conventional antipsychotics. Am J Psychiatry 2001; 158: 266–269.
14. Malla AK, Norman RM, Scholten DJ et al. A comparison of long-term outcome in first-episode schizophrenia following treatment with risperidone or a typical antipsychotic. J Clin Psychiatry 2001; 62(3): 179–184.
15. Baldessarini RJ, Cohen BM, Teicher MH. Significance of neuroleptic dose and plasma level in the pharmacological treatment of psychoses. Arch Gen Psychiatry 1988; 45: 79–90.
16. Harrington M, Lelliott P, Paton C et al. The results of a multi-centre audit of the prescribing of antipsychotic drugs for in-patients in the UK. Psychiatr Bull 2002; 26: 414–418.
17. Geddes J, Freemantle N, Harrison P et al. Atypical antipsychotics in the treatment of schizophrenia: systematic overview and meta-regression analysis. BMJ 2000; 321: 1371–1376.
18. Hogarty GE, McEvoy JP, Munetz M et al. Dose of fluphenazine, familial expressed emotion, and outcome in schizophrenia: results of a two-year controlled study. Arch Gen Psychiatry 1988; 45: 797–805.
19. Marder SR, van Putten T, Mintz J. Low and conventional dose maintenance therapy with fluphenazine decanoate: two-year outcome. Arch Gen Psychiatry 1987; 44: 518–521.
20. Wyatt J. Risks of withdrawing antipsychotic medications. Arch Gen Psychiatry 1995; 52: 196–199.
21. Viguera AC, Baldessarini RJ, Hegarty JD. Clinical risk following abrupt and gradual withdrawal of maintenance neuroleptic treatment. Arch Gen Psychiatry 1997; 54: 49–55.
22. Chouinard G, Bradvejn J, Annable L et al. Withdrawal symptoms after long-term treatment with low-potency neuroleptics. J Clin Psychiatry 1984; 45: 500–502.

Further reading

Bosveld-van Haandel LJM, Slooff CJ, van den Bosch RJ. Reasoning about the optimal duration of prophylactic antipsychotic medication in schizophrenia: evidence arguments. Acta Psychiatr Scand 2001; 103: 335–346.
Csernansky JG, Schuchart EK. Relapse and rehospitalisation rates in patients with schizophrenia: effects of second generation antipsychotics. CNS Drugs 2002; 16: 473–484.

Refractory schizophrenia

Clozapine – dosing regimen

Many of the adverse effects of clozapine are dose-dependent and associated with speed of titration. Adverse effects also tend to be more common at the beginning of therapy. To minimise these problems it is important to start therapy at a low dose and to increase dosage slowly.

Clozapine should be started at a dose of 12.5 mg once a day. Blood pressure should be monitored hourly for 6 hours because of the hypotensive effect of clozapine. This monitoring is not usually necessary if the first dose is given at night. On day 2, the dose can be increased to 12.5 mg twice daily. If the patient is tolerating clozapine, the dose can be increased by 25–50 mg a day, until a dose of 300 mg a day is reached. This can usually be achieved in 2–3 weeks. Further dosage increases should be made slowly in increments of 50–100 mg each week. A plasma level of 350 µg/l should be aimed for to ensure an adequate trial but response may occur at lower plasma level. The dose at which this plasma level is reached varies according to gender and smoking status. The range is approximately 250 mg/day (female non-smoker) to 550 mg/day (male smoker)[1]. The total clozapine dose should be divided and, if sedation is a problem, the larger portion of the dose can be given at night.

The following table is a suggested starting regime for clozapine. This is a cautious regimen more rapid increases have been used in exceptional circumstances. Slower titration may be necessary where sedation is severe. If the patient is not tolerating a particular dose, decrease to one that was tolerated. If the adverse effect resolves, increase the dose again but at a slower rate. If for any reason a patient misses *less than* 2 days' clozapine, restart at the dose prescribed before the event. Do not administer extra tablets to catch up. If more than 2 days are missed, restart at 12.5 mg once daily and increase slowly (but at a faster rate than in drug-naïve patients).

Table	Suggested starting regime for clozapine (in-patients)	
Day	**Morning dose (mg)**	**Evening dose (mg)**
1	–	12.5
2	12.5	12.5
3	25	25
4	25	25
5	25	50
6	25	50
7	50	50
8	50	75
9	75	75
10	75	100
11	100	100
12	100	125
13	125	125
14	125	150
15	150	150
18	150	200
21	200	200
28	200	250

Reference

1. Rostami-Hodjegan A, Amin AM, Spencer EP *et al.* Influence of dose, cigarette smoking, age, sex and metabolic activity on plasma clozapine concentrations: a predictive model and nomograms to aid clozapine dose adjustment and to assess compliance in individual patients. *J Clin Psychopharm* 2004; 24: 70–78.

Optimising clozapine treatment

Optimising clozapine treatment

Target dose *(Note that dose is best adjusted according to patient tolerability)*	• Average dose in UK is around 450 mg/day[1] • Response usually seen in the range 150–900 mg/day[2] • Lower doses required in the elderly, females and non-smokers, and in those prescribed certain enzyme inhibitors[3,4]
Plasma levels	• Most studies indicate that threshold for response is in the range 350–420 µg/l[5,6]. Threshold may be as high as 500 µg/l[7] (see page 4) • Importance of norclozapine levels not established but clozapine/norclozapine ratio may aid assessment of recent compliance.

References

1. Taylor D, Mace S, Mir S *et al.* A prescription survey of the use of atypical antipsychotics for hospital inpatients in the United Kingdom. *Int J Psychiatry Clin Pract* 2000; 4: 41–46.
2. Murphy B, Long C, Paton C. Maintenance doses for clozapine. *Psychiatr Bull* 1998; 22: 12–14.
3. Taylor D. Pharmacokinetic interactions involving clozapine. *Br J Psychiatry* 1997; 171: 109–112.
4. Lane HY, Chang YC, Chang WH *et al.* Effects of gender and age on plasma levels of clozapine and its metabolites: analysed by critical statistics. *J Clin Psychiatry* 1999; 60: 36–40.
5. Taylor D, Duncan D. The use of clozapine plasma levels in optimising therapy. *Psychiatr Bull* 1995; 19: 753–755.
6. Spina E, Avenoso A, Facciolà G *et al.* Relationship between plasma concentrations of clozapine and norclozapine and therapeutic response in patients with schizophrenia resistant to conventional neuroleptics. *Psychopharmacology* 2000; 148: 83–89.
7. Perry PJ. Therapeutic drug monitoring of atypical antipsychotics: is it of potential clinical value? *CNS Drugs* 2000; 13: 167–171.

Optimising clozapine treatment (continued)

The table below shows other suggested options where 3–6 months of clozapine alone has provided unsatisfactory benefit.

Table Augmenting clozapine	
Option	**Comment**
Add sulpiride[1] (400 mg/day)	• May be useful in partial or non-responders. Supported by a randomised, controlled trial
Add lamotrigine[2–4] (25–300 mg/day)	• May be useful in partial or non-responders
Add risperidone[5,6] (2–4 mg/day)	• Increases clozapine plasma levels. May have additive antipsychotic effects. Supported by a randomised, controlled trial
Add omega-3 triglycerides[7,8] (2–3 g EPA daily)	• Modest, if contested, evidence to support efficacy in non- or partial responders to antipsychotics, including clozapine (see page 69)
Add amisulpride[9–11] (400–800 mg/day)	• Developing evidence and experience suggest amisulpride augmentation is worthwhile
Add haloperidol (2 mg/day)	• Anecdotal reports of clinical improvement. No published evidence
Add aripiprazole[12] (15–30 mg/day)	• Very limited evidence that aripiprazole augmentation of clozapine is beneficial

Notes:
- For discussion of augmentation strategies see Chong S-A, Remington G. Clozapine augmentation: safety and efficacy. *Schizophr Bull* 2000; **26**: 421–440.
- Always consider the use of mood stabilisers and/or antidepressants where mood disturbance is thought to contribute to symptoms[13].
- Topiramate has also been suggested, either to augment clozapine or to induce weight loss. It is probably not effective as augmentation and may even worsen psychosis[3,14].
- Other options include adding pimozide[15] and olanzapine[16]. Neither is recommended: pimozide has important cardiac toxicity and the addition of olanzapine is expensive and poorly supported. There is also a single case report of ziprasidone augmentation of clozapine[17].

References

1. Shiloh R, Zemishlany Z, Aizenberg D *et al.* Sulpiride augmentation in people with schizophrenia partially responsive to clozapine. *Br J Psychiatry* 1997; **171**: 569–573.
2. Dursun SM, McIntosh D. Clozapine plus lamotrigine in treatment-resistant schizophrenia. *Arch Gen Psychiatry* 1999; **56**: 950.
3. Dursun SM, Deakin J. Augmenting antipsychotic treatment with lamotrigine or topiramate in patients with treatment-resistant schizophrenia: a naturalistic case-series outcome study. *J Psychopharmacol* 2001; **15**: 297–301.
4. Tiihonen J, Hallikainen T, Ryynanen OP *et al.* Lamotrigine in treatment-resistant schizophrenia: a randomized placebo-controlled crossover trial. *Biol Psychiatry* 2003; **54**: 1241–1248.
5. Joisassen RC, Joseph AJ, Koheggl *et al.* Clozapine augmented with risperidone in the treatment of schizophrenia: a randomised double-blind, placebo-controlled trial. *Am J Psychiatry* 2005; **162**: 130–136.
6. Raskin S, Katz G, Zislin Z *et al.* Clozapine and risperidone: combination/augmentation treatment of refractory schizophrenia: a preliminary observation. *Acta Psychiatr Scand* 2000; **101**: 334–336.
7. McGorry PD, Yung AR, Phillips L *et al.* Double-blind placebo controlled trial of N-3 polyunsaturated fatty acids as an adjunct to neuroleptics. *Schizophr Res* 1998; **29**: 160–161.
8. Puri BK, Richardson AJ. Sustained remission of positive and negative symptoms of schizophrenia following treatment with eicosapentaenoic acid. *Arch Gen Psychiatry* 1998; **55**: 188–189.
9. Mathiasson P, Costa D, Erlandsson K *et al.* The relationship between dopamine D2 receptor occupancy and clinical response in amisulpride augmentation of clozapine non-response. *J Psychopharmacol* 2001; **15**(Suppl.): S41.

10. Munro J, Matthiasson P, Osborne S *et al.* Amisulpride augmentation of clozapine: an open non-randomized study in patients with schizophrenia partially responsive to clozapine. *Acta Psychiatr Scand* 2004; **110**: 292–298.
11. Zink M, Knopf U, Henn FA *et al.* Combination of clozapine and amisulpride in treatment-resistant schizophrenia – case reports and review of the literature. *Pharmacopsychiatry* 2004; **37**: 26–31.
12. Lim S, Pralea C, Schnitt J *et al.* Possible increased efficacy of low-dose clozapine when combined with aripiprazole. *J Clin Psychiatry* 2004; **65**: 9.
13. Citrome L. Schizophrenia and valporate. *Psychopharmacol Bull* 2003; **2**: 74–88.
14. Millson R, Owen J, Lorberg G *et al.* Topiramate for refractory schizophrenia. *Am J Psychiatry* 2002; **159**: 675.
15. Friedman J, Ault K, Powchik P. Pimozide augmentation for the treatment of schizophrenic patients who are partial responders to clozapine. *Biol Psychiatry* 1997; **42**: 522–523.
16. Sonnerberg G, Frank S. Olanzapine augmentation of clozapine. *Ann Clin Psychiatry* 1998; **10**: 113–115.
17. Zink M, Mase E, Dressing H. Combination of ziprasidone and clozapine in treatment-resistant schizophrenia. *Hum Psychopharm* 2004; **19**: 271–273.

Refractory schizophrenia – alternatives to clozapine

The table below lists alternatives to clozapine (where clozapine has proved toxic or is contra-indicated).

Table Alternatives to clozapine
(Treatments are listed in alphabetical order: no preference is implied by position in table.)

Treatment	Comments
Aripiprazole[1] (15–30 mg/day)	Single randomised controlled study indicating moderate effect in patients resistant to risperidone or olanzapine (+ others).
ECT[2-4]	Open studies suggest moderate effect. Often reserved for last-line treatment in practice.
Ginkgo biloba (+ antipsychotic)[5,6]	Possibly effective in combination with haloperidol. Unlikely to give rise to additional adverse effects but clinical experience limited.
Olanzapine[7-12] 5–25 mg/day	Supported by some well-conducted trials but clinical experience disappointing.
Olanzapine[13-16] 30–60 mg/day	Contradictory findings in the literature but possibly effective. Expensive and unlicensed. High-dose olanzapine is not atypical[17] and can be poorly tolerated[18].
Olanzapine + amisulpride[19] (up to 800 mg/day)	Small open study suggests benefit.
Olanzapine + aripiprazole[20]	Single case report suggests benefit.
Olanzapine + glycine[21] (0.8 g/kg/day)	Small, double-blind cross-over trial suggests clinically relevant improvement in negative symptoms.
Olanzapine + lamotrigine[22,23] (up to 400 mg/day)	Reports contradictory and rather unconvincing. Reasonable theoretical basis for adding lamotrigine which is usually well tolerated.
Olanzapine + sulpiride[24] (600 mg/day)	Some evidence that this combination improves mood symptoms.
Omega–3-triglycerides[25,26]	Suggested efficacy but data very limited (see page 69).
Quetiapine[27-29]	Very limited evidence and clinical experience not encouraging.
Risperidone[30,31] 4–8 mg/day	Doubtful efficacy in true treatment-refractory schziophrenia but some supporting evidence. May also be tried in combination with glycine[21] or lamotrigine[22] or indeed with other atypicals[32].
Transcranial magnetic stimulation[33]	Single case report. Included in this table for completeness.

Notes:
- Evidence base is growing: some support for use of some atypicals in partial responders but clozapine remains the drug of choice in true refractory illness.
- Above treatments should be used instead of clozapine only where clozapine cannot be used because of toxicity or very poor tolerability.
- Switching from clozapine to other drug treatments (in clozapine responders) usually destabilises psychotic illness and can have disastrous consequences.

References

1. Modell S, Jody D, Kujawa M *et al.* Efficacy of aripiprazole and perphenazine in severe schizophrenia resistant to treatment with atypical antipsychotics. 17th Congress of the European College of Neuropsychopharmacology, Stockholm, Sweden, 9–13 October 2004.
2. Chanpattana W, Chakrabhand M. Combined ECT and neuroleptic therapy in treatment-refractory schizophrenia: prediction of outcome. *Psychiatry Res* 2001; **105**: 107–115.
3. Tang WK, Ungvari GS. Efficacy of electroconvulsive therapy in treatment resistant schizophrenia: a prospective open trial. *Prog Neuro-Psychopharmacology Bio Psychiatry* 2003; **27**: 373–379.
4. Chanpattana W, Kramer BA. Acute and maintenance ECT with flupenthixol in refractory schizophrenia: sustained improvements in psychopathology, quality of life, and social outcomes. *Schizophr Res* 2003; **63**: 189–193.
5. Zhou D, Zhang X, Su J *et al.* The effects of classic antipsychotic haloperidol plus the extract of *Ginkgo biloba* on superoxide dismutase in patients with chronic refractory schizophrenia. *Chinese Med J-Peking* 1999; **112**(12): 1093–1096.
6. Zhang X, Zhou D, Zhang P *et al.* A double-blind, placebo-controlled trial of extract of *Ginkgo biloba* added to haloperidol in treatment-resistant patients with schizophrenia. *J Clin Psychiatry* 2001; **62**(11): 878–883.
7. Breier A, Hamilton SH. Comparative efficacy of olanzapine and haloperidol for patients with treatment-resistant schizophrenia. *Biol Psychiatry* 1999; **45**: 403–411.
8. Conley RR, Tamminga CA, Bartko JJ *et al.* Olanzapine compared with chlorpromazine in treatment-resistant schizophrenia. *Am J Psychiatry* 1998; **155**: 914–920.
9. Sanders RD, Mossman D. An open trial of olanzapine in patients with treatment-refractory psychoses. *J Clin Psychopharm* 1999; **19**: 62–66.
10. Taylor D, Mir S, Mace S. Olanzapine in practice: a prospective naturalistic study. *Psychiatr Bull* 1999; **23**: 178–180.
11. Bitter I, Dossenbach MRK, Brook S *et al.* Olanzapine versus clozapine in treatment resistant or treatment-intolerant schizophrenia. *Prog Neuro-Psychopharmacology Bio Psychiatry* 2004; **28**: 173–180.
12. Tollefson GD, Birkett MA, Kiesler GM *et al.* Double-blind comparison of olanzapine versus clozapine in schizophrenic patients clinically eligible for treatment with clozapine. *Biol Psychiatry* 2001; **49**: 52–63.
13. Sheitman BB, Lindgren JC, Early J *et al.* High-dose olanzapine for treatment-refractory schizophrenia. *Am J Psychiatry* 1997; **154**: 1626.
14. Fanous A, Lindenmayer JP. Schizophrenia and schizoaffective disorder treated with high doses of olanzapine. *J Clin Psychopharm* 1999; **19**: 275–276.
15. Dursun SM, Gardner DM, Bird DC *et al.* Olanzapine for patients with treatment-resistant schizophrenia: a naturalistic case-series outcome study. *Can J Psychiatry* 1999; **44**: 701–704.
16. Conley RR, Kelly DL, Richardson CM *et al.* The efficacy of high-dose olanzapine versus clozapine in treatment-resistant schizophrenia: a double-blind crossover study. *J Clin Psychopharm* 2003; **23**: 668–671.
17. Bronson BD, Lindenmayer J-P. Adverse effects of high dose olanzapine in treatment-refractory schizophrenia (Letter). *J Clin Psychopharm* 2000; **20**: 382–384.
18. Kelly DL, Conley RR, Richardson CM *et al.* Adverse effects and laboratory parameters of high-dose olanzapine vs. clozapine in treatment-resistant schizophrenia. *Ann Clin Psychiatry* 2003; **15**: 181–186.
19. Zink M, Henn FA, Thome J. Combination of amisulpride and olanzapine in treatment-resistant schizophrenic psychoses. *Eur J Psychiatry* 2004; **19**: 56–58.
20. Duggal HS. Aripiprazole-olanzapine combination for treatment of schizophrenia. *Can J Psychiatry* 2004; **49**: 151.
21. Heresco-Levy U, Ermilov M, Lichtenberg P *et al.* High-dose glycine added to olanzapine and risperidone for the treatment of schizophrenia. *Soc Biol Psychiatry* 2004; **55**: 165–171.
22. Kremer I, Vass A, Gorelik I *et al.* Placebo-controlled trial of lamotrigine added to conventional and atypical antipsychotics in schizophrenia. *Soc Biol Psychiatry* 2004; **56**: 441–446.
23. Dursun SM, Deakin JF. Augmenting antipsychotic treatment with lamotrigine or topiramate in patients with treatment-resistant schizophrenia: a naturalistic case-series outcome study. *J Clin Psychopharm* 2001; **15**: 297–301.
24. Kotler M, Strous RD, Reznik I *et al.* Sulpiride augmentation of olanzapine in the management of treatment-resistant chronic schizophrenia: evidence for improvement of mood symptomatology. *Int Clin Psychopharmacol* 2004; **19**: 23–26.
25. Mellor JE, Laugharne JDE, Peet M. Omega-3 fatty acid supplementation in schizophrenic patients. *Hum Psychopharm* 1996; **11**: 39–46.
26. Puri BK, Steiner R, Richardson AJ. Sustained remission of positive and negative symptoms of schizophrenia following treatment with eicosapentaenoic acid. *Arch Gen Psychiatry* 1998; **55**: 188–189.
27. Reznik I, Benatov R, Sirota P *et al.* Long-term efficacy and safety of quetiapine in treatment-refractory schizophrenia: a case report. *Int J Psychiatry Clin Pract* 2000; **4**: 77–80.
28. Windhager E, Whiteford J, Jones A *et al.* Patients switched to quetiapine demonstrated improved efficacy and tolerability irrespective of previous medication. Poster presented at the 15th European College of Neuropsychopharmacology Congress, Barcelona, Spain, 5–9 October 2002.
29. Nayer A, Jones A, Whiteford J *et al.* Improved efficacy gained from switching to quetiapine in patients with schizophrenia. Poster presented at the 15th European College of Neuropsychopharmacology Congress, Barcelona, Spain, 5–9 October 2002.
30. Breier AF, Malhotra AK, Su TP *et al.* Clozapine and risperidone in chronic schizophrenia: effects on symptoms, Parkinsonian side effects, and neuroendocrine response. *Am J Psychiatry* 1999; **156**: 294–298.
31. Bondolfi G, Dufour H, Patris M *et al.* Risperidone versus clozapine in treatment-resistant chronic schizophrenia: a randomized double-blind study. *Am J Psychiatry* 1998; **155**: 499–504.

32. Lerner V, Libov I, Kotler M *et al.* Combination of 'atypical' antipsychotic medication in the management of treatment-resistant schizophrenia and schizoaffective disorder. *Prog Neuro-Psychopharmacology Bio Psychiatry* 2004; **28**: 89–98.
33. Franck N, Poulet E, Terra JL *et al.* Left temporoparietal transcranial magnetic stimulation in treatment-resistant schizophrenia with verbal hallucinations. *Psychiatry Res* 2003; **120**: 107–109.

Further reading

Henderson DC, Nasrallah RA, Goff DC. Switching from clozapine to olanzapine in treatment-refractory schizophrenia: safety, clinical efficacy, and predictors of response. *J Clin Psychiatry* 1998; **59**: 585–588.
Lindenmayer J-P, Czobar P, Volavka J *et al.* Olanzapine in refractory schizophrenia after failure of typical or atypical antipsychotic treatment: an open-label switch study. *J Clin Psychiatry* 2002; **63**: 931–935.
Still DJ, Dorson PG, Crismon MH *et al.* Effects of switching inpatients with treatment-resistant schizophrenia from clozapine to risperidone. *Psychiatr Serv* 1996; **47**: 1382–1384.

Clozapine – management of common adverse effects

Table

Adverse effect	Timecourse	Action
Sedation	First 4 weeks. May persist, but usually wears off	Give smaller dose in the morning. Reduce dose if necessary
Hypersalivation	First 4 weeks. May persist, but usually wears off. Often very troublesome at night	Give hyoscine 300 µg (Kwells) sucked and swallowed at night. Pirenzepine[1] (not licensed in the UK) up to 50 mg t.d.s. may be tried (see page 63)
Constipation	Usually persists	Recommend high-fibre diet. Bulk forming laxatives ± stimulants may be used. Effective treatment or prevention of constipation is essential
Hypotension	First 4 weeks	Advise patient to take time when standing up. Reduce dose or slow down rate of increase. If severe, consider moclobemide and Bovril[2], or fludrocortisone
Hypertension	First 4 weeks, sometimes longer	Monitor closely and increase dose as slowly as is necessary. Hypotensive therapy (e.g. atenolol 25 mg/day) is sometimes necessary[3]
Tachycardia	First 4 weeks, but sometimes persists	Very common in early stages of treatment but usually benign. Tachycardia, if persistent at rest and associated with fever, hypotension or chest pain, may indicate myocarditis[4,5] (see page 58). Referral to a cardiologist is advised. Clozapine should be stopped if tachycardia occurs in the context of chest pain or heart failure
Weight gain	Usually during the first year of treatment	Dietary counselling is essential. Advice may be more effective if given before weight gain occurs. Weight gain is common and often profound (>10 lb) (see page 83)
Fever	First 3 weeks	Give antipyretic but check FBC. This fever is not usually related to blood dyscrasias[6] but beware myocarditis
Seizures	May occur at any time[7]	Dose-/dose-increase-related. Consider prophylactic valproate* if on high dose or with high plasma level (above 500–600 µg/l). After a seizure: withhold clozapine for 1 day; restart at reduced dose; give sodium valproate. Note that EEG abnormalities are common in those on clozapine[8]
Nausea	First 6 weeks	May give antiemetic. Avoid prochlorperazine and metoclopramide if previous EPSEs
Nocturnal enuresis	May occur at any time	Try manipulating dose schedule. Avoid fluids before bedtime. May resolve spontaneously[9]. In severe cases, desmopressin is usually effective[10]
Neutropenia/ agranulocytosis	First 18 weeks (but may occur at any time)	Stop clozapine; admit to hospital

* Usual dose is 1000–2000 mg/day. Plasma levels may be useful as a rough guide to dosing – aim for 50–100 mg/l. Use of modified-release preparation (Epilim Chrono) may aid compliance: can be given once daily and may be better tolerated.

References

1. Fritze J, Tilmann E. Pirenzepine for clozapine-induced hypersalivation. *Lancet* 1995; **346**: 1034.
2. Taylor D, Reveley A, Faivre F. Clozapine-induced hypotension treated with moclobemide and Bovril. *Br J Psychiatry* 1995; **167**: 409–410.
3. Henderson DC, Daley TB, Kunkel L *et al.* Clozapine and hypertension: a chart review of 82 patients. *J Clin Psychiatry* 2004; **65**: 686–689.
4. Committee on Safety of Medicines. Clozapine and cardiac safety: updated advice for prescribers. *Current Problems in Pharmacovigilance* 2002; **28**: 8–9.
5. Hägg S, Spigset O, Bate A *et al.* Myocarditis related to clozapine treatment. *J Clin Psychopharm* 2001; **21**: 382–388.
6. Tham JC, Dickson RA. Clozapine-induced fevers and 1-year clozapine discontinuation rate. *J Clin Psychiatry* 2002; **63**: 880–884.
7. Pacia SV, Devinsky O. Clozapine-related seizures: experience with 5,629 patients. *Neurology* 1994; **44**: 2247–2249.
8. Centorrino F, Price BH, Tuttle M *et al.* FEG abnormalities during treatment with typical and atypical antipsychotics. *Am J Psychiatry* 2002; **159**: 109–115.
9. Warner MP, Harvey CA, Barnes TRE. Clozapine and urinary incontinence. *Int Clin Psychopharmacol* 1994; **9**: 207–209.
10. Use of desmopressin to treat clozapine-induced nocturnal enuresis (Letter). *J Clin Psychiatry* 1994; **55**: 315–316.

Further reading

Iqbal MM, Rahman A, Husain Z *et al.* Clozapine: a clinical review of adverse effects and management. *Ann Clin Psychiatry* 2003; **15**: 33–48.
Lieberman JA. Maximizing clozapine therapy: managing side effects. *J Clin Psychiatry* 1998; **59**(Suppl. 3): 38–43.

Clozapine – uncommon or unusual adverse effects

Pharmacoepidemiological monitoring of clozapine is more extensive than with any other drug. Our awareness of adverse effects related to clozapine treatment is therefore enhanced. The table below gives brief details of unusual or uncommon adverse effects of clozapine reported since its relaunch in 1990.

Table

Adverse effect	Comment
Agranulocytosis/neutropenia (delayed)[1,2]	Occasional reports of apparent clozapine-related blood dyscrasia even after 1 year of treatment.
Delirium[3]	Reported to be fairly common, but rarely seen in practice if dose is titrated slowly and plasma level determinations are used.
Eosinophilia[4,5]	Reasonably common but significance unclear. Some suggestion that eosinophilia predicts neutropenia but this is disputed.
Heat stroke[6]	Occasional case reported. May be mistaken for NMS.
Hepatic failure/enzyme abnormalities[7,8]	Benign changes in LFTs are common (up to 50% of patients) but worth monitoring because of the very small risk of fulminant hepatic failure.
Pancreatitis[9]	Rare reports of asymptomatic and symptomatic pancreatitis sometimes associated with eosinophilia. Some authors recommend monitoring serum amylase.
Pneumonia[10]	Very rarely results from saliva aspiration. Infections in general may be more common in those on clozapine[11]. Note that respiratory infections may give rise to elevated clozapine levels[12,13]. (Possibly an artefact: smoking usually ceases during an infection.)
Thrombocytopenia[14]	Few data but apparently fairly common. Probably transient and clinically unimportant.

References

1. Thompson A, Castle D, Orr K. Late onset neutropenia with clozapine. *Can J Psychiatry* 2004; **49**: 647–648.
2. Bhanji NH, Margolese HC, Chouinard G *et al.* Late-onset agranulocytosis in a patient with schizophrenia after 117 months of clozapine treatment. *J Clin Psychopharm* 2003; **23**: 522–523.
3. Centorrino F, Albert MJ, Drago-Ferrante G *et al.* Delirium during clozapine treatment: incidence and associated risk factors. *Pharmacopsychiatry* 2003; **36**: 156–160.
4. Hummer M, Sperner-Unterweger B, Kemmler G *et al.* Does eosinophilia predict clozapine induced neutropenia? *Psychopharmacology* 1996;**124**: 201–204.
5. Ames D, Wirshing WC, Baker RW *et al.* Predictive value of eosinophilia for neutropenia during clozapine treatment. *J Clin Psychiatry* 1996; **57**: 579–581.
6. Kerwin RW, Osborne S, Sainz-Fuertes R. Heat stroke in schizophrenia during clozapine treatment: rapid recognition and management. *J Psychopharmacol* 2004; **18**: 121–123.
7. Erdogan A, Kocabasoglu N, Yalug I *et al.* Management of marked liver enzyme increase during clozapine treatment: a case report and review of the literature. *Int J Psychiat Med* 2004; **34**: 83–89.
8. Macfarlane B, Davies S, Mannan K *et al.* Fatal acute fulminant liver failure due to clozapine: a case report and review of clozapine-induced hepatotoxicity. *Gastroenterology* 1997; **112**: 1707–1709.
9. Bergemann N, Ehrig C, Diebold K *et al.* Asymptomatic pancreatitis associated with clozapine. *Pharmacopsychiatry* 1999: **32**: 78–90.
10. Hinkes R, Quesade TV, Currier MB, Gonzalez-Blanco M. Aspiration pneumonia possibly secondary to clozapine-induced sialorrhea. *J Clin Psychopharm* 1996; **16**: 462–463.

11. Landry P, Benaliouad F, Tessier S. Increased use of antibiotics in clozapine-treated patients. *Int Clin Psychopharmacol* 2003; **18**: 297–298.
12. Raaska K, Raitasuo V, Arstila M *et al.* Bacterial pneumonia can increase serum concentration of clozapine. *Eur J Clin Pharmacol* 2002; **58**: 321–322.
13. De Leon J, Diaz FJ. Serious respiratory infections can increase clozapine levels and contribute to side effects: a case report. *Prog Neuro-Psychopharmacology Bio Psychiatry* 2003; **27**: 1059–1063.
14. Jagadheesan K, Agarwal SK, Nizamie SH. Clozapine-induced thrombocytopenia: a pilot study. *Hong Kong Journal of Psychiatry* 2003; **13**: 12–15.

Clozapine – serious adverse effects

Agranulocytosis, thromboembolism, cardiomyopathy and myocarditis

Clozapine clearly and substantially *reduces* overall mortality in schizophrenia, largely because of a considerable reduction in the rate of suicide[1,2]. Nevertheless, clozapine can cause serious, life-threatening adverse effects, of which **agranulocytosis** is the best known. In the UK, there have been three deaths due to clozapine-associated agranulocytosis – a risk of less than 1 in 5000 patients treated. Risk is well managed by the approved clozapine-monitoring systems.

A possible association between clozapine and **pulmonary embolism** has been suggested. Initially, Walker *et al*[1] uncovered a risk of fatal pulmonary embolism of 1 in 4500 – about 20 times the risk in the population as a whole. Following a case report of non-fatal pulmonary embolism possibly related to clozapine[3], data from the Swedish authorities were published[4]. Twelve cases of venous thromboembolism were described, of which five were fatal. The risk of thromboembolism was estimated to be 1 in 2000–6000 patients treated. Thromboembolism may be related to clozapine's observed effect on antiphospholipid antibodies[5]. It seems most likely to occur in the first 3 months of treatment.

It has also been suggested that clozapine is associated with **myocarditis** and **cardiomyopathy**. Australian data identified 23 cases (15 myocarditis, 8 cardiomyopathy), of which 6 were fatal[6]. Risk of death from either cause is estimated from these data to be 1 in 1300. Myocarditis seems to occur within 6–8 weeks of starting clozapine; cardiomyopathy may occur later in treatment. It is notable that other data sources give rather different risk estimates: in Canada the risk of fatal myocarditis was estimated to be 1 in 12,500; in the USA, 1 in 67,000[7]. Despite this uncertainty, patients should be closely monitored for signs of myocarditis especially in the first few months of treatment. Symptoms include tachycardia, fever, flu-like symptoms, fatigue, dyspnoea and chest pain. Signs include ECG changes (ST depression), enlarged heart on radiography and eosinophilia. Many of these symptoms occur in patients on clozapine not developing myocarditis[8]. Nonetheless, signs of heart failure should provoke immediate cessation of clozapine.

Note also that, despite an overall reduction in mortality, younger patients may have an increased risk of sudden death[9], perhaps because of clozapine-induced ECG changes[10]. The overall picture remains very unclear but caution is required. There may, of course, be similar problems with other antipsychotics[11,12].

Summary

- Overall mortality appears to be lower for those on clozapine than in schizophrenia as a whole.
- Risk of fatal agranulocytosis is less than 1 in 5000 patients treated in the UK.
- Risk of fatal pulmonary embolism is estimated to be around 1 in 4500 patients treated.
- Risk of fatal myocarditis or cardiomyopathy may be as high as 1 in 1300 patients.
- Careful monitoring is essential especially during the first 3 months of treatment.

References

1. Walker AM. Mortality in current and former users of clozapine. *Epidemiology* 1997; **8**: 671–677.
2. Munro J, O'Sullivan D, Andrews C *et al.* Active monitoring of 12,760 clozapine recipients in the UK and Ireland: beyond pharmacovigilance. *Br J Psychiatry* 1999; **175**: 576–580.
3. Lacika S, Cooper JP. Pulmonary embolus possibly associated with clozapine treatment (Letter). *Can J Psychiatry* 1999; **44**: 396–397.
4. Hägg S, Spigset O, Söderström TG. Association of venous thromboembolism and clozapine. *Lancet* 2000; **355**: 1155–1156.
5. Davis S. Antiphospholipid antibodies associated with clozapine treatment. *Am J Hematol* 1994; **46**: 166–167.
6. Kilian JG, Kerr K, Lawrence C *et al.* Myocarditis and cardiomyopathy associated with clozapine. *Lancet* 1999; **354**: 1841–1845.
7. Warner B, Alphs L, Schaedelin J *et al.* Myocarditis and cardiomyopathy associated with clozapine (Letter). *Lancet* 2000; **355**: 842–843.
8. Wehmeier PM, Schuler-Springorum M, Heiser P *et al.* Chart review for potential features of myocarditis, pericarditis, and cardiomyopathy in children and adolescents treated with clozapine. *J Child Adolesc Psychopharmacol* 2004; **14**. 267–271.
9. Modal I, Hirschman S, Rava A *et al.* Sudden death in patients receiving clozapine treatment: a preliminary investigation. *J Clin Psychopharm* 2000; **20**: 325–327.
10. Kang UG, Kwon JS, Ahn YM *et al.* Electrocardiographic abnormalities in patients treated with clozapine. *J Clin Psychiatry* 2000; **61**; 441–446.
11. Thomassen R, Vandenbroucke JP, Rosendaal FR. Antipsychotic drugs and thromboembolism (Letter). *Lancet* 2000; **356**: 252.
12. Hägg S, Spigset O. Antipsychotic-induced venous thromboembolism: a review of the evidence. *CNS Drugs* 2002; **16**. 765–776.

Clozapine, neutropenia and lithium

Risk of clozapine-induced neutropenia

Around 2.7% of patients treated with clozapine develop neutropenia. Of these, half do so within the first 18 weeks of treatment and three-quarters by the end of the first year[1]. Risk factors[1] include being Afro-Caribbean (77% increase in risk) and young (17% decrease in risk per decade increase in age), and having a low baseline white cell count (WCC) (31% increase in risk for each 1×10^9/l drop). Risk is not dose-related.

After being released from the bone marrow, neutrophils can either circulate freely in the bloodstream or be deposited next to vessel walls (margination)[2]. All of these neutrophils are available to fight infection. The proportion of marginated neutrophils is greater in people of Afro-Caribbean or African origin than in Caucasians, leading to lower apparent white cell counts (WCC) in the former. This is benign ethnic neutropenia.

Many patients develop neutropenia on clozapine but not all are clozapine-related or even pathological. Benign ethnic neutropenia very probably accounts for a proportion of observed or apparent clozapine-associated neutropenias (hence higher rates among Afro-Caribbeans). Distinguishing between true clozapine toxicity and neutropenia unrelated to clozapine is not possible with certainty but some factors are important. True clozapine-induced neutropenia generally occurs early in treatment. White cell counts are normal to begin with but then fall precipitantly (over 1–2 weeks or less) and recover slowly once clozapine is withdrawn. In benign ethnic neutropenia, WCCs are generally low and may frequently fall below the lower limit of normal. This pattern may be observed before, during and after the use of clozapine. Of course, true clozapine-induced neutropenia can occur in the context of benign ethnic neutropenia. Partly because of this, **any iatrogenic manipulation of WCCs in benign ethnic neutropenia carries significant risk**.

Effect of lithium on the WCC

Lithium increases the neutrophil count and total WCC both acutely[3] and chronically[4]. The magnitude of this effect is poorly quantified, but a mean neutrophil count of 11.9×10^9/l has been reported in lithium-treated patients[3] and a mean rise in neutrophil count of 2×10^9/l in clozapine-treated patients after the addition of lithium[5]. This effect does not seem to be clearly dose related[3,4] although a minimum lithium serum level of 0.4 mmol/l may be required[6]. The mechanism is not completely understood: both stimulation of granulocyte-macrophage colony-stimulating factor (GM-CSF)[7] and demargination[5] have been suggested. Lithium has been successfully used to raise the WCC during cancer chemotherapy[8–10]. White cells are fully formed and function normally – there is no 'left shift'.

Case reports

Lithium has been used to increase the WCC in patients who have developed neutropenia with clozapine, thus allowing clozapine treatment to continue. Four case reports in adults[6,11–13] and two in children[14] have been published. All patients had serum lithium levels of >0.6 mmol/l. Lithium has also been reported to speed the recovery of the WCC when prescribed after the development of clozapine-induced agranulocytosis[6].

Other potential benefits of lithium–clozapine combinations

Combinations of clozapine and lithium may improve symptoms in schizoaffective patients[5] and refractory bipolar illness[15,16]. There are no data pertaining to schizophrenia.

Potential risks

At least 0.7% of clozapine-treated patients develop agranulocytosis, which is potentially fatal. Over 80% of cases develop within the first 18 weeks of treatment[1]. Risk factors include increasing age and Asian race[1]. Some patients may be genetically predisposed[17]. Although the timescale and individual risk factors for the development of agranulocytosis are different from those associated with neutropenia, it is impossible to be certain in any given patient that neutropenia is not a precursor to agranulocytosis. Lithium does not seem to protect against true clozapine induced agranulocytosis: One case of fatal agranulocytosis has occurred with this combination[18] and a second case of agranulocytosis has been reported where the bone marrow was resistant to treatment with GM-CSF[19]. Note also that up to 20% of patients who receive clozapine–lithium combinations develop neurological symptoms typical of lithium toxicity despite lithium levels being maintained well within the therapeutic range[5,20].

The use of lithium to elevate WCC in patients with clear prior clozapine-induced neutropenia is not recommended. Lithium should only be used to elevate WCC where it is strongly felt that prior neutropenic episodes were unrelated to clozapine.

Management of patients with:

1. Low initial WCC (< 4 × 10⁹/l) or neutrophils (< 2.5 × 10⁹/l).
or
2. Clozapine-associated leucopenia (WCC < 3 × 10⁹/l) or neutropenia (neutrophils < 1.5 × 10⁹/l) thought to be linked to benign ethnic neutropenia.

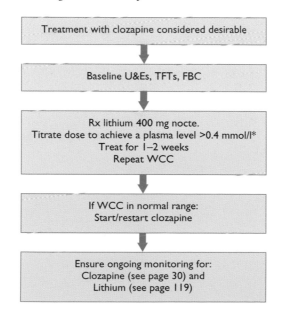

NB: Lithium does not protect against agranulocytosis: if the WCC continues to fall despite lithium treatment, consideration should be given to discontinuing clozapine. Particular vigilance is required in high-risk patients during the first 18 weeks of treatment.

* Higher plasma levels may be appropriate for patients who have an affective component to their illness.

References

1. Munro J, O'Sullivan D, Andrews C *et al.* Active monitoring of 12760 clozapine recipients in the UK and Ireland. *Br J Psychiatry* 1999; **175**: 576–580.
2. Abramson N, Melton B. Leukocytosis: basics of clinical assessment. *Am Fam Physician* 2000; **62**: 2053–2057.
3. Lapierre G, Stewart RB. Lithium carbonate and leukocytosis. *Am J Hosp Pharm* 1980; **37**: 1525–1528.
4. Carmen J, Okafor K, Ike E. The effects of lithium therapy on leukocytes: a 1 year follow-up study. *J Natl Med Assoc* 1993; **85**: 301–303.
5. Small J, Klapper M, Malloy F *et al.* Tolerability and efficacy of clozapine combined with lithium in schizophrenia and schizoaffective disorder. *J Clin Psychopharm* 2003; **23**: 223–228.
6. Blier B, Slater S, Measham T *et al.* Lithium and clozapine-induced neutropenia/agranulocytosis. *Int Clin Psychopharmacol* 1998; **13**: 137–140.
7. Ozdemir MA, Sofuoglu S, Tanrikulu G *et al.* Lithium-induced haematological changes in patients with bipolar affective disorder. *Biol Psychiatry* 1994; **35**: 210–213.
8. Johnke RM, Abernathy RS. Accelerated marrow recovery following total-body irradiation after treatment with vincristine, lithium or combined vincristine-lithium treatment. *Int J Cell Cloning* 1991; **9**: 78–88.
9. Greco FA, Brereton HD. Effect of lithium carbonate on the neutropenia caused by chemotherapy: a preliminary clinical trial. *Oncology* 1977; **34**: 153–155.
10. Ridgeway D, Wolff LJ, Neerhout RC. Enhanced lymphocyte response to PHA among leukopenia patients taking oral lithium carbonate. *Cancer Invest* 1986; **4**: 513–517.
11. Adityanjee M. Modification of clozapine-induced leukopenia and neutropenia with lithium carbonate. *Am J Psychiatry* 1995; **152**: 648–649.
12. Silverstone PH. Prevention of clozapine-induced neutropenia by pretreatment with lithium. *J Clin Psychopharm* 1998; **18**: 86–88.
13. Boshes RA, Manschreck TC, Desrosiers J *et al.* Initiation of clozapine therapy in a patient with pre-existing leucopenia: a discussion of the rationale of current treatment options. *Ann Clin Psychiatry* 2002; **13**: 233–237.
14. Sporn A, Gogtay N, Ortiz AR *et al.* Clozapine-incited neutropenia in children: management with lithium carbonate. *J Child Adolesc Psychopharmacol* 2003; **13**: 401–404.
15. Suppes T, Yang YY. Clozapine treatment of nonpsychotic rapid-cycling bipolar disorder: a report of 3 cases. *Biol Psychiatry* 1994; **36**: 338–340.
16. Puri BK, Taylor DG, Alcock ME. Low-dose maintenance clozapine treatment in the prophylaxis of bipolar affective disorder. *Br J Clin Pract* 1995; **49**: 333–334.
17. Dettling M, Schaub RT, Mueller-Oerlinghausen B *et al.* Further evidence of human leukocyte antigen-encoded susceptibility to clozapine-induced agranulocytosis independent of ancestry. *Pharmacogenetics* 2001; **11**: 135–141.
18. Gerson SL, Lieberman JA, Friedenberg WR *et al.* Polypharmacy in fatal clozapine-associated agranulocytosis. *Lancet* 1991; **338**: 262–263.
19. Valevski A, Modai I, Lahav M *et al.* Clozapine-lithium combined treatment and agranulocytosis. *Int Clin Psychopharmacol* 1993; **8**: 63–65.
20. Blake LM, Marks RC, Luchins DJ. Reversible neurological symptoms with clozapine and lithium. *J Clin Psychopharm* 1992; **12**: 297–299.

Clozapine-related hypersalivation

Clozapine is well known to be causally associated with apparent hypersalivation (drooling, particularly at night). This seems to be chiefly problematic in the early stages of treatment and is probably dose-related. Clinical observation suggests that hypersalivation reduces in severity over time (usually several months) but may persist. Clozapine-induced hypersalivation is socially embarrassing and potentially life-threatening[1], so treatment is a matter of some urgency.

The pharmacological basis of clozapine-related hypersalivation remains unclear. Suggested mechanisms include muscarinic M_4 agonism, adrenergic α_2 antagonism and inhibition of the swallowing reflex[2,3]. The last of these is supported by trials which suggest that saliva production is *not* increased in clozapine-treated patients[4,5].

Whatever the mechanism, drugs which reduce saliva production are likely to diminish the severity of this adverse effect. The table below describes drug treatments so far examined.

References

1. Hinkes R, Quesada TV, Currier MB *et al.* Aspiration pneumonia possibly secondary to clozapine-induced sialorrhea. *J Clin Psychopharm* 1997; **16**: 462–463.
2. Davydov L, Botts SR. Clozapine-induced hypersalivation. *Ann Pharmacother* 2001; **34**: 662–665.
3. Rogers DP, Shramko JK. Therapeutic options in the treatment of clozapine-induced sialorrhea. *Pharmacotherapy* 2000; **20**: 1092–1095.
4. Rabinowitz T, Frankenburg FR, Centorrino F *et al.* The effect of clozapine on saliva flow rate: a pilot study. *Biol Psychiatry* 1996; **40**: 1132–1134.
5. Ben-Aryeh H, Jungerman T, Szargel R *et al.* Salivary flow-rate and composition in schizophrenic patients on clozapine: subjective reports and laboratory data. *Biol Psychiatry* 1996; **39**: 946–949.
6. Fritze J, Elliger T. Pirenzepine for clozapine-induced hypersalivation. *Lancet* 1995; **346**: 1034.
7. Bai Y-M, Lin C-C, Chen J-Y *et al.* Therapeutic effect of pirenzepine for clozapine-induced hypersalivation: a randomized, double-blind, placebo-controlled, cross-over study. *J Clin Psychopharm* 2001; **21**: 608–611.
8. Schneider B, Weigmann H, Hiemke C *et al.* Reduction of clozapine-induced hypersalivation by pirenzepine is safe. *Pharmacopsychiatry* 2004; **37**: 43–45.
9. Spivak B, Adlersberg S, Rosen L *et al.* Trihexyphenidyl treatment of clozapine-induced hypersalivation. *Int Clin Psychopharmacol* 1997; **12**: 213–215.
10. Reinstein MJ, Sirotovskaya LA, Chasanov MA *et al.* Comparative efficacy and tolerability of benzatropine and terazosin in the treatment of hypersalivation secondary to clozapine. *Clin Drug Invest* 1999; **17**: 97–102.
11. Copp P, Lament R, Tennent TG. Amitriptyline in clozapine-induced sialorrhoea. *Br J Psychiatry* 1991; **159**: 166.
12. Calderon J, Rubin E, Sobota WL. Potential use of ipratropium bromide for the treatment of clozapine-induced hypersalivation: a preliminary report. *Int Clin Psychopharmacol* 2000; **15**: 49–52.
13. Freudenreich O, Beebe M, Goff DC. Clozapine-induced sialorrhea treated with sublingual ipratropium spray: a case series. *J Clin Psychopharmacol* 2004; **24**: 98–100.
14. Antonello C, Tessier P. Clozapine and sialorrhea: a new intervention for this bothersome and potentially dangerous side effect. *Rev Psychiatrie Neurosci* 1999; **24**: 250.
15. Grabowski J. Clonidine treatment of clozapine-induced hypersalivation. *J Clin Psychopharm* 1992; **12**: 69.
16. Corrigan FM, Macdonald S. Clozapine-induced hypersalivation and the alpha 2 adrenoceptor. *Br J Psychiatry* 1995; **167**: 412.
17. Kahl KG, Hagenah J, Zapf S *et al.* Botulinum toxin as an effective treatment of clozapine-induced hypersalivation. *Psychopharmacology* 2004; **173**: 229–230.
18. Reinstein MJ, Sonnenberg JG, Mohan SC *et al.* Use of quetiapine to manage patients who experienced adverse effects with clozapine. *Clin Drug Invest* 2003; **23**: 63–67.

Further reading

Cree A, Mir S, Fahy T. A review of the treatment options for clozapine-induced hypersalivation. *Psychiatr Bull* 2001; **25**: 114–116.

Schizophrenia

Table Summary

Treatment	Comments	References*
Pirenzepine 25–100 mg/day	Selective M_1, M_4 antagonist Does not affect clozapine metabolism Extensive clinical experience suggests efficacy in some but randomised trial suggests no effect. Still widely used	6–8
Benzhexol (trihexyphenidyl) 5–15 mg/day	Small, open study suggests useful activity Widely used in some centres but may impair cognitive function	9
Benztropine 2 mg/day + terazosin 2 mg/day	Combination shown to be better than either drug alone Not widely used	10
Amitriptyline 75–100 mg/day	Limited literature support. Adverse effects may be troublesome	11
Ipratropium nasal spray (0.03%) – given sublingually or intranasally	Limited literature support. Rarely used	12, 13
Atropine eye-drops (1%) – given sublingually	Limited literature support. Rarely used	14
Clonidine (0.1 mg patch weekly or 0.1 mg orally at night)	α_2 partial agonist. Limited literature support. May exacerbate psychosis and depression	15
Lofexidine 0.2 mg twice daily	α_2 agonist. Very few data. May exacerbate psychosis and depression	16
Botulinum toxin (Botox)	Effective in treating sialorrhoea associated with neurological disorders. Single case report of success in clozapine-treated patient	17
Quetiapine	May reduce hypersalivation by allowing lower doses of clozapine to be used	18
Propantheline 7.5 mg at night	Peripheral anticholinergic. No central effects. No published data	–
Hyoscine 0.3 mg sucked and swallowed up to 3 times daily	Peripheral and central anticholinergic Very widely used but no published data available May cause cognitive impairment, drowsiness and constipation	–

* References listed on page 63

Guidelines for the initiation of clozapine for patients based in the community

Note: this section provides general guidance – refer to manufacturer's and local policies (where available) for detailed guidance.

Some points to check before starting:

- Is the patient likely to be adherent with oral medication?
- Has the patient understood the need for regular blood tests?
- Is it possible for the patient to be seen every day during the early titration phase?
- Is the patient able to attend the team base or pharmacy to collect medication every week?
- Do patients need medication delivered to their home?

   Mandatory blood monitoring and registration with an approved clozapine monitoring service.

- Register with the relevant monitoring service.
- Perform baseline blood tests (WCC and differential count) before starting clozapine.
- Further blood testing continues weekly for the first 18 weeks and then every 2 weeks for the remainder of the year. After that, the blood monitoring is done monthly.

Dosing (see table on page 47)

Note: other schedules than that described below are possible (e.g. 12-week titration with twice-weekly monitoring).

- Day 1: start at 12.5 mg at night.
- Day 2: increase to 12.5 mg twice a day (unless the dose on day 1 is not tolerated).
- Day 3 and onwards: the dose may be increased by 25–50 mg a day, until a dose of 300 mg is reached. Estimate plasma level of clozapine at this point.
- Further dose increases should be made in increments of 50 mg a week until a dose of 450 mg or level of between 350 and 500 µg/l is achieved (see page 48).
- Doses up to 200 mg may be given as a single dose at night.
- See table for a suggested titration regime.
- Clozapine levels are lower in males, smokers and younger adults (see page 4).

Switching from other antipsychotics

- The switching regime will be largely dependent on the patient's mental state.
- Consider additive side-effects of the antipsychotics (e.g. effect on QTc interval) (see page 87).

- Consider drug interactions (e.g. risperidone may increase clozapine levels).

- All depots, sertindole, pimozide, ziprasidone and thioridazine should be stopped before clozapine is started.

- Other antipsychotics and clozapine may be cross-tapered with varying degrees of caution.

Table Suggested titration regime – clozapine in the community

Day	Day of the week	Morning dose (mg)	Evening dose (mg)	Percentage dose of previous antipsychotic
1	Monday	–	12.5	100
2	Tuesday	12.5	12.5	
3	Wednesday	12.5	25	
4	Thursday	25	25	
5	Friday	25	50	
6	Saturday	25	50	
7	Sunday	25	50	
8	Monday	50	50	75
9	Tuesday	50	75	
10	Wednesday	50	75	
11	Thursday	50	100	
12	Friday	50	100	
13	Saturday	50	100	
14	Sunday	50	100	
15	Monday	75	100	50
16	Tuesday	75	100	
17	Wednesday	75	100	
18	Thursday	100	100	
19	Friday	100	100	
20	Saturday	100	100	
21	Sunday	100	100	
22	Monday	100	125	25
23	Tuesday	100	150	
24	Wednesday	100	175	
25	Thursday	100	200	
26	Friday	100	200	
27	Saturday	100	200	
28	Sunday	100	200	0

Clozapine in the community – acute monitoring requirements

- *Blood pressure (BP), temperature and pulse.* After the first dose, monitor BP, temperature and pulse 1–3 hours afterwards. (This may not be necessary if the first dose is given at bedtime.) Thereafter, the patient should be seen at least once a day, and all three parameters should be monitored before and after the morning dose.

- Continue daily monitoring for at least 2 weeks or until there are no unacceptable adverse effects. Alternate day monitoring may then be undertaken until a stable dose is reached. Thereafter monitor at time of blood testing.

- The formal carer (usually the CPN) should inform the prescriber if:

  - **temperature** rises above **38 °C** (this is very common and is not a good reason, on its own, for stopping clozapine)

  - **pulse** is >**100 bpm** (also common but may rarely be linked to myocarditis)

  - **postural drop** of >**30 mmHg**

  - patient is clearly over-sedated

  - any other **adverse effect is intolerable.**

Additional monitoring requirements (see page 30)

Baseline	1 month	3 months	4–6 months	12 months
Weight, lipids	Weight	Weight, lipids	Weight, lipids	Weight, lipids
HbA$_{1C}$* or plasma glucose*	HbA$_{1C}$* or plasma glucose*		HbA$_{1C}$* or plasma glucose*	HbA$_{1C}$* or plasma glucose*
LFTs			LFTs	
*Perform fasting plasma glucose if HbA$_{1C}$ raised.				

Where available, consider also use of ECG (benefit not established).

Adverse effects

- Sedation and hypotension are common at the start of treatment. These effects can usually be managed by reducing the dose or slowing down the rate of titration.

- Many other adverse effects associated with clozapine can also be managed by dose reduction.

Management of adverse effects

See page 54 et seq.

Serious cardiac adverse effects (see page 58)

Patients who have *persistent* tachycardia at rest, especially during the first 2 months of treatment, should be closely observed for other signs or symptoms of myocarditis or cardiomyopathy. These include palpitations, arrhythmia, symptoms mimicking myocardial infarction, chest pain and other unexplained symptoms of heart failure.

In patients with suspected clozapine-induced myocarditis or cardiomyopathy, the drug must be stopped and the patient referred to a cardiologist. If clozapine-induced myocarditis or cardiomyopathy is confirmed, the patient must not be re-exposed to clozapine.

Fish oils in schizophrenia

Fish oils contain the omega–3 fatty acids, eicosapentanoic acid (EPA) and docosahexanoic acid (DHA). These compounds are thought to be involved in maintaining neuronal membrane structure, in the modulation of membrane proteins and in the production of prostaglandins and leukotrienes[1]. They have been suggested as treatments for a variety of psychiatric illnesses[2] but most research relates to their use in schizophrenia, where case reports[3–5] and prospective trials suggest useful efficacy (see the following table).

Table   A summary of the evidence – fish oils in schizophrenia

References	n	Design	Outcome
Mellor et al. 1995[6]	20	Open label evaluation of fish oil (EPA + DHA) added to usual medication	Significant improvement in symptoms
Peet et al. 2001[7]	45	Double-blind, randomised comparison of EPA (2 g daily), DHA and placebo (12 weeks)	EPA significantly more effective than DHA or placebo
Peet et al. 2001[7]	26	Double-blind, randomised comparison of EPA (2 g daily) or placebo as sole drug treatment (12 weeks)	All 12 patients given placebo required conventional antipsychotic treatment; 8 of 14 given EPA required antipsychotics. EPA more effective
Peet and Horrobin 2002[8]	115	Double-blind, randomised comparison of ethyl-EPA (1, 2 or 4 g/day) and placebo added to antipsychotic treatment (conventional, atypical or clozapine) (12 weeks)	Ethyl-EPA significantly improved response in patients receiving clozapine. 2 g/day most effective dose
Fenton et al. 2001[9]	87	Double-blind, randomised comparison of EPA (3 g daily) and placebo added to standard drug treatment (16 weeks)	No differences between EPA and placebo
Emsley et al. 2002[10]	40	Double-blind, randomised comparison of EPA (3 g daily) and placebo added to standard drug treatment (12 weeks)	EPA associated with significantly greater reduction in symptoms and tardive dyskinesia (9 patients in each group received clozapine)

On balance, evidence suggests that EPA (2–3 g daily) is a worthwhile option in schizophrenia when added to standard treatment, particularly clozapine[11,12]. However, doubt still remains over the true extent of the beneficial effect derived from fish oils. Set against doubts over efficacy are the observations that fish oils are relatively cheap, well tolerated (mild GI symptoms may occur) and may benefit physical health[1].

Fish oils are therefore very tentatively recommended for the treatment of residual symptoms of schizophrenia but particularly in patients responding poorly to clozapine. Careful assessment of response is essential and fish oils should be withdrawn if no effect is observed after 3 months' treatment.

The recommended dose is

Omacor (414 mg EPA) 5 capsules daily

or

Maxepa (170 mg EPA) 10 capsules daily

References

1. Fenton WS, Hibbeln J, Knable M. Fatty acids in schizophrenia. *Biol Psychiatry* 2000; **47**: 821.
2. Freeman MP. Omega–3 fatty acids in psychiatry: a review. *Ann Clin Psychiatry* 2000; **12**: 159–165.
3. Richardson AJ, Easton T, Puri BK. Red cell and plasma fatty acid changes accompanying symptom remission in a patient with schizophrenia treated with eicosapentaenoic acid. *Eur Neuropsychopharm* 2000; **10**: 189–193.
4. Puri BK, Richardson AJ, Horrobin DF *et al.* Eicosapentaenoic acid treatment in schizophrenia associated with symptom remission, normalisation of blood fatty acids, reduced neuronal membrane phospholipid turnover and structural brain changes. *Int J Clin Pract* 2000; **54**: 57–63.
5. Su K-P, Shen W, Huang S-Y. Omega-3 fatty acids as a psychotherapeutic agent for a pregnant schizophrenic patient. *Eur Neuropsychopharm* 2001; **11**: 295–299.
6. Mellor JE, Laugharne JD, Peet M. Schizophrenic symptoms and dietary intake of n3 fatty acids. *Schizophr Res* 1995; **18**: 85–86.
7. Peet M, Brind J, Ramchand CN *et al.* Two double-blind placebo-controlled pilot studies of eicosapentaenoic acid in the treatment of schizophrenia. *Schizophr Res* 2001; **49**: 243–251.
8. Peet M, Horrobin DF. A dose-ranging exploratory study of the effects of ethyl-eicosapentaenoate in patients with persistent schizophrenic symptoms. *J Psychiatry Res* 2002; **36**: 7–18.
9. Fenton WS, Dickerson F, Boronow J *et al.* A placebo-controlled trial of omega-3 fatty acid (ethyl eicosapentaenoic acid) supplementation for residual symptoms and cognitive impairment in schizophrenia. *Am J Psychiatry* 2001; **158**: 2071–2074.
10. Emsley R, Myburgh C, Oosthuizen P *et al.* Randomized, placebo-controlled study of ethyl-eicosapentaenoic acid as supplemental treatment in schizophrenia. *Am J Psychiatry* 2002; **159**: 1596–1598.
11. Emsley R, Oosthuizen P, Van Rensburg SJ. Clinical potential of omega-3 fatty acids in the treatment of schizophrenia. *CNS Drugs* 2003; **17**: 1081–1091.
12. Joy CB, Mumby-Croft R, Joy LA. Polyunsaturated fatty acid supplementation for schizophrenia. *The Cochrane Database of Systematic Reviews* 2003; Issue 2. Art. No. CD001257.DO1: 10.1002/14651858.CD001257.

Further reading

Joy CB, Mumby-Croft R, Joy LA. Polyunsaturated fatty acid (fish or evening primrose oil) for schizophrenia (Cochrane Review). In: The Cochrane Library, Issue 4. Oxford: Update software, 2002.

Extra-pyramidal side-effects (EPSEs)

Table Most common extra-pyramidal side-effects

	Dystonia (uncontrolled muscular contraction)	Pseudo-parkinsonism (tremor, etc.)	Akathisia (restlessness)	Tardive dyskinesia (abnormal movements)
Signs and symptoms[2]	Muscle spasm in any part of the body, e.g. • Eyes rolling upwards (oculogyric crisis) • Head and neck twisted to the side (torticollis) *The patient may be unable to swallow or speak clearly. In extreme cases, the back may arch or the jaw dislocate* Acute dystonia can be both painful and very frightening	• Tremor and/or rigidity • Bradykinesia (decreased facial expression, flat monotone voice, slow body movements, inability to initiate movement) • Bradyphrenia (slowed thinking) • Salivation Pseudo-parkinsonism can be mistaken for depression or the negative symptoms of schizophrenia	A subjectively unpleasant state of inner restlessness where there is a strong desire or compulsion to move • Foot stamping when seated • Constantly crossing/uncrossing legs • Rocking from foot to foot • Constantly pacing up and down Akathisia can be mistaken for psychotic agitation and has been linked with suicide and aggression towards others[3]	A wide variety of movements can occur such as: • Lip smacking or chewing • Tongue protrusion (fly catching) • Choreiform hand movements (pill-rolling or piano-playing) • Pelvic-thrusting Severe orofacial movements can lead to difficulty in speaking, eating or breathing. Movements are worse when under stress
Rating scales	No specific scale Small component of general EPSE scales	Simpson–Angus EPSE Rating Scale[4]	Barnes Akathisia Scale[5]	Abnormal Involuntary Movement Scale[6] (AIMS)
Prevalence (with older drugs)	Approximately 10%[7], but more common in: • In young males • In the neuroleptic-naïve • With high potency drugs (e.g. haloperidol) Dystonic reactions are rare in the elderly	Approximately 20%[9], but more common in: • Elderly females • Those with pre-existing neurological damage (head injury, stroke, etc.)	Approximately 25%[10] Less with typicals. In decreasing order: risperidone, olanzapine, quetiapine and clozapine[11]	5% of patients per year of antipsychotic exposure[12]. More common in: • Elderly women • Those with affective illness • Those who have had acute EPSEs early on in treatment

71

	Dystonia (uncontrolled muscular spasm)	Pseudo-parkinsonism (tremor, etc.)	Akathisia (restlessness)	Tardive dyskinesia (abnormal movements)
Time taken to develop	Acute dystonia can occur within hours of starting antipsychotics (minutes if the IM or IV route is used) Tardive dystonia occurs after months to years of antipsychotic treatment	Days to weeks after antipsychotic drugs are started or the dose is increased	Acute akathisia occurs within hours to weeks of starting antipsychotics or increasing the dose. Tardive akathisia takes longer to develop and can persist after antipsychotics have been withdrawn	Months to years Approximately 50% of cases are reversible[12]
Treatment	Anticholinergic drugs given orally, IM or IV depending on the severity of symptoms[8] • Remember the patient may be unable to swallow • Response to IV administration will be seen within 5 minutes • Response to IM administration takes around 20 minutes	Several options are available depending on the clinical circumstances: • Reduce the antipsychotic dose • Change to an atypical drug (as antipsychotic monotherapy!) • Prescribe an anticholinergic. The majority of patients do not require long-term anticholinergics. Use should be reviewed at least every 3 months	• Reduce the antipsychotic dose • Change to an atypical drug • A reduction in symptoms may be seen with[13]: propranolol 30–80 mg/day, clonazepam (low dose) 5HT$_2$ antagonists such as cyproheptadine[13], mirtazapine[14], trazodone[15], mianserin[16] and cyproheptadine[13] may help, as may diphenhydramine[17] All are unlicensed for this indication Anticholinergics are generally unhelpful[18]	• Stop anticholinergic if prescribed • Reduce dose of antipsychotic • Change to an atypical drug[19] • Clozapine is the most likely antipsychotic to be associated with resolution of symptoms[20] • For other treatment options see page 78[21]

EPSEs are:

- dose-related

- more likely with high-potency typicals

- uncommon with atypicals.

Patients who experience one type of EPSE may be more vulnerable to developing others[22].

References

1. Barnes TRE. The Barnes Akathisia Scale – revisited. *J Psychopharmacol* 2003; **17**: 365–370.
2. Gervin M, Barnes TRE. Assessment of drug-related movement disorders in schizophrenia. *Adv Psychiatric Treat* 2000; **6**: 332–334.
3. Leong GB, Silva JA. Neuroleptic-induced akathisia and violence: a review. *J Forensic Sci* 2003; **48**: 1–3.
4. Simpson GM, Angus JWS. A rating scale for extrapyramidal side-effects. *Acta Psychiatr Scand* 1970; **212**: 11–19.
5. Barnes TRE. A rating scale for drug-induced akathisia. *Br J Psychiatry* 1989; **154**: 672–676.
6. Guy W. *ECDEU Assessment Manual for Psychopharmacology.* Washington, DC: US Department of Health, Education, and Welfare, 1976, pp. 534–537.
7. American Psychiatric Association. Practice guideline for the treatment of schizophrenia. *Am J Psychiatry* 1997; **154**(4 Suppl.): 1–63.
8. van Harten PN, Hoek HW, Kahn RS. Acute dystonia induced by drug treatment. *BMJ* 1999; **319**. 623–626.
9. Bollini P, Pampallona S, Orgam J *et al.* Antipsychotic drugs: is more worse? A meta-analysis of the randomised controlled trials *Psychol Med* 1994; **24**: 307–316.
10. Halstead SM, Barnes TRE, Speller JC. Akathisia: prevalence and associated dysphoria in an in-patient population with chronic schizophrenia. *Br J Psychiatry* 1994; **164**: 177–183.
11. Hirose S. The causes of underdiagnosing akathisia. *Schizophr Bull* 2003; **29**: 547–558.
12. American Psychiatric Association. *Tardive Dyskinesia: A Task Force Report of the American Psychiatric Association.* Washington, DC. American Psychiatric Association, 1992.
13. Miller CH, Fleischaker WW. Managing antipsychotic induced acute and chronic akathisia. *Drug Safety* 2000; **22**: 73–81.
14. Poyurovsky M, Ephstein E, Fuchs C *et al.* Efficacy of low-dose mirtazepine in neuroleptic-induced akathisia: a double-blind randomized placebo-controlled pilot study. *J Clin Psychopharm* 2003; **23**: 305–308.
15. Stryjer R, Strous RD, Bar F et al. Treatment of neuroleptic-induced akathisia with the 5-HT2a antagonist trazodone. *Clin Neuropharmacol* 2003; **26**: 137–141.
16. Stryjer R, Grupper D, Strous R. Mianserin for the rapid improvement of chronic akathisia in a schizophrenia patient. *Eur Psychiatry* 2004; **19**: 237–240.
17. Vinson DR. Diphenhydramine in the treatment of akathisia induced by prochlorperazine. *J Emerg Med* 2003; **26**: 265–270.
18. Lima AR, Weiser KVS, Bacaltchuk J *et al.* Anticholinergics for neuroleptic-induced acute akathisia. Cochrane Database of Systematic Reviews, 2003.
19. Glazer W. Expected incidence of tardive dyskinesia associated with atypical antipsychotics. *J Clin Psychiatry* 2000; **61**(Suppl. 4): 21–26.
20. Simpson GM. The treatment of tardive dyskinesia and tardive dystonia. *J Clin Psychiat* 2000; **61**(Suppl. 4): 39–44.
21. Duncan D, McConnell H, Taylor D. Tardive dyskinesia: how is it prevented and treated? *Psychiatr Bull* 1997; **21**: 422–425.
22. Jong-Hoon K, Hee Jung B. Prevalence and characteristics of subjective akathisia, objective akathisia, and mixed akathisia in chronic schizophrenic subjects. *Clin Neuropharmacol* 2003; **26**: 312–316.

Hyperprolactinaemia

Because dopamine inhibits prolactin release, dopamine antagonists can be expected to increase prolactin plasma levels. All antipsychotics cause measurable changes in prolactin but some do not increase prolactin above the normal range at standard doses. These drugs are clozapine, olanzapine, quetiapine, aripiprazole and ziprasidone[1-3].

Hyperprolactinaemia is often superficially asymptomatic (i.e. the patient does not spontanteously report problems) and there is evidence that hyperprolactinaemia does not affect subjective quality of life[4]. Nonetheless, persistent elevation of plasma prolactin is associated with a number of adverse consequences. These include sexual dysfunction[5-8] (but note that other pharmacological activites also give rise to sexual dysfunction), reductions in bone mineral density[9-12], menstrual disturbances[2,13], breast growth and galactorrhoea[13], suppression of the hypothalamic-pituitary-gonadal axis[14] and a possible increase in the risk of breast cancer[2,15,16].

Treatment

For most patients with symptomatic hyperprolactinaemia, a switch to a non prolactin-elevating drug is the first choice[2,8,17,18]. Symptoms resolve slowly and symptom severity does not always reflect prolactin changes[17]. Genetic differences may play a part[19].

For patients who need to remain on a prolactin-elevating antipsychotic, dopamine agonists may be effective[3,17,20]. Amantadine, carbergoline and bromocriptine have all been used, but each has the potential to worsen psychosis (although this has not been reported in trials).

References

1. David SR, Taylor CC, Kinon BJ et al. The effects of olanzapine, risperidone, and haloperidol on plasma prolactin levels in patients with schizophrenia. Clin Ther 2000; 22: 1085–1095.
2. Haddad PM, Wieck A. Antipsychotic-induced hyperprolactinaemia mechanisms, clinical features and management. Drugs 2004; 64: 2291–2314.
3. Hammer MB, Arana GW. Hyperprolactinaemia in antipsychotic-treated patients: guidelines for avoidance and management. CNS Drugs 1998; 209–222.
4. Kaneda Y. The impact of prolactin elevation with antipsychotic medications on subjective quality of life in patients with schizophrenia. Clin Neuropharmacol 2003; 26: 182–184.
5. Bobes J, Garcia-Portilla MP, Rejas J et al. Frequency of sexual dysfunction and other reproductive side-effects in patients with schizophrenia treated with risperidone, olanzapine, quetiapine, or haloperidol: the results of the EIRE study. J Sex Marital Ther 2003; 29: 125–147.
6. Smith S. Effects of antipsychotics on sexual and endocrine function in women: implications for clinical practice. J Clin Psychopharm 2003; 23: S27–S32.
7. Spollen JJ, Wooten RG, Cargile C et al. Prolactin levels and erectile function in patients treated with risperidone. J Clin Psychopharm 2004; 24: 161–166.
8. Knegtering R, Castelein S, Bous H et al. A randomized open-label study of the impact of quetiapine versus risperidone on sexual functioning. J Clin Psychopharm 2004; 24: 56–61.
9. Halbreich U, Palter S. Accelerated osteoporosis in psychiatric patients: possible pathophysiological processes. Schizophr Bull 1996; 22: 447–454.
10. Becker D, Liver O, Mester R et al. Risperidone, but not olanzapine decreases bone mineral density in female premenopausal schizophrenia patients. J Clin Psychopharm 2003; 64: 761–766.
11. Meaney AM, O'Keane V. Reduced bone mineral density in patients with schizophrenia receiving prolactin raising anti-psychotic medication. J Psychopharmacol 2003; 17: 455–458.
12. Meaney AM, Smith S, Howes OD et al. Effects of long-term prolactin-raising antipsychotic medication on bone mineral density in patients with schizophrenia. Br J Psychiatry 2004; 184: 503–508.
13. Wieck A, Haddad PM. Antipsychotic-induced hyperprolactinaemia in women: pathphysiology, severity and consequences: selective literature review. Br J Psychiatry 2003; 182: 199–204.
14. Smith S, Wheeler MJ, Murrey R et al. The effects of antipsychotic-induced hyperprolactinaemia on the hypothalamic-pituitary-gonadal axis. J Clin Psychopharm 2002; 22: 109–114.

15. Halbreich U, Shen J, Panaro V. Are chronic psychiatric patients at increased risk for developing breast cancer? *Am J Psychiatry* 1996; **153**: 559–560.
16. Wang PS, Walker AM, Tsuang MT *et al.* Dopamine antagonists and the development of breast cancer. *Arch Gen Psychiatry* 2002; **59**: 1147–1154.
17. Duncan D, Taylor D. Treatment of psychotropic-induced hyperprolactinaemia. *Psychiatr Bull* 1995; **19**: 755–757.
18. Anghelesu I, Wolf J. Successful switch to aripiprazole after induction of hyperprolactinaemia by ziprasidone: a case report. *J Clin Psychiatry* 2004; **65**: 1286–1287.
19. Young R, Lawford BR, Barnes M *et al.* Prolactin levels in antipsychotic treatment of patients with schizophrenia carrying the DRD2*A1 allele. *Br J Psychiatry* 2004; **185**: 147–151.
20. Cavallaro R, Cocchi F, Angelone SM *et al.* Cabergoline treatment of risperidone-induced hyperprolactinaemia: a pilot study. *J Clin Psychiatry* 2004; **65**: 187–190.

Schizophrenia

Algorithm for the treatment of antipsychotic-induced akathisia

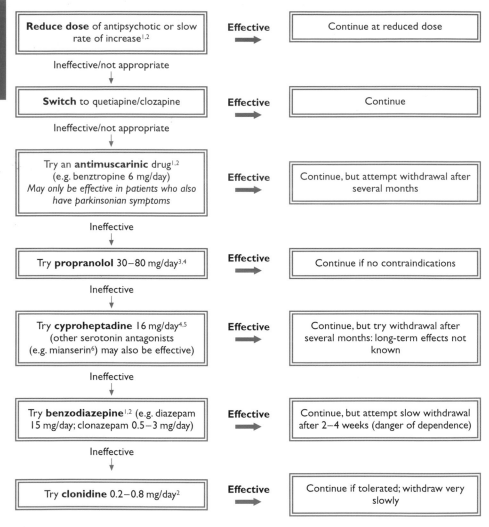

Notes:

- Akathisia is sometimes difficult to diagnose with certainty. A careful history of symptoms, medication and illicit substance use is essential. Note that severe akathisia may be linked to violent or suicidal behaviour[7–9].
- Evaluate efficacy of each treatment option over at least 1 month. Some effect may be seen after a few days but it may take much longer to become apparent in those with chronic akathisia.
- Withdraw previously ineffective treatments before starting the next option in the algorithm.
- Combinations of treatment may be used in refractory cases if carefully monitored.
- Consider tardive akathisia in patients on long-term therapy.

References

1. Fleischhacker WW, Roth SD, Kane JM. The pharmacologic treatment of neuroleptic-induced akathisia. *J Clin Psychopharm* 1990; **10**: 12–21.
2. Sachdev P. The identification and management of drug-induced akathisia. *CNS Drugs* 1995; **4**: 28–46.
3. Adler L, Angrist B, Peselow E, *et al.* A controlled assessment of propranolol in the treatment of neuroleptic-induced akathisia. *Br J Psychiatry* 1986; **149**: 42–45.
4. Fischel T, Hermesh H, Aizenberg D *et al.* Cyproheptadine versus propranolol for the treatment of acute neuroleptic-induced akathisia: a comparative double-blind study. *J Clin Psychopharm* 2001; **21**: 612–615.
5. Weiss D, Aizenberg D, Hermesh H *et al.* Cyproheptadine treatment of neuroleptic-induced akathisia. *Br J Psychiatry* 1995; **167**: 483–486.
6. Poyurovsky M, Shadorodsky M, Fuchs M *et al.* Treatment of neuroleptic-induced akathisia with the 5HT$_2$ antagonist mianserin. *Br J Psychiatry* 1999; **174**: 238–242.
7. Drake RE, Ehrlich J. Suicide attempts associated with akathisia. *Am J Psychiatry* 1985; **142**: 499–501.
8. Azhar MZ, Varma SL. Akathisia-induced suicidal behaviour. *Eur Psychiatry* 1992; **7**: 239–241.
9. Hansen L. A critical review of akathisia, and its possible association with suicidal behaviour. *Hum Psychopharm* 2001; **16**: 495–505.

Further reading

Maidment I. Use of serotonin antagonists in the treatment of neuroleptic-induced akathisia. *Psychiatr Bull* 2000; **24**: 348–351.

Schizophrenia

Treatment of tardive dyskinesia (TD)

TD remains a commonly encountered problem despite the introduction and widespread use of so-called atypical antipsychotics[1]. Treatment of established TD is often unsuccessful, so prevention and early detection are essential. There is now fairly good evidence that some newer 'atypical' antipsychotics are less likely to cause TD[2–5] although TD certainly does occur with these drugs[6–9]. The observation that atypicals produce less TD than typical drugs is consistent with the long-held belief that early acute movement disorders and akathisia predict later TD[10]. Note, also, that TD can occur after miniscule doses of conventional drugs and in the absence of portentious acute movement disorder[11].

Treatment – first steps

Most authorities recommend the withdrawal of anticholinergic drugs and a reduction in the dose of antipsychotic as initial steps in those with early signs of TD[12,13] (dose reduction may initially worsen TD). However, it has become common practice to withdraw the antipsychotic prescribed when TD was first observed and to substitute another drug. The use of clozapine[12] is probably best supported in this regard, but quetiapine, another weak striatal dopamine antagonist, is also effective[14–19]. Olanzapine is also an option[20,21] while there are a few supporting data for risperidone[22] and aripiprazole[23].

Treatment – additional agents

Switching or withdrawing antipsychotics is not always effective and so additional agents are often used. The table below describes the most frequently prescribed add-on drugs for TD.

Drug	Comments
Tetrabenazine[24]	Only licensed treatment for TD in UK. Has antipsychotic properties but reported to be depressogenic. Dose is 25–200 mg/day.
Benzodiazepines[12,13]	Widely used and considered effective but Cochrane suggests benzodiazepines are 'experimental'[25]. Intermittent use may be necessary to avoid tolerance to effects. Most used are clonazepam 1–4 mg/day and diazepam 6–25 mg/day.
Vitamin E[26,27]	Numerous studies but efficacy remains to be conclusively established. Dose is in the range 400–1600 IU/day.

Treatment – other possible options

The large number of proposed treatments for TD undoubtedly reflects the somewhat limited effectiveness of standard remedies. The following table lists some of these putative treatments in alphabetical order. Supporting evidence is slim in each case.

Drug	Comments
Amino acids[28]	Use is supported by a small randomised, placebo-controlled trial. Low risk of toxicity. No evidence of effect in women.
Calcium antagonists[29]	A few published studies but not widely used. Cochrane is dismissive.
Donepezil[30]	Supported by a single study. Dose is 10 mg/day.
Gabapentin[31]	Data derived almost entirely from a single research group. Adds weight to theory that GABAergic mechanisms improve TD. Dose is 900–1200 mg/day.
Levetiracetam[32]	Single case report. Dose was 1000 mg/day.
Melatonin[33]	Use is supported by a well-conducted trial. Usually well tolerated. Dose is 10 mg/day.
Naltrexone[34]	May be effective when added to benzodiazepines. Well tolerated. Dose is 200 mg/day.
Ondansetron[35,36]	Limited evidence but low toxicity. Dose – up to 12 mg/day.
Pyridoxine[37]	Supported by a well-conducted trial. Dose – up to 400 mg/day.
Quercetin[38]	Plant compound which is thought to be an antioxidant. No human studies in TD but widely used in other conditions.
Transcranial magnetic stimulation[39] (rTMS)	Single case report.

Note: Botulinum toxin may have a role in tardive dystonia.[40,41]

References

1. Halliday J, Farrington S, MacDonald S et al. Nithsdale schizophrenia surveys 23: movement disorders – 20-year review. Br J Psychiatry 2002; 181: 422–427.
2. Beasley CM, Dellva MA, Tamura RN. Randomised double-blind comparison of the incidence of tardive dyskinesia in patients with schizophrenia during long-term treatment with olanzapine or haloperidol. Br J Psychiatry 1999; 174: 23–30.
3. Glazer WM. Expected incidence of tardive dyskinesia associated with atypical antipsychotics. J Clin Psychiatry 2000; 61(Suppl. 4): 21–26.
4. Correll CU, Leucht S, Kane JM. Lower risk for tardive dyskinesia associated with second-generation antipsychotics: a systematic review of 1-year studies. Am J Psychiatry 2004; 161: 414–425.
5. Dolder CR, Jeste DV. Incidence of tardive dyskinesia with typical versus atypical antipsychotics in very high risk patients. Soc Biol Psychiatry 2003; 53: 1142–1145.
6. Karama S, Lal S. Tardive dyskinesia following brief exposure to risperidone – a case study (Letter). Eur Psychiatry 2004; 19: 391–392.
7. Gafoor R, Brophy J. Three case reports of emergent dyskinesia with clozapine. Eur Psychiatry 2003; 18: 260–261.
8. Bhanji MH, Margolese HC. Tardive dyskinesia associated with olanzapine in a neuroleptic-naïve patient with schizophrenia (Letter). Can J Psychiatry 2004; 49: 343.
9. Keck ME, Muller MB, Binder EB et al. Ziprasidone-related tardive dyskinesia (Letter). Am J Psychiatry 2004; 161: 175–176.
10. Sachdev P. Early extrapyramidal side-effects as risk factors for later tardive dyskinesia: a prospective study. Aust NZ J Psychiatry 2004; 38: 445–449.
11. Oosthuizen PP, Emsley RA, Maritz JS et al. Incidence of tardive dyskinesia in first-episode psychosis patients treated with low-dose haloperidol. J Clin Psychiatry 2003; 64: 1075–1108.
12. Duncan D, McConnell H, Taylor D. Tardive dyskinesia – how is it prevented and treated? Psychiatr Bull 1997; 21: 422–425.
13. Simpson GM. The treatment of tardive dyskinesia and tardive dystonia. J Clin Psychiatry 2000; 61(Suppl. 4): 39–44.
14. Vesely C, Küfferle B, Brücke T et al. Remission of severe tardive dyskinesia in a schizophrenic patient treated with the atypical antipsychotic substance quetiapine. Int Clin Psychopharmacol 2000; 15: 57–60.

15. Alptekin K, Kivircik AK. Quetiapine-induced improvement of tardive dyskinesia in three patients with schizophrenia. *Int Clin Psychopharmacol* 2002; **17**: 263–264.
16. Nelson MW, Reynolds RR, Kelly DL *et al.* Adjunctive quetiapine decreases symptoms of tardive dyskinesia in a patient taking risperidone. *Clin Neuropharmacol* 2003; **26**: 297–298.
17. Emsley R, Turner HJ, Schronen J *et al.* A single-blind, randomized trial comparing quetiapine and haloperidol in the treatment of tardive dyskinesia. *J Clin Psychiatry* 2004; **65**: 676–701.
18. Bressan RA, Jones HM, Pilowsky LS. Atypical antipsychotic drugs and tardive dykinesia: relevance of D_2 receptor affinity. *J Psychopharmacol* 2004; **18**: 124–127.
19. Sacchetti E, Valsecchi P. Quetiapine, clozapine, and olanzapine in the treatment of tardive dyskinesia induced by first-generation antipsychotics: a 124-week case report. *Int Clin Psychopharmacol* 2003; **18**: 357–359.
20. Soutullo CA, Keck PE, McElroy SL. Olanzapine in the treatment of tardive dyskinesia: a report of two cases (Letter). *J Clin Psychopharm* 1999; **19**: 100–101.
21. Kinon BJ, Jeste DV, Kollack-Walker S *et al.* Olanzapine treatment for tardive dyskinesia in schizophrenia patients: a prospective clinical trial with patients randomized to blinded dose reduction periods. *Prog Neuro-Psychopharmacology Bio Psychiatry* 2004; **28**: 985–996.
22. Bai YM, Yu SC, Lin CC. Risperidone for severe tardive dyskinesia: a 12-week randomized, double-blind, placebo-controlled study. *J Clin Psychiatry* 2003; **64**: 1342–1348.
23. Duggal HS. Aripiprazole-induced improvement in tardive dyskinesia (Letter). *Can J Psychiatry* 2003; **48**: 771–772.
24. Jankovic J, Beach J. Long-term effects of tetrabenazine in hyperkinetic movement disorders. *Neurology* 1997; **48**: 358–362.
25. Walker P, Soares KVS. Benzodiazepines for neuroleptic-induced tardive dyskinesia. *Cochrane Database of Systematic Reviews* 2003, Issue 2. Art. No. CD000205. DOI: 10.1002/14651858.
26. Adler LA, Rotrosen J, Edson R *et al.* Vitamin E treatment for tardive dyskinesia. *Arch Gen Psychiatry* 1999; **56**: 836–841.
27. Zhang XY, Zhou DF, Cao LY *et al.* The effect of vitamin E treatment on tardive dyskinesia and blood superoxide dismutase: a double-blind placebo-controlled trial. *J Clin Psychopharm* 2004; **24**: 83–86.
28. Richardson MA, Bevans ML, Read LL *et al.* Efficacy of the branched-chain amino acids in the treatment of tardive dyskinesia in men. *Am J Psychiatry* 2003; **160**: 1117–1124.
29. Soares-Weiser K, Rathbone J. Calcium channel blockers for neuroleptic-induced tardive dyskinesia. *Cochrane Database of Systematic Reviews* 2004, Issue 1. Art. No. CD000206.pub2. DOI: 10.1002/14651858.
30. Caroff SN, Campbell EC, Havey JC *et al.* Treatment of tardive dyskinesia with donepezil. *J Clin Psychiatry* 2001; **62**: 128–129.
31. Hardoy MC, Carta MG, Carpiniello B *et al.* Gabapentin in antipsychotic-induced tardive dyskinesia: results of 1-year follow-up. *J Affect Disorders* 2003; **75**: 125–130.
32. McGavin CL, John V, Musser WS. Levetiracetam as a treatment for tardive dyskinesia: a case report. *Neurology* 2003; **61**: 419–420.
33. Shamir E, Barak Y, Shalman I *et al.* Melatonin treatment for tardive dyskinesia: a double-blind, placebo-controlled, crossover study. *Arch Gen Psychiatry* 2001; **58**: 1049–1052.
34. Wonodi I, Adami H, Sherr J *et al.* Naltrexone treatment of tardive dyskinesia in patients with schizophrenia. *J Clin Psychopharm* 2004; **24**: 441–445.
35. Sirota P, Mosheva T, Shabtay H *et al.* Use of the selective serotonin 3 receptor antagonist ondansetron in the treatment of neuroleptic-induced tardive dyskinesia. *Am J Psychiatry* 2000; **157**: 287–289.
36. Naidu PS, Kulkarni SK. Reversal of neuroleptic-induced orofacial dyskinesia by 5-HT3 receptor antagonists. *Eur J Pharmacol* 2001; **420**: 113–117.
37. Lerner V, Miodownik C, Kaptsan A *et al.* Vitamin B_6 in the treatment of tardive dyskinesia: a double-blind, placebo-controlled, crossover study. *Am J Psychiatry* 2001; **158**: 1511–1514.
38. Naidu PS, Singh A, Kulkarni SK. Reversal of haloperidol-induced orofacial dyskinesia by quercetin, a bioflavonoid. *Psychopharmacology* 2003; **167**: 418–423.
39. Brambilla P, Perez J, Monchieri S *et al.* Transient improvement of tardive dyskinesia induced with rTMS. *Neurology* 2003; **61**: 1155.
40. Tarsy D, Kaufman D, Sethi KD *et al.* An open study of botulinum toxin A for treatment of tardive dystonia. *Clin Neuropharmacol* 1997; **20**: 90–93.
41. Brashear A, Ambrosins WT, Eckert GJ *et al.* Comparison of treatment of tardive dystonia and idiopathic cervical dystonia with botulinum type A. *Movement Disord* 1998; **13**: 158–161.

Further reading

Paleacu D, Giladi N, Moore O *et al.* Tetrabenazine treatment in movement disorders. *Clin Neuropharmacol* 2004; **27**: 230–233.

Neuroleptic malignant syndrome (NMS)

NMS is a rare but potentially serious even fatal adverse effect of all antipsychotics. NMS is a syndrome largely of sympathetic hyperactivity occurring as a result of dopaminergic antagonism in the context of psychological stressors and genetic predisposition[1]. Although widely seen as an acute, severe syndrome, NMS may, in many cases, have few signs and symptoms; 'full-blown' NMS may thus represent the extreme of a range of non-malignant related symptoms[2]. Certainly, asymptomatic rises in plasma creatine kinase (CK) are fairly common[3].

The incidence and mortality of NMS are difficult to establish and probably vary as drug use changes and recognition increases. It has been estimated that less than 1% of all patients treated with conventional antipsychotics will experience NMS[4]. Incidence figures for atypical drugs are not

Table Neuroleptic malignant syndrome	
Signs and symptoms[1,4,19,20]	Rigidity, fever, diaphoresis, confusion, fluctuating consciousness
	Fluctuating blood pressure, tachycardia
	Elevated creatine kinase, leucocytosis, altered liver function tests
Risk factors[19–23]	High-potency typical drugs, recent or rapid dose increase, rapid dose reduction, abrupt withdrawal of anticholinergics
	Psychosis, organic brain disease, alcoholism, Parkinson's disease, hyperthyroidism, psychomotor agitation, mental retardation
	Agitation, dehydration
Treatments[4,19,24–26]	In the psychiatric unit: Withdraw antipsychotics, monitor temperature, pulse, BP
	In the medical/A&E unit: Rehydration, bromocriptine + dantrolene, sedation with benzodiazepines, artificial ventilation if required
	L-dopa and carbamazepine have also been used, among many other drugs. Consider ECT for treatment of psychosis
Restarting antipsychotics[19,24,27]	Antipsychotic treatment will be required in most instances and rechallenge is associated with acceptable risk
	Stop antipsychotics for at least 5 days, preferably longer. Allow time for symptoms and signs to resolve completely
	Begin with very small dose and increase very slowly with close monitoring of temperature, pulse and blood pressure. CK monitoring may be used, but is controversial[20]. Close monitoring of physical and biochemical parameters is effective in reducing progression to full-blown NMS[28,29]
	Consider using an antipsychotic structurally unrelated to that associated with NMS or a drug with low dopamine affinity (quetiapine or clozapine)
	Avoid depots and high-potency conventional antipsychotics

available, but all have been reported to be associated with the syndrome[5–10], even newer drugs like ziprasidone[11] and aripiprazole[12,13]. Mortality may be lower with atypicals[14]. NMS is also very rarely seen with other drugs such as antidepressants[15–17] and lithium[18].

References

1. Gurrera RJ. Sympathoadrenal hyperactivity and the etiology of neuroleptic malignant syndrome. *Am J Psychiatry* 1999; **156**: 169–180.
2. Bristow MF, Kohen D. How 'malignant' is the neuroleptic malignant syndrome? In early mild cases it may not be malignant at all. *BMJ* 1993; **307**: 1223–1224.
3. Meltzer HY, Cola PA, Parsa M. Marked elevations of serum creatine kinase activity associated with antipsychotic drug treatment. *Neuropsychopharmacology* 1996; **15**: 395–405.
4. Guzé BH, Baxter LR. Neuroleptic malignant syndrome. *New Engl J Med* 1995; **313**: 163–165.
5. Hasan S, Buckley P. Novel antipsychotics and the neuroleptic malignant syndrome: a review and critique. *Am J Psychiatry* 1998; **155**: 1113–1116.
6. Sierra-Biddle D, Herran A, Diez-Aja S *et al.* Neuroleptic malignant syndrome and olanzapine. *J Clin Psychopharm* 2000; **20**: 704–705.
7. Stanley AK, Hunter J. Possible neuroleptic malignant syndrome with quetiapine. *Br J Psychiatry* 2000; **176**: 497.
8. Gallarda T, Olié J-P. Neuroleptic malignant syndrome in a 72-year-old man with Alzheimer's disease: a case report and review of the literature. *Eur Neuropsychopharm* 2000; **10**(Suppl. 3): 357.
9. Suh H, Bronson B, Martin R. Neuroleptic malignant syndrome and low-dose olanzapine (Letter). *Am J Psychiatry* 2003; **160**: 796.
10. Jangbahadoor Sing K, Ramaekers GMGI, Van Harten P. Neuroleptic malignant syndrome and quetiapine (Letter). *Am J Psychiatry* 2002; **159**: 149–150.
11. Leibold J, Patel V, Hasan RA. Neuroleptic malignant syndrome associated with ziprasidone in an adolescent. *Clin Ther* 2004; **26**: 1105–1108.
12. Spalding S, Alessi NE, Radwan K. Aripiprazole and atypical neuroleptic malignant syndrome. *J Am Acad Child Psychiat* 2004; **43**: 1457–1458.
13. Chakraborty N, Johnston T. Aripirazole and neuroleptic malignant syndrome. *Int Clin Psychopharmacol* 2004; **19**: 351–353.
14. Ananth J, Parameswaran S, Gunatilake S *et al.* Neuroleptic malignant syndrome and atypical antipsychotic drugs. *J Clin Psychiatry* 2004; **65**: 464–470.
15. June R, Yunus M, Gossman W. Neuroleptic malignant syndrome associated with nortriptyline. *Am J Emerg Med* 1999; **17**: 736–737.
16. Young C. A case of neuroleptic malignant syndrome and serotonin disturbance. *J Clin Psychopharm* 1997; **17**: 65–66.
17. Kontaxakis VP, Havaki-Kontaxakis BJ, Pappa DA *et al.* Neuroleptic malignant syndrome after addition of paroxetine to olanzapine. *J Clin Psychopharm* 2003; **23**: 671–672.
18. Gill J, Singh H, Nugent K. Acute lithium intoxication and neuroleptic malignant syndrome. *Pharmacotherapy* 2003; **23**: 811–815.
19. Levenson JL. Neuroleptic malignant syndrome. *Am J Psychiatry* 1985; **142**: 1137–1145.
20. Hermesh H, Manor I, Shiloh R *et al.* High serum creatinine kinase level: possible risk factor for neuroleptic malignant syndrome. *J Clin Psychopharm* 2002; **22**: 252–256.
21. Spivak B, Gonen N, Mester R *et al.* Neuroleptic malignant syndrome associated with abrupt withdrawal of anticholinergic agents. *Int Clin Psychopharmacol* 1996; **11**: 207–209.
22. Spivak B, Weizman A, Wolovick L *et al.* Neuroleptic malignant syndrome during abrupt reduction of neuroleptic treatment. *Acta Psychiatr Scand* 1990; **81**: 168–169.
23. Viejo LF, Morales V, Punal P *et al.* Risk factors in neuroleptic malignant syndrome. A case-control study. *Acta Psychiatr Scand* 2003; **107**: 45–49.
24. Olmsted TR. Neuroleptic malignant syndrome: guidelines for treatment and reinstitution of neuroleptics. *Southern Med J* 1988; **81**: 888–891.
25. Shoop SA, Cernek PK. Carbidopa/levodopa in the treatment of neuroleptic malignant syndrome (Letter). *Ann Pharmacother* 1997; **31**: 119.
26. Terao T. Carbamazepine in the treatment of neuroleptic malignant syndrome (Letter). *Biol Psychiatry* 1999; **45**: 378–382.
27. Wells AJ, Sommi RW, Chrismon ML. Neuroleptic rechallenge after neuroleptic malignant syndrome: case report and literature review. *DICP Ann Pharmacother* 1988; **22**: 475–480.
28. Shiloh R, Valevski A, Bodinger L *et al.* Precautionary measures reduce risk of definite neuroleptic malignant syndrome in newly typical neuroleptic-treated schizophrenia inpatients. *Int Clin Psychopharmacol* 2003; **18**: 147–179.
29. Hatch CD, Lund BC, Perry PJ. Failed challenge with quetiapine after neuroleptic malignant syndrome with conventional antipsychotics. *Pharmacotherapy* 2001; **21**: 1003–1006.

Antipsychotic-induced weight gain

Antipsychotics have long been recognised as weight-inducing agents. Suggested mechanisms include $5HT_{2C}$ antagonism, H_1 antagonism, hyperprolactinaemia and increased serum leptin (leading to leptin desensitisation)[1-3]. There is no evidence that drugs exert any direct metabolic effect: weight gain seems to result from increased food intake and, in some cases, reduced energy expenditure[4]. Risk of weight gain appears to be related to clinical response[5] and may also have a genetic basis[6,7].

All available antipsychotics have been associated with weight gain, although mean weight gained varies substantially between drugs. With all drugs, some patients gain no weight. Assessment of relative risk is made difficult by the poor quality of available data and the scarcity of long-term data. The following table suggests approximate relative risk of weight gain and mean weight gain (based on two systematic reviews[8,9]).

(See also page 84 for advice of treating drug-induced weight gain and page 27 for switching strategies.)

Table	Drug-induced weight gain
Drug	**Risk/extent of weight gain**
Clozapine Olanzapine	**High**
Zotepine Thioridazine	**Moderate/high**
Chlorpromazine Quetiapine Risperidone	**Moderate**
Amisulpride Aripiprazole Haloperidol Trifluoperazine Ziprasidone	**Low**

References

1. McIntyre RS, Mancini DA, Basile VS. Mechanisms of antipsychotic-induced weight gain. *J Clin Psychiatry* 2001; **62**(Suppl. 23): 23–29.
2. Herran A, Garcia Unzueta MT, Amado JA *et al.* Effects of long-term treatment with antipsychotics on serum leptin levels. *Br J Psychiatry* 2001; **179**: 59–62.
3. Monteleone P, Fabrazzo M, Tortorella A *et al.* Pronounced early increase in circulating leptin predicts lower weight gain during clozapine treatment. *J Clin Psychopharm* 2002; **22**: 424–426.
4. Virkkunen M, Wahlbeck K, Rissanen A *et al.* Decrease of energy expenditure causes weight increase in olanzapine treatment – a case study. *Pharmacopsychiatry* 2002; **35**: 124–126.
5. Czobor P, Volavka J, Sheitman B *et al.* Antipsychotic-induced weight gain and therapeutic response: a differential association. *J Clin Psychopharm* 2002; **22**: 244–251.
6. Basile VS, Masellis M, McIntyre RS *et al.* Genetic dissection of atypical antipsychotic-induced weight gain: novel preliminary data on the pharmacogenetic puzzle. *J Clin Psychiatry* 2001; **62**(Suppl. 23): 45–66.
7. Reynolds GP, Zhang Z, Zhang X. Polymorphism of the promotor region of the serotonin $5-HT_{2C}$ receptor gene and clozapine-induced weight gain. *Am J Psychiatry* 2003; **160**: 677–679.
8. Allison DB, Mentore JL, Moonseong H *et al.* Antipsychotic-induced weight gain: a comprehensive research synthesis. *Am J Psychiatry* 1999; **156**: 1686–1696.
9. Taylor DM, McAskill R. Atypical antipsychotics and weight gain – a systematic review. *Acta Psychiatr Scand* 2000; **101**: 416–432.

Further reading

Consensus Development Conference on Antipsychotic Drugs and Obesity and Diabetes. *Diabetes Care* 2004; **27**: 596–601.

Treatment of drug-induced weight gain

Weight gain is an important adverse effect of nearly all antipsychotics with obvious consequences for self-image, morbidity and mortality. Prevention and treatment are therefore matters of clinical urgency.

Patients starting antipsychotic treatment or changing drugs should, as an absolute minimum, be weighed and their weight clearly recorded. Estimates of body mass index and waist circumference should, ideally, also be made at baseline and then every 6 months[1]. There is evidence that very few UK patients have anywhere near adequate monitoring of weight[2]. Clearly, monitoring of weight parameters is essential to assess the value of preventative and remedial measures. (Cont.)

Drug	Comments
Amantadine[15–18] (100–300 mg/day)	May attenuate olanzapine-related weight gain. Seems to be well tolerated.
Bupropion[19,20] (amfebutamone)	Seems to be effective in obesity when combined with calorie-restricted diets. Few data of its effects on drug-induced weight gain. Note that pharmacology is essentially that of a dual-acting antidepressant. Caution in patients with bipolar illness.
Fluoxetine[21,22] (and other SSRIs)	Probably not effective.
H$_2$ antagonists[23–26] (e.g. nizatidine 300 mg b.d. or famotidine 40 mg/day)	Some positive studies but most negative. Effect, if any, is small. Few data supporting a reversal of weight gain.
Metformin[27,28] (500 mg t.d.s.)	Limited data in drug-related weight gain but has weak weight-reducing properties in other populations. Ideal for those with weight gain and diabetes.
Methylcellulose (1500 mg)	Old-fashioned and rather unpalatable preparation. No data in drug-induced weight gain but fairly widely used. Also acts as a laxative so may be suitable for clozapine-related weight gain.
Orlistat[29–31] (120 mg t.d.s. a.c./p.c.)	Reliable effect in obesity, especially when combined with calorie restriction. Few published data in drug-induced weight gain but fairly widely used with some success. Failure to adhere to a low-fat diet will result in fatty diarrhoea and possible malabsorption of orally administered medication.
Phenylpropanolamine[32]	Probably not effective.
Reboxetine[33] (4 mg daily)	Attenuates olanzapine-induced weight gain. No data on weight reduction.
Sibutramine[31,34] (10–15 mg daily)	Effective but few data in drug-induced obesity. Tachycardia and hypertension may be problematic. Note that the SPC lists 'psychiatric illness' as a contraindication. Panic[35] and psychosis[36] have both been reported.
Topiramate[37–42] (up to 150 mg daily)	Reliably reduces weight even when drug-induced, but data are mainly observational. Problems may arise because of topiramate's propensity for causing sedation, confusion and cognitive impairment.
Zonisamide[43] (400–600 mg/day)	Newer antiepileptic drug with weight-reducing properties. No data on drug-induced weight gain.

Most of the relevant literature in this area relates to attempts at reversing antipsychotic-related weight gain. There are relatively few data suggesting that early interventions can prevent weight gain[3] although this seems a more sensible approach.

When weight gain occurs, initial options involve switching drugs or instituting behavioural programmes (or both). Switching is not well researched but there is support for switching to aripiprazole[4] or ziprasidone[5] as a method for reversing weight gain. It is possible that switching to other drugs with a low propensity for weight gain is equally beneficial[6,7].

A variety of behavioural methods have been proposed and evaluated with fairly good results[8]. Methods include calorie restriction[9], low glycaemic index diet[10], Weight Watchers[11] and diet/exercise programmes[12–14].

Pharmacological methods should be considered only where behavioural methods have failed or where obesity presents clear, immediate physical risk to the patient. Some options are described in the table above (alphabetical order – no preference implied by position in table).

References

1. Marder SR, Essock SM, Miller AL et al. Physical health monitoring of patients with schizophrenia. Am J Psychiatry 2004; 161: 1334-1349.
2. Paton C, Esop R, Young C et al. Obesity, dyslipidaemias and smoking in an inpatient population treated with antipsychotic drugs. Acta Psychiatr Scand 2004; 110: 299–305.
3. Littrell KH, Hilligoss NM, Kirshner CD et al. The effects of an educational intervention on antipsychotic-induced weight gain. J Nurs Scholarship 2003; 35: 237–241.
4. Casey DE, Carson WH, Saha AR et al. Switching patients to aripiprazole from other antipsychotic agents: a multicenter randomized study. Psychopharmacology (Berl) 2003; 166: 391-399.
5. Weiden PJ, Daniel DG, Simpson G et al. Improvement in indices of health status in outpatients with schizophrenia switched to ziprasidone. J Clin Psychopharm 2003; 23: 595–600.
6. Gupta S, Masand PS, Virk S et al. Weight decline in patients switching from olanzapine to quetiapine. Schizophr Res 2004; 70: 57–62.
7. Ried LD, Renner BT, Bengston MA et al. Weight change after an atypical antipsychotic switch. Ann Pharmacother 2003; 37: 1381-1386.
8. Werneke U, Taylor D, Sanders TAB et al. Behavioural management of antipsychotic-induced weight gain: a review. Acta Psychiatr Scand 2003; 108: 252–259.
9. Cohen S, Glazewski R, Khan S et al. Weight gain with risperidone among patients with mental retardation: effect of calorie restriction. J Clin Psychiatry 2001; 62: 114–116.
10. Smith H, White T. Low glycaemic index in patients prescribed clozapine: pilot study. Psychiatr Bull 2004; 28: 292–294.
11. Ball P, Coons VB, Buchanan RW. A program for treating olanzapine-related weight gain. Psychiatr Serv 2001; 52: 967-969.
12. Pendlebury J, Ost D. Cromwell house weight management programme for patients with severe enduring mental illness: preliminary results. Poster presented at ECNP Annual Congress, Barcelona, Spain, 5–9 October 2002.
13. Vreeland B, Minsky S, Menza M et al. A program for managing weight gain associated with atypical antipsychotics. Psychiatr Serv 2003; 54: 1155–1157.
14. Ohlsen RI, Treasure J, Pilowsky LS. A dedicated nurse-led service for antipsychotic-induced weight gain. Psychiatr Bull 2004; 28: 164–166.
15. Floris M, Lejeune J, Deberdt W. Effect of amantadine on weight gain during olanzapine treatment. Eur Neuropsychopharm 2001; 11: 181–182.
16. Gracious BL, Krysiak TE, Youngstrom EA. Amantadine treatment of psychotropic-induced weight gain in children and adolescents: case series. J Child Adolesc Psychopharmacol 2002; 12: 249–257.
17. Bahk WM, Lee KU, Chae JH et al. Open label study of the effect of amantadine on weight gain induced by olanzapine. Psychiat Clin Neurosci 2004; 58: 163–167.
18. Deberdt W, Winokur A, Cavazzoni PA et al. Amantadine for weight gain associated with olanzapine treatment. Eur Neuropsychopharm 2005; 15: 13–21.
19. Gadde KM, Parker CB, Maner LG et al. Bupropion for weight loss: an investigation of efficacy and tolerability in overweight and obese women. Obes Res 2001; 9: 544–551.
20. Jain AK, Kaplan RA, Gadde KM et al. Bupropion SR vs. placebo for weight loss in obese patients with depressive symptoms. Obes Res 2002; 10: 1049–1056.
21. Poyurovsky M, Pashinian A, Gil-Ad I et al. Olanzapine-induced weight gain in patients with first-episode schizophrenia: a double-blind, placebo-controlled study of fluoxetine addition. Am J Psychiatry 2002; 159: 1058–1060.

22. Bustillo JR, Lauriello J, Parker K et al. Treatment of weight gain with fluoxetine in olanzapine-treated schizophrenic outpatients. Neuropsychopharmacology 2003; 28: 527–529.

23. Cavazzoni P, Tanaka Y, Roychowdhury SM et al. Nizatidine for prevention of weight gain with olanzapine: a double-blind placebo-controlled trial. Eur Neuropsychopharm 2003; 13: 81–85.

24. Pae CU, Kim JJ, Lee KU et al. Effect of nizatidine on olanzapine-associated weight gain in schizophrenic patients in Korea: a pilot study. Hum Psychopharm 2003; 18: 453–456.

25. Poyurosky M, Tal V, Maayan R et al. The effect of famotidine addition on olanzapine-induced weight gain in first-episode schizophrenia patients: a double-blind placebo-controlled pilot study. Eur Neuropsychopharm 2004; 14: 332–336.

26. Atmaca M, Kuloglu M, Tezcan E et al. Nizatidine for the treatment of patients with quetiapine-induced weight gain. Hum Psychopharm 2004; 19: 37–40.

27. Morrison JA, Cottingham EM, Barton BA. Metformin for weight loss in pediatric patients taking psychotropic drugs. Am J Psychiatry 2002; 159: 655–657.

28. Mogul HR, Peterson SJ, Weinstein BI et al. Long-term (2–4 year) weight reduction with metformin plus carbohydrate-modified diet in euglycemic, hyperinsulinemic, midlife women (syndrome W). Heart Disease 2003; 5: 384–392.

29. Sjostrom L, Rissanen A, Andersen T et al. Randomised placebo-controlled trial of orlistat for weight loss and prevention of weight regain in obese patients. Lancet 1998; 352: 167–172.

30. Hilger E, Quiner S, Ginzel MD et al. The effect of orlistat on plasma levels of psychotropic drugs in patients with long-term psychopharmacotherapy. J Clin Psychopharm 2002; 22: 68–70.

31. Werneke U, Taylor D, Sanders TAB. Options for pharmacological management of obesity in patients treated with atypical antipsychotics. Int Clin Pyschopharmacol 2002; 17: 145–159.

32. Borovicka MC, Fuller MA, Konicki PE et al. Phenylpropanolamine appears not to promote weight loss in patients with schizophrenia who have gained weight during clozapine treatment. J Clin Psychiatry 2002; 63: 345–348.

33. Poyurovsky M, Isaacs I, Fuchs C et al. Attenuation of olanzapine-induced weight gain with reboxetine in patients with schizophrenia: a double-blind, placebo-controlled study. Am J Psychiatry 2003; 160: 297–302.

34. Arterburn DE, Crane PK, Veenstra DL. The efficacy and safety of sibutramine for weight loss. Arch Intern Med 2004; 164: 994–1003.

35. Binkley K, Knowles SR. Sibutramine and panic attacks. Am J Psychiatry 2002; 159: 1793–1794.

36. Taflinski T, Chojnacka J. Sibutramine-associated psychotic episode. Am J Psychiatry 2000; 157: 2057–2058.

37. Dursun SM, Devarajan S. Clozapine weight gain plus topiramate weight loss. Can J Psychiatry 2000; 45: 198.

38. Levy E, Margolese HC, Chouinard G. Topiramate produced weight loss following olanzapine-induced weight gain in schizophrenia. J Clin Psychiatry 2002; 63: 1045.

39. Van Ameringen M, Mancini C, Campbell M et al. Topiramate treatment for SSRI-induced weight gain in anxiety disorders. J Clin Psychiatry 2002; 63: 981–984.

40. Appolinario JC, Fontenelle LF, Papelbaum M et al. Topiramate use in obese patients with binge eating disorder: an open study. Can J Psychiatry 2002; 47: 271–273.

41. Chengappa KN, Chalasani L, Brar JS et al. Changes in body weight and body mass index among psychiatric patients receiving lithium, valporate, or topiramate: an open-label nonrandomized chart review. Clin Ther 2002; 24: 1576–1584.

42. Pavuluri MN, Janicak PG, Carbray J. Topiramate plus risperidone for controlling weight gain and symptoms in preschool mania. J Child Adolesc Psychopharmacol 2002; 12: 271–273.

43. Gadde KM, Francisy DM, Eagner HR 2nd et al. Zonisamide for weight loss in obese adults: a randomized controlled trial. JAMA 2003; 289: 1820–1825.

Further reading

Appolinario JC, Bueno JR, Coutinho W. Psychotropic drugs in the treatment of obesity. What promise? CNS Drugs 2004; 18: 629–651.

Psychotropic-related QT prolongation

Introduction

Many psychotropic drugs are associated with ECG changes and it is possible that certain drugs are linked to serious ventricular arrhythmia and sudden cardiac death. Specifically, some agents are linked to prolongation of the cardiac QT interval, a risk factor for the ventricular arrhythmia torsade de pointes, which is occasionally fatal. Recent case-control studies have suggested that the use of some antipsychotics is associated with an increase in the rate of sudden cardiac death[1–4]. Overall risk, however, remains extremely low.

ECG monitoring of drug-induced changes in a mental health trust is complicated by a number of factors. Psychiatrists may have limited expertise in ECG interpretation, for example. (Self-reading, computerised ECG devices are available and to some extent compensate for some lack of expertise.) In addition, ECG machines may not be as readily available in all clinical areas as they are in general medicine. Also, time for ECG determination may not be available in many areas (e.g. out-patients). Lastly, ECG determination may be difficult to perform in acutely disturbed, physically uncooperative patients.

ECG monitoring of all patients is therefore impracticable and, given that risks are probably very small, of dubious benefit. This section sets out a pragmatic strategy for risk reduction and should be seen as guidance on minimising the *possible* risk associated with some drugs.

QT prolongation

- The cardiac QT interval (usually cited as QTc – QT corrected for heart rate) is a useful, but imprecise indicator of risk of torsade de pointes and of increased cardiac mortality[5]. Different correction factors and methods may give markedly different values[6].

- There is considerable controversy over the exact association between QTc and risk of arrhythmia. Very limited evidence suggests that risk is exponentially related to the extent of prolongation beyond normal limits (440 ms for men; 470 ms for women), although there are well-known exceptions which appear to disprove this theory[7]. Rather stronger evidence links QTc values over 500 ms to a clearly increased risk of arrhythmia[8].

- QTc measurements and evaluation are complicated by:
  - difficulty in determining the end of the T wave, particularly where U waves are present (this applies both to manual and self-reading ECG machines)[8]
  - normal physiological variation in QTc interval: QT varies with gender, time of day, food intake, alcohol intake, menstrual cycle, ECG lead, etc.[6,7]
  - variation in the extent of drug-induced prolongation of QTc because of changes in plasma levels. QTc prolongation is most prominent at peak drug plasma levels and least obvious at trough levels[6,7].

Other ECG changes

Other reported drug-induced changes include atrial fibrillation, giant P waves, T-wave changes and heart block[7]. These occur much less commonly than QTc changes (with the possible exception of changes in T-wave morphology).

Quantifying risk

Drugs are categorised here according to data available on their effects on the cardiac QTc interval (as calculated by Bazett's correction formula). 'No-effect' drugs are those with which QTc prolongation has not been reported either at therapeutic doses or in overdose. 'Low-effect' drugs are those for which severe QTc prolongation has been reported *only* following overdose or where only small average increases (<10 ms) have been observed at clinical doses. 'Moderate-effect' drugs are those which have been observed to prolong QTc by >10 ms on average when given at normal clinical doses or where ECG monitoring is officially recommended in some circumstances. 'High-effect' drugs are those for which extensive average QTc prolongation (usually >20 ms at normal clinical doses) has been noted or where ECG monitoring is mandated by the manufacturer's data sheet.

Note that effect on QTc may not necessarily equate to risk of torsade de pointes or sudden death[9], although this is often assumed. Note also that categorisation is inevitably approximate given the problems associated with QTc measurements.

Table   Psychotropics – effect on QTc[6,7,10–21]

No effect	Moderate effect
Amisulpride	Chlorpromazine
Aripiprazole	Quetiapine
	Ziprasidone
	Zotepine
SSRIs (except citalopram)	
Reboxetine	TCAs
Mirtazapine	
MAOIs	
	High effect
Carbamazepine	Any intravenous antipsychotic
Gabapentin	Methadone (see page 241)
Lamotrigine	Thioridazine
Valproate	Pimozide
	Sertindole
Benzodiazepines	
	Any drug or combination of drugs used in doses exceeding recommended maximum
Low effect	**Unknown effect**
Clozapine	Loxapine
Flupentixol	Pipothiazine
Fluphenazine	Trifluoperazine
Haloperidol	Zuclopenthixol
Olanzapine*	
Risperidone	Anticholinergic drugs (procyclidine, benzhexol, etc.)
Sulpiride	
Citalopram	
Venlafaxine	
Trazodone	
Lithium	

*Single case of QTc prolongation[14], all other data suggest no effect[7,12,13].

Other risk factors

A number of physiological/pathological factors are associated with an increased risk of QT changes and of arrhythmia (Table 1) and many non-psychotropic drugs are linked to QT prolongation (Table 2)[8].

Table I   Physiological risk factors for QTc prolongation and arrhythmia
Cardiac   Long QT syndrome   Bradycardia   Ischaemic heart disease   Myocarditis   Myocardial infarction   Left ventricular hypertrophy
Metabolic   Hypokalaemia   Hypomagnesaemia   Hypocalcaemia
Others   Extreme physical exertion   Stress or shock   Anorexia nervosa   Extremes of age – children and elderly may be more susceptible to QT changes   Female gender
Note: Hypokalaemia-related QTc prolongation is more commonly observed in acute psychotic admissions[22]. Also be aware that there are several physical and genetic factors which may not be discovered on routine examination but which probably predispose patients to arrhythmia[23,24].

Table 2 Non-psychotropics associated with QT prolongation	
Antibiotics Erythromycin Clarithromycin Ampicillin Co-trimoxazole Pentamidine (Some 4-quinolones affect QTc – see manufacturers' literature)	**Antiarrhythmics** Quinidine Disopyramide Procainamide Sotalol Amiodarone Bretylium
Antimalarials Chloroquine Mefloquine Quinine	**Others** Amantadine Cyclosporin Diphenhydramine Hydroxyzine Nicardipine Tamoxifen
Note: β_2 agonists and sympathomimetics may provoke torsade de pointes in patients with prolonged QTc.	

ECG monitoring recommendations

Generally, prescribing should be such that the need for ECG monitoring is minimised: alternative drugs are usually available and so ECG monitoring should be avoided whenever possible.

Table	ECG monitoring recommendations (*authors' opinion*)		
	No other risk factors	**Physiological/ pathological risk factors***	**When co-administered with other QT-prolonging drugs****
'No-effect' drugs	None	None	None
'Low-effect' drugs	None	None	Baseline ECG, then 6-monthly; consider referral to cardiologist
'Moderate-effect' drugs	None	Correct risk factors if possible, if not baseline ECG, then 6 monthly; consider referral to cardiologist	Avoid or refer to cardiologist
'High-effect' drugs	Baseline ECG then 6-monthly; consider referral to cardiologist	Correct risk factors if possible, if not – avoid	Avoid
'Unknown-effect' drugs	None	Correct risk factors if possible, if not baseline ECG then 6-monthly; consider referral to cardiologist	Avoid or refer to cardiologist

Notes

* Many conditions necessitate close cardiac monitoring, regardless of drugs prescribed. Recommendations in this column therefore represent additional requirements to those already mandated by the patient's condition.

** Defined as any drug listed in Table 2 on page 89 or psychotropics of moderate or high effect. The use of some of these drugs may necessitate cardiac monitoring. Recommendations in this column therefore represent *additional* requirements to those already mandated by the use of these drugs alone.

Actions to be taken

- **QTc <440 ms (men) or <470 ms (women)**
  No action required unless abnormal T-wave morphology – consider referral to cardiologist if in doubt.
- **QTc >440 ms (men) or >470 ms (women) but <500 ms**
  Consider switch to drug of lower effect; reperform ECG and consider referral to cardiologist.
- **QTc >500 ms**
  Stop suspected causative drug(s) and switch to drug of lower effect; refer to cardiologist immediately.
- **Abnormal T-wave morphology**
  Review treatment. Consider switch to drug of lower effect. Refer to cardiologist immediately.

Metabolic inhibition

The effect of drugs on the QTc interval is plasma level-dependent. Drug interactions are therefore important, especially when metabolic inhibition results in increased plasma levels of the drug affecting QTc. Commonly used metabolic inhibitors include fluvoxamine, fluoxetine, paroxetine, nefazodone and valproate. This is a complex area with an expanding database.

Other cardiovascular risk factors

The risk of drug-induced arrhythmia and sudden cardiac death with psychotropics is very small with a few drugs and probably non-existent with many others. Of much greater concern are other patient-related risk factors for cardiovascular disease. These include smoking, obesity and impaired glucose tolerance, and present a much greater risk to patient mortality than the uncertain outcome of QT changes. See relevant sections for discussion of these problems.

References

1. Reilly JG, Ayis SA, Ferrier IN et al. Thioridazine and sudden unexplained death in psychiatric in-patients. Br J Psychiatry 2002; 180: 515–522.
2. Ray WA, Meredith S, Thapa PB et al. Antipsychotics and the risk of sudden cardiac death. Arch Gen Psychiatry 2001; 58: 1161–1167.
3. Hennessy S, Bilker WB, Knauss JS et al. Cardiac arrest and ventricular arrhythmia in patients taking antipsychotic drugs: cohort study using administrative data. BMJ 2002; 325: 1070–1072.
4. Straus SM, Bleumink GS, Dieleman JP et al. Antipsychotics and the risk of sudden cardiac death. Arch Intern Med 2004; 164: 1293–1297.
5. Malik M, Camm AJ. Evaluation of drug-induced QT interval prolongation. Implications for drug approval and labelling. Drug Safety 2001; 24(5): 323–351.
6. Haddad PM, Anderson IM. Antipsychotic-related QTc prolongation, torsade de pointes and sudden death. Drugs 2002; 62: 1649–1671.
7. Taylor DM. Antipsychotics and QT prolongation. Acta Psychiatr Scand 2003; 107: 85–95.
8. Botstein P. Is QT interval prolongation harmful? A regulatory perspective. Am J Cardiol 1993; 72(6): 50B–52B.
9. Witchel HJ, Hancox JC, Nutt DJ. Psychotropic drugs, cardiac arrhythmia, and sudden death. J Clin Psychopharm 2003; 23: 58–77.
10. Glassman AH, Bigger JT. Antipsychotic drugs – prolonged QTc interval, torsade de pointes and sudden death. Am J Psychiatry 2001; 158: 1774–1782.
11. Warner B, Hoffman P. Investigation of the potential of clozapine to cause torsade de pointes. Adverse Drug React Toxicol Rev 2002; 21: 189–203.
12. Harrigan EP, Miceli JJ, Anziano R et al. A randomized evaluation of the effects of six antipsychotic agents on QTc, in the absence and presence of metabolic inhibition. J Clin Psychopharm 2004; 24: 62–69.
13. Lindborg SR, Beasley CM, Alaka K et al. Effects of intramuscular olanzapine vs. haloperidol and placebo QTc intervals in acutely agitated patients. Psychiatry Res 2003; 119: 113–123.
14. Dineen S, Withrow K, Voronovitch L et al. QTc prolongation and high-dose olanzapine (Letter). Psychosomatics 2003; 44: 174–175.
15. Gupta S, Nienhaus K, Shah S. Quetiapine and QTc issues: a case report (Letter). J Clin Psychiatry 2003; 64: 612–613.
16. Su KP, Shen WW. A pilot cross-over design study on QTc interval prolongation associated with sulpiride and haloperidol (Letter). Schizophr Res 2002; 59: 93–94.
17. Lin CH, Chen MC, Wang SY et al. Predictive factors for QTc prolongation in schizophrenia patients taking antipsychotics. J Formos Med Assoc 2004; 103: 437–441.
18. Chong SA, Mythily LA, Lum A et al. Prolonged QTc intervals in medicated patients with schizophrenia. Hum Psychopharm 2003; 18: 647–649.
19. Krantz MJ, Kutinsky IB, Robertson AD et al. Dose-related effects of methadone on QT prolongation in a series of patients with torsade de pointes. Pharmacotherapy 2003; 23: 802–805.
20. Gil M, Sala M, Anguera I et al. QT prolongation and torsade de pointes in patients infected with human immunodeficiency virus and treated with methadone. Am J Cardiol 2004; 93: 952.
21. Piquet V, Desmeules J, Ehret G et al. QT interval prolongation in patients on methadone with concomitant drugs. J Clin Psychopharm 2004; 24: 446–448.
22. Hatta K, Takahashi T, Nakamura H et al. Prolonged QT interval in acute psychotic patients. Psychiatry Res 2000; 94: 279–285.
23. Priori SG, Napolitano C, Schwartz PJ. Low penetrance in the long-QT syndrome clinical impact. Circulation 1999; 99: 529–533.
24. Frassati D, Tabib A, Lachaux B et al. Hidden cardiac lesions and psychotropic drugs as a possible cause of sudden death in psychiatric patients: a report of 14 cases and review of the literature. Can J Psychiatry 2004; 49: 100–105.

Further reading

Titier K, Girodet P-O, Verdoux H. Atypical antipsychotics – from potassium channels to torsade de pointes and sudden death. Drug Safety 2005; 28: 35–51.

Schizophrenia

Antipsychotics, diabetes and impaired glucose tolerance

Schizophrenia

Schizophrenia seems to be associated with relatively high rates of insulin resistance and diabetes[1,2] – an observation that predates the discovery of effective antipsychotics[3–5].

Antipsychotics

Data relating to diabetes and antipsychotic use are numerous but less than perfect[6–8]. The main problem is that incidence and prevalence studies assume full or uniform screening for diabetes. Neither is likely to be correct[6]. The following should be read with this in mind.

Typical antipsychotics

Phenothiazine derivatives have long been associated with impaired glucose tolerance and diabetes[9]. Diabetes prevalence rates have been reported to have substantially increased following the introduction and widespread use of conventional drugs[10]. Prevalence of impaired glucose tolerance seems to be higher with aliphatic phenothiazines than with fluphenazine or haloperidol[11]. Hyperglycaemia has also been reported with other conventional drugs, such as loxapine[12], and more recent data confirm an association with haloperidol[13].

Atypical antipsychotics

Clozapine
Clozapine has been strongly linked to hyperglycaemia, impaired glucose tolerance and diabetic ketoacidosis[14]. The risk of diabetes appears to be higher with clozapine than with other atypical and conventional drugs, especially in younger patients[15–17], although this is not a consistent finding[18,19].

As many as a third of patients may develop diabetes after 5 years of treatment[20]. Many cases of diabetes are noted in the first 6 months of treatment and some occur within 1 month[21], some after many years[19]. Death from ketoacidosis has also been reported[21]. Diabetes associated with clozapine is not necessarily linked to obesity or to family history of diabetes[14,22].

Clozapine appears to increase plasma levels of insulin in a clozapine level-dependent fashion[23,24]. It has been shown to be more likely than typical drugs to increase plasma glucose and insulin following oral glucose challenge[25]. Much clozapine-related diabetes may go unnoticed[26].

Olanzapine
Like clozapine, olanzapine has been strongly linked to impaired glucose tolerance, diabetes and diabetic ketoacidosis[27]. Risk of diabetes has also been reported to be higher than with typical drugs[28], again with a particular risk in younger patients[16]. The time course of development of diabetes has

not been established but impaired glucose tolerance seems to occur even in the absence of obesity and family history of diabetes[14,22]. Olanzapine may be more diabetogenic than risperidone[29-31].

It appears that olanzapine is associated with plasma levels of glucose and insulin higher than those seen with conventional drugs (after oral glucose load)[25,32].

Risperidone
Risperidone has been linked mainly in case reports to impaired glucose tolerance[33], diabetes[34] and ketoacidosis[35]. The number of reports of such adverse effects is substantially smaller than with either clozapine or olanzapine[36]. At least one study has suggested that changes in fasting glucose are significantly less common with risperidone than with olanzapine[29].

Risperidone seems no more likely than typical drugs to be associated with diabetes[16,28,30], although there may be an increased risk in patients under 40 years of age[16]. Risperidone has, however, been observed adversely to affect fasting glucose and plasma glucose (following glucose challenge) compared with levels seen in healthy volunteers (but not compared with patients taking typical drugs)[25].

Quetiapine
Like risperidone, quetiapine has been linked to cases of new-onset diabetes and ketoacidosis[37,38]. Again, the number of reports is much fewer than with olanzapine or clozapine. Quetiapine appears to be more likely than conventional drugs to be associated with diabetes[16,39]. Inexplicably, quetiapine may ameliorate clozapine-related diabetes when given in conjunction with clozapine[40].

Other atypicals

There are relatively few data relating to other atypical drugs. Amisulpride appears not to elevate plasma glucose[41] and seems not to be associated with diabetes[42]. Early data for aripiprazole[43,44] and ziprasidone[45] suggest that neither drug alters glucose homeostasis. These three drugs are cautiously recommended for those with a history of or predispostion to diabetes mellitus.

Monitoring

Diabetes is a growing problem in western society and has a strong association with obesity, (older) age, (lower) educational achievement and certain racial groups[46,47]. Diabetes markedly increases cardiovascular mortality, largely as a consequence of atherosclerosis[48]. Intervention to reduce plasma glucose levels and minimise other risk factors (obesity, hypercholesterolaemia) is therefore essential[49].

There is no clear consensus on diabetes-monitoring practice for those receiving antipsychotics. Given the known parlous state of testing for diabetes in the UK[6], arguments over precisely which tests are done and when seem redundant. There is an overwhelming need to improve monitoring by any means and so any tests for diabetes are supported – urine glucose and random plasma glucose included.

Ideally, though, all patients should have baseline fasting plasma glucose (FPG) tests performed[50]. This is often difficult to achieve in acutely ill, disorganised patients so measurement of glycosylated haemoglobin (HbA_{1C}) may also be used (fasting not required). Frequency of monitoring should then be determined by physical factors (e.g. weight gain) and known risk factors (e.g. family history of diabetes). The absolute minimum is yearly testing for diabetes for all patients.

Recommended monitoring		
	Ideally	**Minimum**
Baseline	FPG or HbA$_{1C}$	Urine glucose (UG) Random plasma glucose (RPG)
Continuation	All drugs: FPG or HbA$_{1C}$ every 12 months For clozapine and olanzapine or if other risk factors present: FPG or HbA$_{1C}$ after one month, then every 4–6 months	UG or RPG every 12 months

References

1. Schimmelbusch WH, Mueller PS, Sheps J. The positive correlation between insulin resistance and duration of hospitalization in untreated schizophrenia. *Br J Psychiatry* 1971; **118**: 429–436.
2. Waitzkin L. A survey of unknown diabetes in a mental hospital. I. Men under age fifty. *Diabetes* 1966; **15**: 97–104.
3. Kasanin J. The blood sugar curve in mental disease. *Arch Neuro Psychiatr* 1926; **16**: 414–419.
4. Braceland FJ, Meduna LJ, Vaichulis JA. Delayed action of insulin in schizophrenia. *Am J Psychiatry* 1945; **102**: 108–110.
5. Kohen D. Diabetes mellitus and schizophrenia: historical perspective. *Br J Psychiatry* 2004; **184**:S64–S66.
6. Taylor D, Young C, Esop R *et al.* Testing for diabetes in hospitalised patients prescribed antipsychotic drugs. *Br J Psychiatry* 2004; **185**: 152–156.
7. Haddad PM. Antipsychotics and diabetes: review of non-prospective data. *Br J Psychiat* 2004; **184**: S80–S86.
8. Bushe C, Leonard B. Association between atypical antipsychotic agents and type 2 diabetes: review of prospective clinical data. *Br J Psychiatry* 2004; **184**: S87–S93.
9. Arneson GA. Phenothiazine derivatives and glucose metabolism. *J Neuropsychiatry* 1964; **5**: 181.
10. Lindenmayer J-P, Nathan A-M, Smith RC. Hyperglycemia associated with the use of atypical antipsychotics. *J Clin Psychiatry* 2001; **62**(Suppl. 23): 30–38.
11. Keskiner A, el-Toumi A, Bousquet T. Psychotropic drugs, diabetes and chronic mental patients. *Psychosomatics* 1973; **14**: 176–181.
12. Tollefson G, Lesar T. Nonketotic hyperglycemia associated with loxapine and amoxapine: case report. *J Clin Psychiatry* 1983; **44**: 347–348.
13. Lindenmayer JP, Czobor P, Volavka J *et al.* Changes in glucose and cholesterol levels in patients with schizophrenia treated with typical and atypical antipsychotics. *Am J Psychiatry* 2003; **160**: 290–296.
14. Mir S, Taylor D. Atypical antipsychotics and hyperglycaemia. *Int Clin Psychopharmacol* 2001; **16**: 63–74.
15. Lund BC, Perry PJ, Brooks JM *et al.* Clozapine use in patients with schizophrenia and the risk of diabetes, hyperlipidemia, and hypertension: a claims based approach. *Arch Gen Psychiatry* 2001; **58**: 1172–1176.
16. Sernyak MJ, Leslie DL, Alarcon RD *et al.* Association of diabetes mellitus with use of atypical neuroleptics in the treatment of schizophrenia. *Am J Psychiatry* 2002; **159**: 561–566.
17. Gianfrancesco FD, Grogg AL, Mahmoud RA *et al.* Differential effects of risperidone, olanzapine, clozapine, and conventional antipsychotics on type 2 diabetes: findings from a large health plan database. *J Clin Psychiatry* 2002; **63**: 920–930.
18. Wang PS, Glynn RJ, Ganz DA *et al.* Clozapine use and risk of diabetes mellitus. *J Clin Psychopharm* 2002; **22**: 236–243.
19. Sumiyoshi T, Roy A, Anil AE *et al.* A comparison of incidence of diabetes mellitus between atypical antipsychotic drugs. A survey of clozapine, risperidone, olanzapine and quetiapine (Letter). *J Clin Pyschopharm* 2004; **24**: 345–348.
20. Henderson DC, Cagliero E, Gray C *et al.* Clozapine, diabetes mellitus, weight gain, and lipid abnormalities: a five-year naturalistic study. *Am J Psychiatry* 2000; **157**: 975–981.
21. Koller E, Schneider B, Bennett K *et al.* Clozapine-associated diabetes. *Am J Med* 2001; **111**: 716–723.
22. Sumiyoshi T, Roy A, Jayathilake K *et al.* The effect of hypertension and obesity in the development of diabetes mellitus in patients treated with atypical antipsychotic drugs (Letter). *J Clin Psychopharm* 2004; **24**: 452–454.
23. Melkersson KI, Hulting A-L, Brismar KE. Different influences of classical antipsychotics and clozapine on glucose-insulin homeostasis in patients with schizophrenia or related psychoses. *J Clin Psychiatry* 1999; **60**: 783–791.
24. Melkersson K. Clozapine and olanzapine, but not conventional antipsychotics, increase insulin release in vitro. *Eur Neuropsychopharm* 2004; **14**: 115–119.
25. Newcomer JW, Haupt DW, Fucetola R *et al.* Abnormalities in glucose regulation during antipsychotic treatment of schizophrenia. *Arch Gen Psychiatry* 2002; **59**: 337–345.
26. Sernyak MJ, Gulanski B, Leslie DL *et al.* Undiagnosed hyperglycemia in clozapine-treated patients with schizophrenia. *J Clin Psychiatry* 2003; **64**: 605–608.
27. Wirshing DA, Spellberg BJ, Erhart SM *et al.* Novel antipsychotics and new onset diabetes. *Biol Psychiatry* 1998; **44**: 778–783.

28. Koro CE, Fedder DO, L'Italien GJ *et al.* Assessment of independent effect of olanzapine and risperidone on risk of diabetes among patients with schizophrenia: population based nested case-control study. *BMJ* 2002; **325**: 243–245.

29. Meyer JM. A retrospective comparison of weight, lipid, and glucose changes between risperidone- and olanzapine-treated inpatients: metabolic outcomes after 1 year. *J Clin Psychiatry* 2002; **63**: 425–433.

30. Gianfrancesco F, White R, Wang RH *et al.* Antipsychotic-induced type 2 diabetes: evidence from a large health plan database. *J Clin Psychopharm* 2003; **23**: 328–335.

31. Leslie DL, Rosenheck RA. Incidence of newly diagnosed diabetes attributable to atypical antipsychotic medications. *Am J Psychiatry* 2004; **161**: 1709–1711.

32. Ebenbichler CF, Laimer M, Eder U *et al.* Olanzapine induces insulin resistance: results from a prospective study. *J Clin Psychiatry* 2003; **64**: 1436–1439.

33. Mallya A, Chawla P, Boyer SK *et al.* Resolution of hyperglycemia on risperidone discontinuation: a case report. *J Clin Psychiatry* 2002; **63**: 453–454.

34. Wirshing DA, Pierre JM, Eyeler J *et al.* Risperidone-associated new-onset diabetes. *Biol Psychiatry* 2001; **50**: 148–149.

35. Hine TJ, Pitchford NJ, Kingdom FAA *et al.* Diabetic ketoacidosis associated with risperidone treatment? *Psychomasomatics* 2000; **41**: 369–371.

36. Koller EA, Cross JT, Doraiswamy PM *et al.* Risperidone-associated diabetes mellitus. *Pharmacotherapy* 2003; **23**: 735–744.

37. Henderson DC. Atypical antipsychotic-induced diabetes mellitus: how strong is the evidence? *CNS Drugs* 2002; **16**: 77–89.

38. Koller EA, Weber J, Doraiswamy PM *et al.* A survey of reports of quetiapine-associated hyperglycemia and diabetes mellitus. *J Clin Psychiatry* 2004; **65**: 857–863.

39. Citrome L, Jaffe A, Levine J *et al.* Relationship between antipsychotic medication treatment and new cases of diabetes among psychiatric inpatients. *Psychiatr Serv* 2004; **55**: 1006–1013.

40. Reinstein MJ, Sirotovskaya LA, Jones LE. Effect of clozapine-quetiapine combination therapy on weight and glycaemic control. *Clin Drug Invest* 1999; **18**: 99–104.

41. Vanelle JM, Douki S. Metabolic control in patients with comorbid schizophrenia and depression treated with amisulpride or olanzapine. *European College of Neuropsychopharmacology*, Stockholm, Sweden, 9–13 October 2004.

42. Hermans G, De Hert M, Van Eyck D *et al.* The metabolic syndrome in schizophrenic patients treated with antipsychotics. Poster presented at 17th Congress of the European College of Neuropsychopharmacology, Stockholm, Sweden, 9–13 October 2004.

43. Keck PE Jr, McElroy SL. Aripiprazole: a partial dopamine D2 receptor agonist antipsychotic. *Expert Opin Inv Drug* 2003; **12**: 655–662.

44. Pigott TA, Carson WH, Saha AR *et al.* Aripiprazole for the prevention of relapse in stabilized patients with chronic schizophrenia: a placebo-controlled 26-week study. *J Clin Psychiatry* 2003; **64**: 1048–1056.

45. Simpson GM, Glick ID, Weiden PJ *et al.* Randomized, controlled, double-blind multicenter comparison of the efficacy and tolerability of ziprasidone and olanzapine in acutely ill inpatients with schizophrenia or schizoaffective disorder. *Am J Psychiatry* 2004; **161**: 1837–1847.

46. Mokdad AH, Ford ES, Bowman BA *et al.* The continuing increase of diabetes in the U.S. *Diabetes Care* 2001; **24**: 412.

47. Mokdad AH, Ford ES, Bowman BA *et al.* Diabetes trends in the U.S.: 1990–1998. *Diabetes Care* 2000; **23**: 1278.

48. Beckman JA, Creager MA, Libby P. Diabetes and atherosclerosis epidemiology, pathophysiology, and management. *JAMA* 2002; **287**: 2570–2581.

49. Haupt DW, Newcomer JW. Hyperglycemia and antipsychotic medications. *J Clin Psychiatry* 2001; **62**(Suppl. 27): 15–26.

50. Marder SR, Essock SM, Miller AL *et al.* Physical health monitoring of patients with schizophrenia. *Am J Psychiatry* 2004; **161**: 1334–1349.

Antipsychotics and hyperlipidaemia

Morbidity and mortality from cardiovascular disease are higher in people with schizophrenia than in the general population[1]. Hyperlipidaemia is an established risk factor for cardiovascular disease along with obesity, hypertension, smoking, diabetes and sedentary lifestyle. The majority of patients with schizophrenia have several of these risk factors and can be considered at 'high risk' of developing cardiovascular disease. Hyperlipidaemia is treatable and intervention is known to reduce morbidity and mortality[2].

Effect of antipsychotic drugs on lipids

Typicals: Phenothiazines are known to be associated with increases in triglycerides and low-density lipoprotein (LDL) cholesterol and decreases in high-density lipoprotein (HDL)[3] cholesterol, but the magnitude of these effects is poorly quantified[4]. Haloperidol seems to have minimal effect on lipid profiles[3].

Atypicals: Although there are more data pertaining to some atypicals, they are derived from a variety of sources and are reported in different ways, making it difficult to compare drugs directly. While cholesterol levels can rise, the most profound effect of these drugs seems to be on triglycerides. Raised triglycerides are in general, associated with obesity and diabetes. From the available data, olanzapine would seem to have the greatest propensity to increase lipids; quetiapine, moderate propensity; and risperidone, minimal or no propensity. Data for other atypicals are scarce.

Olanzapine has been shown to increase triglyceride levels by 40% over the short (12 weeks) and medium (16 months) terms[5,6]. Levels may continue to rise for up to a year[7]. Up to two-thirds of olanzapine-treated patients have raised triglycerides[8] and just under 10% may develop severe hypertriglyceridaemia[9]. While weight gain with olanzapine is generally associated with both increases in cholesterol[6,10] and triglycerides[9], severe hypertriglyceridaemia can occur independently of weight gain[9]. In one study, patients treated with olanzapine and risperidone gained a similar amount of weight, but in olanzapine patients serum triglyceride levels increased by four times as much (80 mg/dl) as in risperidone patients (20 mg/dl)[9]. Quetiapine[11] seems to have more modest effects than olanzapine.

A case-control study conducted in the UK found that patients with schizophrenia who were treated with olanzapine were five times more likely to develop hyperlipidaemia than controls and three times more likely to develop hyperlipidaemia than patients receiving typical antipsychotics[12]. Risperidone-treated patients could not be distinguished from controls.

Clozapine: Mean triglyceride levels have been shown to double and cholesterol levels to increase by at least 10% after 5 years' treatment with clozapine[13]. Patients treated with clozapine have triglyceride levels that are almost double those of patients who are treated with typical antipsychotics[14,15]. Cholesterol levels do not seem to be significantly different.

Particular care should be taken before prescribing clozapine, olanzapine, quetiapine and possibly phenothiazines for patients who are obese, diabetic or known to have pre-existing hyperlipidaemia[16].

Screening

All patients should have their lipids measured at baseline. Those prescribed clozapine, olanzapine, quetiapine or phenothiazines should have their serum lipids measured every 3 months for the first year of treatment[7]. Those prescribed other antipsychotics should have their lipids measured after 3 months then annually.

Treatment of hyperlipidaemia

If moderate to severe hyperlipidaemia develops during antipsychotic treatment, a switch to another antipsychotic less likely to cause this problem should be considered in the first instance. Although not recommended as a strategy in patients with treatment-resistant illness, clozapine-induced hyper-triglyceridaemia has been shown to reverse after a switch to risperidone[17]. This may hold true with other switching regimens but data are scarce.

Patients with raised cholesterol may benefit from dietary advice and/or treatment with statins. Risk tables and treatment guidelines can be found in the *British National Formulary (BNF)*. Evidence supports the treatment of cholesterol concentrations as low as 4 mmol/l in high-risk patients[18]. Coronary heart disease and stroke risk can be reduced by a third by reducing cholesterol to as low as 3.5 mmol/l[2]. When triglycerides alone are raised, diets low in saturated fats, fish oil and fibrates are effective treatments[7]. Such patients should be screened for IGT and diabetes (see page 92). Note the effective use of fish oils in some psychiatric conditions.

Summary

Monitoring	
Drug	**Suggested monitoring**
Clozapine Quetiapine Olanzapine Phenothiazines	Fasting lipids and cholesterol at baseline then every 3 months for a year, then annually
Other antipsychotics	Fasting lipids and cholesterol at baseline and at 3 months, and then annually

References

1. Brown S, Inskip H, Barraclough B. Causes of the excess mortality of schizophrenia. *Br J Psychiatry* 2000; **177**: 212–217.
2. Durrington P. Dyslipidaemia. *Lancet* 2003; **362**: 717–731.
3. Sasaki J, Funakoshi M, Arakawa K. Lipids and apolipoproteins in patients treated with major tranquilisers. *Clin Pharmacol Ther* 1985; **37**: 684–687.
4. Henkin Y, Como JA, Oberman A. Secondary dyslipidaemia: inadvertent effects of drugs in clinical practice. *JAMA* 1992; **267**: 961–968.
5. Sheitman BB, Bird PM, Binz W *et al.* Olanzapine-induced elevation of plasma triglyceride levels. *Am J Psychiatry* 1999; **156**: 1471–1472.
6. Osser DN, Najarian DM, Dufresne RL. Olanzapine increases weight and serum triglyceride levels. *J Clin Psychiatry* 1999; **60**: 767–770.
7. Meyer JM. Effects of atypical antipsychotics on weight and serum lipid levels. *J Clin Psychiatry* 2001; **62**(Suppl. 27): 27–34.
8. Melkersson KI, Hulting AL, Brismar KE. Elevated levels of insulin, leptin and blood lipids in olanzapine treated patients with schizophrenia or related psychoses. *J Clin Psychiatry* 2000; **61**: 742–749.
9. Mayer JM. Novel antipsychotics and severe hyperlipidaemia. *J Clin Psychopharm* 2001; **21**: 369–374.
10. Kinon BJ, Basson BR, Gilmore JA *et al.* Long term olanzapine treatment: weight change and weight-related health factors in schizophrenia. *J Clin Psychiatry* 2001; **62**: 92–100.
11. Atmaca M, Kuloglu M, Tezcan E. Serum leptin and triglyceride levels in patients on treatment with atypical antipsychotics. *J Clin Psychiatry* 2003; **64**: 598–604.
12. Koro CE, Fedder DO, L'Italien GJ. An assessment of the independent effects of olanzapine and risperidone exposure on the risk of hyperlipidaemia in schizophrenic patients. *Arch Gen Psychiatry* 2002; **59**: 1021–1026.

13. Henderson DC. Clozapine: diabetes mellitus, weight gain and lipid abnormalities. *J Clin Psychiatry* 2001; **62**(Suppl. 23): 39–44.
14. Ghaeli P, Dufresne RL. Serum triglyceride levels in patients treated with clozapine. *Am J Health Syst Pharm* 1996; **53**: 2079–2081.
15. Spivak B, Roitman S, Vered Y *et al.* Diminished suicidal and aggressive behaviour, high plasma norepinephrine levels, and serum triglyceride levels in chronic neuroleptic-resistant schizophrenic patients maintained on clozapine. *Clin Neuropharmacol* 1998; **21**: 245–250.
16. Trino B, Kin NY, Beaulieu S. Novel antipsychotics and severe hyperlipidaemia: comments on the Meyer paper. *J Clin Psychopharm* 2002; **22**: 536–537.
17. Ghaeli P, Dufresne RL. Elevated serum triglycerides on clozapine resolve with risperidone. *Pharmacotherapy* 1995; **15**: 382–385.
18. Heart Protection Study Collaborative Group. MRC/BHF heart protection study of cholesterol lowering with simvastatin in 20536 high risk individuals: a randomised placebo controlled trial. *Lancet* 2002; **360**: 7–72.

Further reading

American Diabetes Association, American Psychiatric Association, American Association of Clinical Endocrinologists *et al.* Consensus development conference on antipsychotic drugs and obesity and diabetes. *J Clin Psychiatry* 2004; **65**: 267–272.

Koponen H, Saari K, Savolainen M *et al.* Weight gain and glucose and lipid metabolism disturbances during antipsychotic medication. *Eur Arch Psychiatry Clin Neurosci* 2002; **252**: 294–298.

Paton C, Esop R, Young C *et al.* Obesity, dyslipidaemias and smoking in an in-patient population treated with antipsychotic drugs. *Acta Psychiatr Scand* 2004; **110**: 299–305.

Antipsychotics and sexual dysfunction

Primary sexual disorders are common, although reliable normative data are lacking[1]. Reported prevalence rates vary depending on the method of data collection (low numbers with spontaneous reports, increasing with confidential questionnaires and further still with direct questioning[2]). Physical illness, psychiatric illness, substance misuse and prescribed drug treatment can all cause sexual dysfunction[2].

Baseline sexual functioning should be determined if possible (questionnaires may be useful) because sexual function can affect quality of life and affect compliance with medication (sexual dysfunction is one of the major causes of treatment dropout)[3]. Complaints of sexual dysfunction may also indicate progression or inadequate treatment of underlying medical or psychiatric conditions. It may also be due to drug treatment, and intervention may greatly improve quality of life[4].

The human sexual response

There are four phases of the human sexual response, as detailed in the table below[2,5-7].

Table	The human sexual response
Desire	• Related to testosterone levels in men • Possibly increased by dopamine and decreased by prolactin • Psychosocial context and conditioning significantly affect desire
Arousal	• Influenced by testosterone in men and oestrogen in women • Other potential mechanisms include: central dopamine stimulation, modulation of the cholinergic/adrenergic balance, peripheral α_1 agonism and nitric oxide • Physical pathology such as hypertension or diabetes can have a significant effect
Orgasm	• May be related to oxytocin • Inhibition of orgasm may be caused by an increase in serotonin activity, as well as α_1 blockade
Resolution	• Occurs passively after orgasm
Note: Many other hormones and neurotransmitters may interact in a complex way at each phase.	

Effects of psychosis

Up to 82% of men and 96% of women with schizophrenia report problems with sexual dysfunction[8]. Men[8] complain of reduced desire, inability to achieve an erection and premature ejaculation whereas women complain more generally about reduced enjoyment[8,9]. Women with psychosis are known to have reduced fertility[10]. People with psychosis are less able to develop good psychosexual relationships and, for some, treatment with an antipsychotic can improve sexual functioning[11]. Assessment of sexual functioning can clearly be difficult in someone who is psychotic.

Effects of antipsychotic drugs

Sexual dysfunction has been reported as a side-effect of all antipsychotics[4], and up to 45% of people taking typical antipsychotics experience sexual dysfunction[12]. Individual susceptibility varies and all effects are reversible. Antipsychotics decrease dopaminergic transmission, which in itself can decrease libido but may also increase prolactin levels via negative feedback. This can cause amenorrhoea in women and a lack of libido, breast enlargement and galactorrhoea in both men and women[13]. Anticholinergic effects can cause disorders of arousal[14] and drugs that block peripheral α_1 receptors cause particular problems with erection and ejaculation in men[4]. Drugs that are antagonists at both peripheral α_1 receptors and cholinergic receptors can cause priapism[15]. Antipsychotic-induced sedation and weight gain may reduce sexual desire[15]. These principles can be used to predict the sexual side-effects of different antipsychotic drugs (see table below).

Table Sexual adverse effects of antipsychotics	
Drug	**Type of problem**
Phenothiazines	• Hyperprolactinaemia and anticholinergic effects. Reports of delayed orgasm at lower doses followed by normal orgasm but without ejaculation at higher doses[9] • Most problems occur with thioridazine (which can also reduce testosterone levels)[16] • Priapism has been reported with thioridazine, risperidone and chlorpromazine (probably due to α_1 blockade)[17–19]
Thioxanthenes	• Arousal problems and anorgasmia[11]
Haloperidol	• Similar problems to the phenothiazines[20] but anticholinergic effects reduced[17]
Olanzapine	• Possibly less sexual dysfunction due to relative lack of prolactin-related effects[20] • Priapism reported rarely[21]
Risperidone	• Potent elevator of serum prolactin • Less anticholinergic • Specific peripheral α_1 adrenergic blockade leads to a moderately high reported incidence of ejaculatory problems such as retrograde ejaculation[22,23] • Priapism reported rarely[15]
Sulpiride/amisulpride	• Potent elevators of serum prolactin[12]
Quetiapine	• No effect on serum prolactin[24] • Possibly associated with the lowest risk of sexual dysfunction[25–27]
Clozapine	• Significant α_1 adrenergic blockade and anticholinergic effects[28]. No effect on prolactin[29] • Probably fewer problems than with typical antipsychotics[30]
Aripiprazole	• Few data but problems not expected

Treatment

Before attempting to treat sexual dysfunction, a thorough assessment is essential to determine the most likely cause. Assuming that physical pathology has been excluded, the following principles apply.

Spontaneous remission may occasionally occur[15]. The most obvious first step is to decrease the dose or discontinue the offending drug where appropriate. The next step is to switch to a different drug that is less likely to cause the specific sexual problem experienced (see table above). If this fails or is not practicable, 'antidote' drugs can be tried: for example, cyproheptadine (a $5HT_2$ antagonist at doses of 4–16 mg/day) has been used to treat SSRI-induced sexual dysfunction but sedation is a common side-effect. Amantadine, buproprion, buspirone, bethanechol and yohimbine have all been used with varying degrees of success but have a number of unwanted side-effects and interactions with other drugs (see opposite).

Table Remedial treatments for psychotropic-induced sexual dysfunction

Drug	Pharmacology	Potential treatment for	Side-effects
Alprostadil[1,6]	Prostaglandin	Erectile dysfunction	Pain, fibrosis, hypotension, priapism
Amantadine[1,33]	Dopamine agonist	Prolactin-induced reduction in desire and arousal (dopamine increases libido and facilitates ejaculation)	Return of psychotic symptoms, GI effects, nervousness, insomnia
Bethanechol[34]	Cholinergic or cholinergic potentiation of adrenergic neurotransmission	Anticholinergic-induced arousal problems and anorgasmia (from TCAs, antipsychotics, etc.)	Nausea and vomiting, colic, bradycardia, blurred vision, sweating
Bromocriptine[4]	Dopamine agonist	Prolactin-induced reduction in desire and arousal	Return of psychotic symptoms, GI effects
Bupropion[35]	Noradrenaline and dopamine reuptake inhibitor	SSRI-induced sexual dysfunction (evidence poor)	Concentration problems, reduced sleep, tremor
Buspirone[31]	$5HT_{1a}$ partial agonist	SSRI-induced sexual dysfunction, particularly decreased libido and anorgasmia	Nausea, dizziness, headache
Cyproheptadine[1,31,36]	$5HT_2$ antagonist	Sexual dysfunction caused by increased serotonin transmission (e.g. SSRIs), particularly anorgasmia	Sedation and fatigue. Reversal of the therapeutic effect of antidepressants
Sildenafil[6,37–39]	Phosphodiesterase inhibitor	Erectile dysfunction of any aetiology Anorgasmia in women	Mild headaches, dizziness
Yohimbine[1,6,40–42]	Central and peripheral α_2 adrenoceptor antagonist	SSRI-induced sexual dysfunction, particularly erectile dysfunction, decreased libido and anorgasmia (evidence poor)	Anxiety, nausea, fine tremor, increased BP, sweating, fatigue

Note: The use of the drugs listed above should ideally be under the care or supervision of a specialist in sexual dysfunction.

The evidence base supporting the use of 'antidotes' is poor[15].

Drugs such as sildenafil (Viagra) or alprostadil (Caverject) are effective only in the treatment of erectile dysfunction. In the UK they are available for prescription by GPs for a limited number of medical indications, not including psychosis or antipsychotic-induced impotence[32]. The psychological approaches used by sexual dysfunction clinics may be difficult for clients with mental health problems to engage in[4].

References

1. Baldwin DS, Thomas SC, Birtwistle J. Effects of antidepressant drugs on sexual function. *Int J Psychiatr Clin Pract* 1997; 1: 47–58.
2. Pollack MH, Reiter S, Hammerness P. Genitourinary and sexual adverse effects of psychotropic medication. *Int J Psychiatry Med* 1992; 22: 305–327.
3. Montejo AL, Llorca G, Izquierdo JA *et al.* Incidence of sexual dysfunction associated with antidepressant agents: a prospective multicentre study of 1022 outpatients. *J Clin Psychiatry* 2001; 62: 10–20.
4. Segraves RT. Effects of psychotropic drugs on human erection and ejaculation. *Arch Gen Psychiatry* 1989; 46: 275–284.
5. Stahl SM. The psychopharmacology of sex. I. Neurotransmitters and the 3 phases of the human sexual response. *J Clin Psychiatry* 2001; 62: 80–81.
6. Garcia-Reboll L, Mulhall JP, Goldstein I. Drugs for the treatment of impotence. *Drugs Aging* 1997; 11: 140–151.
7. DeGroat WC, Booth AM. Physiology of male sexual functioning. *Ann Intern Med* 1980; 92: 329–331.
8. MacDonald S, Halliday J, MacEwan T *et al.* Nithsdale Schizophrenia Surveys 24: sexual dysfunction. *Br J Psychiatry* 2003; 182: 50–56.
9. Smith S. Effects of antipsychotics on sexual and endocrine function in women: implications for clinical practice. *J Clin Psychopharm* 2003; 23(Suppl 1): 27–32.
10. Howard LM, Kumar C, Leese M *et al.* The general fertility rate in women with psychotic disorders. *Am J Psychiatry* 2002; 159: 991–997.
11. Aizenberg D, Zemishlany Z, Dorfman-Etrog P *et al.* Sexual dysfunction in male schizophrenic patients. *J Clin Psychiatry* 1995; 56: 137–141.
12. Smith S, O'Keane V, Murray R. Sexual dysfunction in patients taking conventional antipsychotic medication. *Br J Psychiatry* 2002; 181: 49–55.
13. Meltzer HY, Casey DE, Garver DL *et al.* Adverse effects of the atypical antipsychotics. *J Clin Psychiatry* 1998; 59(Suppl. 12): 17–22.
14. Aldridge SA. Drug-induced sexual dysfunction. *Clin Pharmacy* 1982; 1: 141–147.
15. Baldwin D, Mayers A. Sexual side-effects of antidepressant and antipsychotic drugs. *Adv Psychiatric Treat* 2003; 9: 202–210.
16. Kotin J, Wilbert DE, Verburg D *et al.* Thioridazine and sexual dysfunction. *Am J Psychiatry* 1976; 133: 82–85.
17. Mitchell JE, Popkin MK. Antipsychotic drug therapy and sexual dysfunction in men. *Am J Psychiatry* 1982; 139: 633–637.
18. Loh C, Leckband SG, Meyer JM *et al.* Risperidone-induced retrograde ejaculation: case report and review of the literature. *Int Clin Psychopharmacol* 2004; 19: 111–112.
19. Thompson JW, Ware MR, Blashfield RK. Psychotropic medication and priapism: a comprehensive review. *J Clin Psychiatry* 1990; 51: 430–433.
20. Crawford A, Beasley C, Tollefson G. The acute and long term effect of olanzapine compared with placebo and haloperidol on serum prolactin concentrations. *Schizophr Res* 1997; 26: 41–54.
21. Olanzapine UK summary of product characteristics.
22. Tran PV, Hamilton SH, Kuntz AJ. Double-blind comparison of olanzapine versus risperidone in the treatment of schizophrenia and other psychotic disorders. *J Clin Psychopharm* 1997; 17: 407–418.
23. Raja M. Risperidone-induced absence of ejaculation. *J Clin Psychopharm* 1999; 14: 317–319.
24. Peuskens J, Link CGG. A comparison of quetiapine and chlorpromazine in the treatment of schizophrenia. *Acta Psychiatr Scand* 1997; 96: 265–273.
25. Bobes J, Garcia-Portilla MP. Frequency of sexual dysfunction and other reproductive side effects in patients with schizophrenia treated with risperidone, olanzapine, quetiapine or haloperidol: the results of the EIRE study. *J Sex Marital Ther* 2003; 29: 124–147.
26. Byerly MJ, Lescouflair E, Weber MT *et al.* An open-label trial of quetiapine for antipsychotic induced sexual dysfunction. *J Sex Marital Ther* 2004; 30: 325–332.
27. Knegtering R, Castelein S, Bous H et al. A randomised open-label study of the impact of quetiapine versus risperidone on sexual functioning. *J Clin Psychopharm* 2004; 24: 56–61.
28. Coward DM. General pharmacology of clozapine. *Br J Psychiatry* 1992; 160(Suppl. 17): 5–11.
29. Meltzer HY, Goode DJ, Schyve PM *et al.* Effect of clozapine on human serum prolactin levels. *Am J Psychiatry* 1979; 136: 1550–1555.
30. Aizenberg D, Modai I, Landa A *et al.* Comparison of sexual dysfunction in male schizophrenic patients maintained on treatment with classical antipsychotics versus clozapine. *J Clin Psychiatry* 2001; 62: 541–544.

31. Rothschild AJ. Sexual side-effects of antidepressants. *J Clin Psychiatry* 2000; **61**: 28–36.
32. UK HNS Health Service Circular, HSC 1999/177.
33. Valevski A, Modai I, Zbarski E *et al.* Effect of amantadine on sexual dysfunction in neuroleptic-treated male schizophrenic patients. *Clin Neuropharmacol* 1998; **21**: 355–357.
34. Gross MD. Reversal by bethanechol of sexual dysfunction caused by anticholinegic antidepressants. *Am J Psychiatry* 1982; **139**: 1193–1294.
35. Masand PS, Ashton AK, Gupta S *et al.* Sustained-release bupropion for selective serotonin reuptake inhibitor-induced sexual dysfunction: a randomised, double blind, placebo controlled, parallel group study. *Am J Psychiatry* 2001; **158**: 805–807.
36. Lauerma H. Successful treatment of citalopram-induced anorgasmia by cyproheptadine. *Acta Psychiatr Scand* 1996; **93**: 69–70.
37. Nurnberg HG, Hensley PL, Lauriello J *et al.* Sildenafil for women patients with antidepressant-induced sexual dysfunction. *Psychiatr Serv* 1999; **50**: 1076–1078.
38. Salerian AJ, Deibler WE, Vittone BJ *et al.* Sildenafil for psychotropic-induced sexual dysfunction in 31 women and 61 men. *J Sex Marital Ther* 2000; **26**: 133–140.
39. Nurnberg HG, Hensley PL, Gelenberg AJ *et al.* Treatment of antidepressant-associated sexual dysfunction with sildenafil: a randomized controlled trial. *JAMA* 2003; **289**: 56–64.
40. Jacobsen FM. Fluoxetine-induced sexual dysfunction and an open trial of yohimbine. *J Clin Psychiatry* 1992; **53**: 119–122.
41. Michelson D, Kociban K, Tamura R *et al.* Mirtazapine, yohimbine or olanzapine augmentation therapy for serotonin reuptake-associated female sexual dysfunction: a randomised, placebo controlled trial. *J Psychiatr Res* 2002; **36**: 147–152.
42. Woodrum ST, Brown CS. Management of SSRI-induced sexual dysfunction. *Ann Pharmacother* 1998; **32**: 1209–1215.

Schizophrenia

Antipsychotic-induced hyponatraemia

Hyponatraemia can occur in the context of

1. **Water intoxication** where water consumption exceeds the maximal renal clearance capacity. Serum and urine osmolality are low. The prevalence of water intoxication is estimated to be 5% in chronically ill, hospitalised, psychiatric patients[1,2]. The primary aetiology is poorly understood. It has been postulated that it may be driven, at least in part, by an extreme compensatory response to the anticholinergic side-effects of antipsychotic drugs[3].

2. Drug-induced syndrome of inappropriate antidiuretic hormone (**SIADH**) where the kidney retains an excessive quantity of solute-free water. Serum osmolality is low and urine osmolality relatively high. The prevalence of SIADH is estimated to be as high as 11% in acutely ill psychiatric patients[4]. Risk factors for antidepressant-induced SIADH (increasing age, female gender, medical co-morbidity and polypharmacy) seem to be less relevant in the population of patients treated with antipsychotic drugs[5]. SIADH usually develops in the first few weeks of treatment with the offending drug. Phenothiazines, haloperidol, pimozide, risperidone, quetiapine, olanzapine and clozapine have all been implicated[5]. Note, however, that the literature consists entirely of case reports and case series.

3. Severe **hyperlipidaemia** and/or **hyperglycaemia** lead to secondary increases in plasma volume and 'pseudohyponatraemia'[3]. Both are more common in people treated with antipsychotic drugs than in the general population and should be excluded as causes.

Mild to moderate hyponatraemia presents as confusion, nausea, headache and lethargy. As the plasma sodium falls, these symptoms become increasingly severe and seizures and coma can develop.

References

1. DeLeon J, Verghese C, Tracy JI *et al.* Polydipsia and water intoxication in psychiatric patients: a review of the epidemiological literature. *Biol Psychiatry* 1994; **35**: 408–419.
2. Patel JK. Polydipsia, hyponatraemia and water intoxication among psychiatric patients. *Hosp Community Psychchiatry* 1994; **45**: 1073–1074.
3. Siegel AJ, Baldessarini RJ, Klepser MB *et al.* Primary and drug induced disorders of water homeostasis in psychiatric patients: principles of diagnosis and management. *Harv Rev Psychiatry* 1998; **6**: 190–200.
4. Siegler EL, Tamres D, Berlin JA *et al.* Risk factors for the development of hyponatraemia in psychiatric inpatients. *Arch Intern Med* 1995; **155**: 953–957.
5. Madhusoodanan S, Bogunovic OJ, Moise D *et al.* Hyponatraemia associated with psychotropic medications: a review of the literature and spontaneous reports. *Adverse Drug React Toxicol Rev* 2002; **21**: 17–29.
6. Canuso CM, Goldman MB. Clozapine restores water balance in schizophrenic patients with polydipsia-hyponatraemia syndrome. *J Neuropsychiatry Clin Neurosci* 1999; **11**: 86–90.
7. Spears NM, Leadbetter RA, Shutty MS. Clozapine treatment in polydipsia and intermittent hyponatraemia. *J Clin Psychiatry* 1996; **57**: 123–128.
8. Littrell KH, Johnson CG, Littrell SH *et al.* Effects of olanzapine on polydipsia and intermittent hyponatraemia. *J Clin Psychiatry* 1997; **58**: 549.
9. Kawai N, Baba A, Suzuki T. Risperidone failed to improve polydipsia-hyponatraemia of the schizophrenic patients. *Psychiat Clin Neurosci* 2002; **56**: 107–110.
10. Montgomery JH, Tekell JL. Adjunctive quetiapine treatment of the polydipsia, intermittent hyponatraemia and psychosis syndrome: a case report. *J Clin Psychiatry* 2003; **64**: 339–341.
11. Canuso CM, Goldman MB. Does minimising neuroleptic dosage influence hyponatraemia? *Psychiatry Res* 1996; **63**: 227–229.

Table Treatment[3,4]

Cause of hyponatraemia	Antipsychotic drugs implicated	Treatment
Water intoxication (serum and urine osmolality low)	Only very speculative evidence to support drugs as a cause. Core part of illness in a minority of patients (e.g. psychotic polydypsia)	• **Fluid restriction** with careful monitoring of serum sodium, particularly diurnal variation (Na drops as the day progresses). Refer to specialist medical care if Na < 125 mmol/l. • Consider treatment with **clozapine**: shown to increase plasma osmolality into the normal range and increase urine osmolality (not usually reaching the normal range)[6]. These effects are consistent with reduced fluid intake. This effect is not clearly related to improvements in mental state[7]. • There are both[5] positive and negative reports for olanzapine[8] and risperidone[9] and one positive case report for quetiapine[10]. Compared with clozapine, the evidence base is weak. • There is no evidence that either reducing or increasing the dose of an antipsychotic results in improvements in serum sodium in water-intoxicated patients[11]. • Demeclocycline should not be used (exerts its effect by interfering with ADH and increasing water excretion, already at capacity in these patients).
SIADH (serum osmolality low and urine osmolality relatively high)	All antipsychotic drugs	• If mild, **fluid restriction** with careful monitoring of serum sodium. Refer to specialist medical care if Na < 125 mmol/l. • **Switch to a different antipsychotic drug.** There are insufficient data available to guide choice. Be aware that cross-sensitivity may occur (the individual may be predisposed and the choice of drug is unimportant). • Consider **demeclocycline** (see *BNF* for details). • Lithium may be effective[5] but is a potentially toxic drug. Remember that hyponatraemia predisposes to lithium toxicity.

Antipsychotics: relative adverse effects – a rough guide

Drug	Sedation	Extra-pyramidal	Anti-cholinergic	Hypotension	Prolactin elevation
Amisulpride	–	+	–	–	+++
Aripiprazole	–	+/–	–	–	–
Benperidol	+	+++	+	+	+++
Chlorpromazine	+++	++	++	+++	+++
Clozapine	+++	–	+++	+++	–
Flupentixol	+	++	++	+	+++
Fluphenazine	+	+++	++	+	+++
Haloperidol	+	+++	+	+	+++
Loxapine	++	+++	+	++	+++
Olanzapine	++	+/–	+	+	+
Perphenazine	+	+++	+	+	+++
Pimozide	+	+	+	+	+++
Pipothiazine	++	++	++	++	+++
Promazine	+++	+	++	++	++
Quetiapine	++	–	+	++	–
Risperidone	+	+	+	++	+++
Sertindole	–	–	–	+++	+/–
Sulpiride	–	+	–	–	+++
Thioridazine	+++	+	+++	+++	++
Trifluoperazine	+	+++	+/–	+	+++
Ziprasidone	+	+/–	–	+	+/–
Zotepine	+++	+	+	++	+++
Zuclopenthixol	++	++	++	+	+++

Key: +++ high incidence/severity   ++ moderate
     + low   – very low

Note: the table above is made up of approximate estimates of relative incidence and/or severity, based on clinical experience, manufacturers' literature and published research. This is a rough guide – see individual sections for more precise information.

Other side effects not mentioned in this table do occur. Please see dedicated sections on other side effects included in this book for more information.

chapter 3

Bipolar disorder

Valproate

Valproate is available in the UK in three forms: sodium valproate (Epilim) and valproic acid (Convulex), licensed for the treatment of epilepsy, and semisodium valproate (Depakote), licensed for the acute treatment of mania. Both semisodium and sodium valproate are metabolised to valproic acid, which is apparently responsible for the pharmacological activity of all three preparations. Clinical studies of the treatment of affective disorders variably use sodium valproate, semisodium valproate, 'valproate' or valproic acid. The great majority have used valproate semisodium.

Randomised, controlled trials (RCTs) have shown valproate to be effective in the treatment of mania[1,2]. Approximately 50% of patients respond during the acute phase[1]. Freeman et al.[2] found lithium to be more effective overall than valproate, while Swann et al.[3] found that patients who had depressive symptoms at baseline were more likely to respond to valproate than lithium. Patients who have experienced 10 or more episodes of mania may also respond better to valproate (as semisodium) than lithium[4], although this study may have preselected lithium-resistant patients. In a further double-blind, placebo-controlled study of valproate in 36 patients who had failed to respond to or could not tolerate lithium, the median decrease in Young Mania Rating Scale scores was 54% in the valproate group and 5% in the placebo group[5]. Open studies suggest that valproate may be effective in bipolar depression.

Although open-label studies suggest that valproate is effective in the prophylaxis of bipolar affective disorder[6,7], only two RCTs have been published to date[8,9]. In the first[8], no difference was found between lithium, valproate semisodium and placebo in the primary outcome measure, time to any mood episode, although divalproex was superior to lithium and placebo on some secondary outcome measures. This study could be criticised for including patients who were 'not ill enough' and for not lasting 'long enough' (1 year). In the second RCT[9], which lasted for 47 weeks, there was no difference in relapse rates between divalproex (valproate semisodium) and olanzapine. This study had no placebo arm, so is difficult to interpret. Valproate is sometimes used to treat aggressive behaviour of variable aetiology[10].

Plasma levels

Valproate has a complex pharmacokinetic profile, following a three-compartment model and showing protein-binding saturation. Plasma level monitoring is supposedly, therefore, of more limited use than with carbamazepine or lithium. A dose of at least 1000 mg/day and a serum level of at least 50 mg/l may be robustly associated with response[11]. Achieving therapeutic plasma levels rapidly using a loading dose regime is well tolerated but not proven to provide a more rapid response in the treatment of mania[12]. (This study was not powered to detect any difference in efficacy.) Plasma levels can perhaps more reliably detect non-compliance or predict or confirm toxicity.

Adverse effects[13]

Sodium valproate causes both hyperammonaemia and gastric irritation, which can sometimes lead to intense nausea. Lethargy and confusion can occasionally occur with starting doses of above 200–300 mg b.d. Weight gain can be significant[14], particularly when valproate is used in conjunction with clozapine. Hair loss with curly regrowth, and peripheral oedema can also occur. Sodium valproate may very rarely cause fulminant hepatic failure[15]. All cases reported to date have occurred in children, often receiving multiple anticonvulsants and with family histories of hepatic problems. It would seem wise to evaluate clinically any patient with raised LFTs and to also monitor other markers of hepatic function such as albumin and prothrombin time. Valproate can cause hyper-androgenism in women and polycystic ovaries[16]. It is also associated with thrombocytopenia, leuco-penia, red cell hypoplasia and pancreatitis. Many side-effects of valproate are dose-related (peak plasma level-related) and increase in frequency and severity when the plasma level is >100 mg/l. The once-daily 'chrono' form of sodium valproate does not produce as high peaks as the conventional forms of valproate and may be better tolerated. There is also a suggestion that valproate semisodium may be better tolerated in some.

Use of valproate in women of childbearing age

Valproate is an established teratogen. The risk of foetal malformations is 7.2%[17], much of which is due to neural tube defects. NICE recommends that alternative anticonvulsants are to be preferred in women with epilepsy[17].

The SPCs[18] for sodium and semisodium valproate state that:

- These drugs should not be initiated in women of childbearing potential without specialist advice (from a neurologist or psychiatrist).
- Women who are trying to conceive and require valproate, should be prescribed prophylactic folate.

Women who have mania are likely to be sexually disinhibited. The risk of unplanned pregnancy is likely to be above population norms (where 50% of pregnancies are unplanned). Adequate contraception should be ensured and prophylactic folate prescribed.

Interactions with other drugs[19,20]

Valproate is highly protein-bound (up to 94%): other drugs that are highly protein-bound can displace valproate from albumin and precipitate toxicity (e.g. *aspirin*[21]). Other, less strongly protein-bound drugs, can be displaced by valproate, leading to higher free levels and increased therapeutic effect or toxicity (e.g. *warfarin*). Valproate is hepatically metabolised: drugs that inhibit CYP enzymes can increase valproate levels (e.g. *erythromycin*, *fluoxetine* and *cimetidine*). Valproate can increase the plasma levels of some drugs, possibly by inhibition/competitive inhibition of their metabolism. Examples include *TCAs* (particularly clomipramine[22]), *lamotrigine*[23] and *phenobarbitone*.

Pharmacodynamic interactions also occur. The anticonvulsant effect of valproate is antagonised by drugs that lower the seizure threshold (e.g. antipsychotics and antidepressants). Weight gain can be exacerbated by other drugs that have this effect (e.g. antipsychotics, particularly clozapine and olanzapine).

References

1. Bowden CL, Brugger AM, Swann AC *et al.* Efficacy of divalproex sodium vs lithium and placebo in the treatment of mania. *JAMA* 1994; **271**: 918–924.
2. Freeman TW, Clothier JL, Pazzaglia P. A double-blind comparison of valproate and lithium in the treatment of acute mania. *Am J Psychiatry* 1992; **149**: 108–111.
3. Swann AC, Bowden CL, Morris D *et al.* Depression during mania: treatment response to lithium or divalproex. *Arch Gen Psychiatry* 1997; **54**: 37–42.
4. Swann AC, Bowden CL, Calabrese JR. Differential effect of number of previous episodes of affective disorder on response to lithium or divalproex in acute mania. *Am J Psychiatry* 1999; **156**: 1264–1266.
5. Pope HG, McElroy SL, Keck PE *et al.* Valproate in the treatment of acute mania: a placebo-controlled study. *Arch Gen Psychiatry* 1991; **48**: 62–68.
6. Calabrese JR, Delucchi GA. Spectrum of efficacy of valproate in 55 patients with rapid-cycling bipolar disorder. *Am J Psychiatry* 1990; **147**: 431–434.
7. McElroy SL, Keck PE, Pope HG. Sodium valproate: its use in primary psychiatric disorders. *J Clin Psychopharm* 1987; **7**: 16–24.

Bipolar disorder

8. Bowden CL, Calabrese JR, McElroy SL *et al.* A randomised, placebo-controlled 12-month trial of divalproex and lithium in the treatment of outpatients with bipolar 1 disorder. *Arch Gen Psychiatry* 2000; 57: 481–489.

9. Tohen M, Ketter TA, Zarate CA *et al.* Olanzapine versus divalproex sodium for the treatment of acute mania and maintenance of remission: a 47 week study. *Am J Psychiatry* 2003; **160**: 1263–1271.

10. Lindenmayer JP, Kotsaftis A.Use of sodium valproate in violent and aggressive behaviours: a critical review. *J Clin Psychiatry* 2000; **61**: 123–128.

11. Taylor D, Duncan D. Doses of carbamazepine and valproate in bipolar affective disorder. *Psychiatr Bull* 1997; **21**: 221–223.

12. Hirschfeld RMA, Allen MH, McEvoy JP. Safety and tolerability of oral loading divalproex sodium in acutely manic bipolar patients. *J Clin Psychiatry* 1999; **60**: 815–818.

13. Summary of product characteristics for sodium valproate, semi-sodium valproate and valproic acid. Data Sheet Compendium, ABPI Data Sheet Compendium 2004.

14. Vanina Y, Podolskaya A, Sedky K *et al.* Body weight changes associated with psychopharmacology. *Psychiatr Serv* 2002; **53**: 842–847.

15. Rimmer EM, Richens A. An update on sodium valproate. *Pharmacotherapy* 1985; **5**: 171–184.

16. Piontec CM, Wisner KL. Appropriate clinical management of women taking valproate. *J Clin Psychiatry* 2000; **61**: 161–163.

17. National Institute for Clinical Excellence. Newer drugs for epilepsy in adults. Technology Appraisal 76. 2004. www.nice.org.uk

18. Summary of product characteristics (Epilim & Depakote). www.medicines.org.uk

19. Spina E, Perucca E. Clinical significance of pharmacokinetic interactions between antiepileptic and psychotropic drugs. *Epilepsia* 2002; **43**: 37–44.

20. Patsalos PN, Froscher W, Pisani F *et al.* The importance of drug interactions in epilepsy therapy. *Epilepsia* 2002; **43**: 365–385.

21. Goulden KJ, Dooley JM, Camfield PR *et al.* Clinical valproate toxicity induced by acetylsalicylic acid. *Neurology* 1987; **37**: 1392–1394.

22. Fehr C, Grunder G, Hiemke C *et al.* Increase in serum clomipramine concentrations caused by valproate. *J Clin Psychopharm* 2000; **20**: 493–494.

23. Morris R, Black A, Lam E *et al.* Clinical study of lamotrigine and valproic acid in patients with epilepsy: using a drug interaction to advantage? *Ther Drug Monit* 2000; **22**: 656–660.

Lithium

History

The use of lithium in medicine goes back some 150 years, and the most significant developments are listed below[1]:

1845–1860: Lithium was used in the treatment of gout.

1865–1880: Mania and melancholia were incorporated into the group of gouty diseases and were therefore treated with lithium-containing salts.

1880: Carl Lange described periodic depression (thought to be another gouty disease) and treated patients prophylactically for many years with 'alkaline salts', resulting in the ingestion of 5–25 mmol lithium/day, although he never recognised lithium as the active ingredient of these salts.

1920s: A Danish psychiatrist, H.J. Schou, described the same depressive illness as Carle Lange but was against the latter's prophylactic therapy of alkaline salts, thus ending an era. Ironically his son, Mogens Schou, later emerged as a major advocate of lithium therapy.

Early 1950s: Lithium salts were used widely in the USA as a salt substitute in cardiac patients, with disastrous results, leading to the discovery of their renal toxicity, especially in sodium-depleted patients. Around the same time, John Cade first used lithium to treat various psychiatric disorders; he noted a very good response in manic patients and some improvement in patients with schizophrenia. Many of these patients showed signs of lithium toxicity (the pharmacokinetics of lithium were not fully understood).

Early 1970s: A double-blind discontinuation study was published by Hartigan Baastrup, which demonstrated beyond doubt the efficacy of lithium therapy. Standardised testing of serum lithium was also introduced around this time.

1977: A paper was published which showed that long-term lithium treatment might induce slight, chronic, irreversible kidney damage with accompanying reduction of renal concentrating ability. The acceptable therapeutic range for lithium has fallen steadily since, in order to maximise therapeutic response while minimising unwanted side-effects. It is now accepted as being 0.6 -1.0 mmol/l, with the lower part of the range being appropriate for prophylaxis and for elderly patients, and the upper part being appropriate for acute treatment and the prophylaxis of unstable bipolar affective disorder. Interestingly, lithium salts are still freely available in some parts of the world as remedies for rheumatoid and gouty diseases.

1990s: Clinical utility reexamined. Doubts expressed.

Use

Lithium is widely used for the prophylaxis and treatment of mania and hypomania, recurrent depression and bipolar affective disorder. Its use in the treatment of acute mania[2] is limited by the fact that it usually takes at least a week to achieve a response[3] and that the co-administration of high doses of potent antipsychotics may increase the risk of neurological side-effects. It can also be difficult to achieve therapeutic serum levels rapidly and monitoring can be problematic if the patient is unco-operative.

Lithium and antidepressants are probably equally effective in the prophylaxis of recurrent depressive illness[4]. Lithium is a useful addition to an antidepressant in a patient with an acute depressive episode that is proving difficult to treat[3].

Lithium is also used in the prophylaxis of bipolar affective disorder where it reduces both the number and the severity of relapses[2,5]. The NNT to prevent relapse into mania or depression has been calculated to be 10 and 14 respectively[6]. Lithium also offers some protection against antidepressant-induced hypomania. It is accepted clinical practice to consider starting treatment with a mood-stabiliser if two episodes of mania or depression have occurred in a 3-year period[3]. Although numerous factors have been studied in an attempt to identify patients who are likely to respond to lithium, an empirical trial is still the best predictor of long-term outcome. Relapse within 1 year of starting lithium prophylaxis is highly suggestive of a poor long-term response. Clinical features associated with a favourable response include marked psychomotor retardation and endogenous and psychotic features. In addition, some evidence points to the previous pattern of illness as a predictor of response to lithium[7]: patients whose illness shows a pattern of mania followed by depression followed by a euthymic interval, or those whose illness shows an irregular pattern, are more likely to respond to lithium prophylaxis than those who show a pattern of depression – mania – euthymia or have a rapidly cycling illness (four or more episodes/year)[8].

Intermittent treatment with lithium may worsen the natural course of bipolar illness (a much greater than expected incidence of manic relapse is seen in the first few months after discontinuing lithium[9–11], even in patients who have been symptom-free for as long as 5 years[12]). There is a suggestion that depressive relapses may also increase[11]. This has led to recommendations that lithium treatment should not be started unless there is a clear intention to continue it for at least 3 years[13]. This advice has obvious implications for initiating lithium treatment against a patient's will (or in someone known to be non-compliant) during a period of acute illness. The risk of relapse may be reduced by decreasing the dose of lithium gradually over a period of 1 month[14]. Intermittent treatment with lithium does not seem to have the same detrimental effect on the course of unipolar depressive illness.

It is estimated that 15% of those with bipolar illness take their own life[15]. Mortality from physical illness is also increased. Chronic treatment with lithium reduces mortality from suicide to the same level as that seen in the general population[8,16,17]. There is no convincing evidence that mortality from other causes is altered.

Lithium is used in combination with antipsychotics in the treatment of schizo-affective illness[18], and is also used to treat aggressive[19] and self-mutilating behaviour and in steroid-induced psychosis[20]. The neuropharmacology of lithium[21] is not clearly understood but its therapeutic effect is thought to be related, among other things, to its ability to block neuronal calcium channels, and its effects on GABA pathways. The efficacy of lithium does not go unchallanged. For a review, see Moncrieff[22].

Plasma levels

Lithium is rapidly absorbed from the gastrointestinal tract, but has a long distribution phase. Blood should ideally be taken 12 hours after the last dose was administered. Pharmacokinetic data show that the level, for any given individual, is reproducible if blood is taken 10–14 hours postdose (for once-daily dosing with modified-release preparations)[23]. On average, the serum level can be expected to fall by 0.2 mmol/l between 12 and 24 hours postdose[24].

Lithium should be started at a dose of 400 mg at night: lower in the elderly or in renal impairment. The serum level should be measured after 5–7 days, and then weekly until the desired level has been achieved. Once the serum level is stable, it should be checked 3–6 monthly: more often if problems are suspected or the patient is elderly or is co-prescribed interacting drugs. Full guidance on monitoring can be found on pages 120–121. Serum levels of 0.6–1.0 mmol/l are usually aimed for, although in some individuals further benefit can be gained by going slightly higher[25]. A re-analysis of the original lithium clinical trials cast doubt on this 'conventional wisdom': the authors concluded that the absolute level used for maintenance may be less important than the rapid reduction in serum lithium level that occurred in these trials when patients were switched from one treatment group to another[26]. Children and adolescents may require higher serum levels than adults to ensure that an adequate brain concentration is achieved[27].

Formulations of lithium

There is no significant difference in the pharmacokinetics of the two most widely prescribed brands of lithium: Priadel and Camcolit[3]. Not all preparations are bio-equivalent, however, and care must be taken to make sure that the patient receives the same preparation each time a new prescription is supplied.

- Lithium carbonate 400 mg tablets each contain 10.8 mmol lithium.

- Lithium citrate 564 mg tablets each contain 6 mmol lithium. Lithium citrate liquid is available in two strengths; it should be administered twice daily:
  – 5.4 mmol/5 ml equivalent to 200 mg lithium carbonate.
  – 10.8 mmol/5 ml equivalent to 400 mg lithium carbonate.

Lack of clarity over which preparation is intended when prescribing can lead to the patient receiving a subtherapeutic or toxic dose.

Adverse effects

Side-effects tend to be directly related to plasma levels and their frequency increases dramatically at levels above 1 mmol/l. Mild gastrointestinal symptoms can occur when therapy is initiated and are usually transient. Fine hand tremor may occur, as may mild thirst and polyuria. Polyuria may occur more frequently with twice-daily dosing[28]. Propranolol can be useful in the treatment of lithium-induced tremor. Certain skin conditions, such as psoriasis and acne, can be aggravated by lithium therapy.

In the longer term, hypothyroidism may occur, although this should not be a reason for stopping lithium treatment: thyroxine replacement therapy is indicated. TFTs usually return to normal when lithium is discontinued. The risk of developing hypothyroidism is probably very much higher than is commonly believed, particularly in middle-aged women (prevalence up to 20%[29]). There is a strong case for testing for thyroid autoantibodies in this group before starting lithium (to better estimate risk) and for measuring TFTs more frequently in the first year of treatment[29]. Lithium treatment also increases the risk of hyperparathyroidism, and patients receiving long-term lithium should have their serum calcium level monitored[30].

Some patients complain that lithium 'curbs creativity' or produces 'mental dulling'. A study of artists and writers found that for the majority creativity actually increased with lithium treatment, because of thoughts and actions being more organised. A small minority reported diminished creativity (those who felt inspired by high mood)[31].

The long term complication that has received the most attention is nephrotoxicity. A small reduction in glomerular filtration rate is seen in 20% of patients[23]. In the vast majority of patients this effect is benign[32]. A very small number of lithium-treated patients may develop interstitial nephritis. Lithium can also cause a reduction in urinary concentrating capacity (nephrogenic diabetes insipidus – hence occurrence of thirst and polyuria), which is reversible in the short-to-medium term but may be irreversible after long-term treatment (>15 years)[23,32].

Lithium toxicity

Toxic effects reliably occur at levels >1.5 mmol/l and usually consist of gastrointestinal effects (increasing anorexia, nausea and diarrhoea) and CNS effects (muscle weakness, drowsiness, ataxia, coarse tremor and muscle twitching). Above 2 mmol/l, increased disorientation and seizures are seen, which can progress to coma and death. In the presence of more severe symptoms, osmotic diuresis or forced alkaline diuresis should be initiated[33] (*Note:* not thiazide or loop diuretics under any circumstances). Above 3 mmol/l, peritoneal or haemodialysis is often used[33]. These plasma levels are only a guide and individuals can vary in their susceptibility to symptoms of toxicity.

Before prescribing lithium

Before prescribing lithium, renal, cardiac and thyroid function should be checked[23]. Women of childbearing age should be advised to use reliable contraception. Patients should be informed about symptoms of toxicity: why they might occur and what to do. Bouts of vomiting/diarrhoea or any form of dehydration will lead to sodium depletion and therefore to increased plasma lithium levels. Similarly, a salt-free diet is contraindicated. It is also wise to ensure that the patient is aware of the importance of maintaining an adequate fluid balance and of the need not to double today's dose because yesterday's was forgotten. Basic information about lithium and how to minimise the risk of toxicity is contained in the *Patient Information Leaflet* found inside each box of lithium tablets.

Interactions with other drugs

Because of lithium's relatively narrow therapeutic index, interactions with other drugs can be very important. The most commonly encountered interactions are as follows.

Diuretics can increase serum lithium levels markedly by reducing its clearance. Thiazides are the worst culprits, while loop diuretics are somewhat safer. Initial thiazide diuresis is accompanied by the loss of sodium. This loss is compensated for within a few days by an increase in sodium reabsorption in the proximal tubule. As the kidney cannot distinguish between sodium and lithium at this site, it follows that there is also an increase in lithium reabsorption, leading to decreased renal clearance.

Non-steroidal anti-inflammatory drugs (NSAIDs) can increase serum lithium levels by up to 40%[34]. The mechanism of this interaction is not clearly understood, although it is thought to be related to the effects of NSAIDs on fluid balance, and is particularly important if PRN NSAIDs are added to a long-standing regular prescription of lithium. Lithium toxicity secondary to NSAID co-prescription has led to legal cases where substantial damages have been awarded against psychiatrists. One case in 1999 was settled for £600,000[35]. Some NSAIDs can be obtained without a prescription. Patients should be aware of the potential interaction. Lithium toxicity has also been reported with the COX 2 inhibitors rofecoxib (now withdrawn) and celecoxib[36]. There is one case report of lithium toxicity in a patient stabilised on lithium and ibuprofen when celecoxib was added[37]. Caution is required with all COX 2 inhibitors.

Haloperidol: following the famous publication by Cohen and Cohen[38] reporting severe neurotoxicity, widespread anxiety set in about using the combination of lithium and haloperidol. It is important to put this interaction into perspective; if the lithium levels are in the therapeutic range (0.6–1.0 mmol/l) and the haloperidol dose is not increased rapidly to heroic heights, the chance of inducing a toxic state is very low indeed. Haloperidol and lithium is a widely prescribed and very useful combination[39].

Carbamazepine, in combination with lithium, has been reported to cause neurotoxic reactions. Again, higher (>1 mmol/l) plasma lithium levels were involved than are now thought acceptable, and most of the references state that a previous neurotoxic reaction to lithium alone is a risk factor! Carbamazepine and lithium are often combined in patients with refractory illness[40].

SSRIs have been linked to an increased incidence of CNS toxicity when used with lithium. Although the mechanism of this interaction is not completely understood, it is likely to be mediated through serotonin pathways. It is prudent to be aware and to check lithium levels soon after starting treatment with an SSRI (although it must be noted that some reports claim neurotoxic reactions in the absence of raised lithium levels). Clinical experience has shown this combination to be useful and any interaction rare[41].

ACE inhibitors decrease the excretion of lithium. They can also precipitate renal failure, so extra care is needed in monitoring both serum creatinine and lithium, if these drugs are prescribed together. Care is also required with **angiotensin 2 antagonists**[42] (losartan, valsartan, candesartan, eprosartan, irbesartan and telmisartan).

Summary table – lithium

Indications	Mania, hypomania; prophyaxis in bipolar disorder and recurrent depression. Also effective in schizo-affective disorder and aggression
Pre-lithium work-up	ECG, thyroid function tests, renal function tests (serum creatinine and urea), U&Es
Monitoring	Start at 400 mg once daily (200 mg in the elderly). Plasma level after 5–7 days, then every 5–7 days until the required level is reached (0.6–1.0 mmol/l). Blood should be taken 12 hours after the last dose. Once stable, check level every 3–6 months. Check U&Es and TFTs every 6 months
Stopping	Slowly reduce over at least 1 month

Bipolar disorder

References

1. Amdisen A. Historical origins. In: Johnson FN (ed). *Depression and Mania: Modern Lithium Therapy*. Oxford: IRL Press, 1987, Ch. 6, pp. 24–28.
2. Cookson J. Lithium: balancing risks and benefits. *Br J Psychiatry* 1997; **178**: 120–124.
3. Ferrier IN, Tyrer SP, Bell AJ. Lithium therapy. *Adv Psychiatric Treat* 1995; **1**: 102–110.
4. Souza FGM, Goodwin GM. Lithium treatment and prophylaxis in unipolar depression: a meta-analysis. *Br J Psychiatry* 1991; **158**: 666–675.
5. Tondo L, Baldessarini RJ, Floris G. Long term clinical effectiveness of lithium maintenance treatment in types I and II bipolar disorder. *Br J Psychiatry* 2001; **178**(Suppl. 41): 184–190.
6. Geddes JR, Burgess S, Hawton K. Long-term lithium therapy for bipolar disorder: systematic review and meta-analysis of randomised controlled trials. *Am J Psychiatry* 2004; **161**: 217–222.
7. Faedda GL, Baldessarini RJ, Tohen M *et al*. Episode sequence in bipolar disorder and response to lithium treatment. *Am J Psychiatry* 1991; **148**: 1237–1239.
8. Tondo L, Hennen J, Baldessarini RJ. Lower suicide risk with long-term lithium treatment in major affective illness: a meta-analysis. *Acta Psychiatr Scand* 2001; **103**: 163–172.
9. Mander AJ, Loudon JB. Rapid recurrence of mania following abrupt discontinuation of lithium. *Lancet* 1988; **ii**: 15–17.
10. Suppes T, Baldessarini R, Faedda GL *et al*. Risk of recurrence following discontinuation of lithium treatment for bipolar disorder. *Arch Gen Psychiatry* 1991; **48**: 1082–1085.
11. Cavanagh J, Smyth R, Goodwin GM. Relapse into mania or depression following lithium discontinuation: a 7 year follow up. *Acta Psychiatr Scand* 2004; **109**: 91–95.
12. Yazici O, Kora K, Polat A *et al*. Controlled lithium discontinuation in bipolar patients with good response to long-term lithium prophylaxis. *J Affect Disorders* 2004; **80**: 269–271.
13. Goodwin GM. Recurrence of mania after lithium withdrawal. *Br J Psychiatry* 1994; **164**: 149–152.
14. Baldessarini RJ, Tondo L, Faeda GL *et al*. Effects of the rate of discontinuing lithium maintenance treatment in bipolar disorders. *J Clin Psychiatry* 1996; **57**: 441–448.
15. Harris EC, Barraclough B. Excess mortality of mental disorder. *Br J Psychiatry* 1998; **173**: 11–53.
16. Schou M, Mult HC. Forty years of lithium treatment. *Arch Gen Psychiatry* 1997; **54**: 9–13.
17. Stat PR, Frank E, Kostelnik B. Suicide attempts in patients with bipolar 1 disorder during acute and maintenance phases of intensive treatment with pharmacotherapy and adjunctive psychotherapy. *Am J Psychiatry* 2002; **159**: 1160–1164.
18. Jefferson JW. Lithium: the present and the future. *J Clin Psychiatry* 1990; **51**(Suppl.): 4–8.
19. Tyrer SP. Lithium and treatment of aggressive behaviour. *Eur Neuropsychopharm* 1994; **4**: 234–236.
20. Falk WE, Mahnke MW, Poskanzer DC. Lithium prophylaxis with corticotropin-induced psychosis. *JAMA* 1979; **241**: 1011–1012.
21. Peet M, Pratt JP. Lithium. Current status in psychiatric disorder. *Drugs* 1993; **46**: 7–17.
22. Moncrieff J. Lithium: evidence reconsidered. *Br J Psychiatry* 1997; **171**: 113–119.
23. Using lithium safely. *Drug Ther Bull* 1999; **37**: 22–24.
24. *Priadel: Psychiatrist's Handbook*. Delandale Laboratories, 1986.
25. Gelenberg AJ, Kane JM, Keller MB *et al*. Comparison of standard and low serum levels of lithium for maintenance treatment of bipolar disorder. *New Engl J Med* 1989; **21**: 1489–1493.
26. Perlis RH, Sachs GS, Lafer B. Effect of abrupt change from standard to low serum levels of lithium: a re-analysis of double-blind lithium maintenance data. *Am J Psychiatry* 2002; **159**: 1155–1159.

27. Moore CM, Demopulos CM, Henry ME. Brain-to-serum lithium ratio and age: an in vivo magnetic resonance spectroscopy study. *Am J Psychiatry* 2002; **159**: 1240–1242.
28. Bowen RC, Grof P, Grof E. Less frequent lithium administration and lower urine volume. *Am J Psychiatry* 1991; **148**: 189–192.
29. Johnson EM, Eagles JM. Lithium associated clinical hypothyroidism: prevalence and risk factors. *Br J Psychiatry* 1999; **175**: 336–339.
30. Bendz H, Sjodin I, Toss G *et al.* Hyperparathyroidism and long-term lithium therapy – a cross-sectional study and the effect of lithium withdrawal. *J Intern Med* 1996; **240**: 357–365.
31. Muller-Oerlinghausen B. Mental functioning. In: Johnson FN (ed.). *Depression and Mania: Modern Lithium Therapy.* Oxford: IRL Press, 1987, Ch. 68, pp. 246–252.
32. Gitlin M. Lithium and the kidney: an updated review. *Drug Safety* 1999; **20**: 231–243.
33. Tyrer SP. Lithium intoxication: appropriate treatment. *CNS Drugs* 1996; **6**: 426–439.
34. Reimann IW, Diener U, Frolich C. Indomethacin but not aspirin increases plasma lithium ion levels. *Arch Gen Psychiatry* 1983; **40**: 283–286.
35. Nicholson J, Fitzmaurice B. Monitoring patients on lithium – a good practice guideline. *Psychiatr Bull* 2002; **26**: 348–351.
36. Phelan KM, Mosholder AD, Lu S. Lithium interaction with the cyclooxygenase 2 inhibitors rofecoxib and celecoxib and other nonsteroidal anti-inflammatory drugs. *J Clin Psychiatry* 2003; **64**: 1328–1334.
37. Slordal L, Samstad S, Bathen J *et al.* A life-threatening interaction between lithium and celecoxib. *Br J Clin Pharmacol* 2003; **55**: 413–414.
38. Cohen WJ, Cohen NH. Lithium carbonate, haloperidol and irreversible brain damage. *JAMA* 1974; **230**: 1283–1287.
39. Goldney RD, Spence ND. Safety of the combination of lithium and neuroleptic drugs. *Am J Psychiatry* 1996; **143**: 882–884.
40. Freeman MP, Stoll AL. Mood stabiliser combinations: a review of efficacy and safety. *Am J Psychiatry* 1998; **155**: 12–22.
41. Hawley CJ, Loughlin PJ, Quick SJ *et al.* Efficacy, safety and tolerability of combined administration of lithium and selective serotonin reuptake inhibitors: a review of the current evidence. *Int Clin Psychopharmacol* 2000; **15**: 197–206.
42. Zwanger P, Marcuse A, Boerner RJ. Lithium intoxication after administration of AT$_1$ blockers. *J Clin Psychiatry* 2001; **62**: 208–209.

Further reading

Schou M. Lithium prophylaxis: myths and realities. *Am J Psychiatry* 1989; **146**: 573–576.
Various. Lithium in the treatment of manic-depressive illness: an update. Proceedings of a meeting. *J Clin Psychiatry* 1998; **59**(Suppl. 6).
Young AH. Treatment of bipolar affective disorder. *BMJ* 2000; **321**: 1302–1303.

Carbamazepine

Carbamazepine is primarily used as an anticonvulsant in the treatment of grand mal and focal seizures. It is also used in the management of trigeminal neuralgia and, in the UK, is licensed for the prophylaxis of bipolar illness in patients who do not respond to lithium. Carbamazepine monotherapy is effective in acute mania[1], with open studies showing a response rate of 50–60%[2]. It is probably as effective as lithium[3] (direct comparative studies have not been powered to detect a difference[4]). Carbamazepine also appears to usefully augment the effects of antipsychotics in acute mania[5].

Open studies also suggest that monotherapy is effective in bipolar depression[6]: carbamazepine has a similar molecular structure to TCAs, but without possessing their ability to induce mania in bipolar depression. Carbamazepine may also usefully augment antidepressants or other mood-stabilisers in refractory unipolar depression[7,8]. Although carbamazepine is generally considered to be as effective as lithium in the prophylaxis of bipolar illness[9], several published studies report a very low response rate and high drop-out rate[3,10]. A recent blinded, randomised trial of lithium versus carbamazepine found lithium to be the superior prophylactic agent[11]. Most of the lithium treatment failures occurred in the first 3 months of treatment whereas relapses on carbamazepine occurred at a rate of 40% per year.

It is 'perceived wisdom' that carbamazepine is more effective than lithium in rapid-cycling illness (four or more episodes/year). Although some evidence supports this view[12], negative studies have also been published[13].

There are also reports of carbamazepine being successful in treating aggressive behaviour in patients with schizophrenia[14]. This is apparently not a result of its anticonvulsant effect, as patients with normal EEGs may respond. A trial of carbamazepine is often thought worthwhile, as a last resort, in various psychiatric illnesses (such as panic disorder, borderline personality disorder and episodic dyscontrol syndrome) where no other drug is specifically indicated. The literature consists primarily of case reports and open case series. Carbamazepine is also used in the management of alcohol withdrawal symptoms[15], although the high doses required initially are often poorly tolerated.

Plasma levels

When carbamazepine is used as an anticonvulsant the therapeutic range is stated as being 4–12 mg/l, although the supporting evidence is not strong. A dose of at least 600 mg/day and a serum level of at least 7 mg/l seem to be required in affective illness[16], although some studies do not support this view[17].

Carbamazepine serum levels vary significantly within a dosage interval. It is important to sample at a point in time where levels are likely to be reproducible for any given individual. The most appropriate way of monitoring is to take a trough level before the first dose of the day. Carbamazepine is an hepatic-enzyme inducer that induces its own metabolism as well as that of other drugs. An initial plasma half-life of around 30 hours is reduced to around 12 hours on chronic dosing. For this reason, plasma levels should be checked 2–4 weeks after an increase in dose to ensure that the desired level is still being obtained.

The published clinical trials that demonstrate the efficacy of carbamazepine as a mood-stabiliser used doses that are significantly higher (usually in the order of 800–1200 mg/day) than those prescribed in everyday UK clinical practice[18].

Adverse effects

The main problems encountered with carbamazepine therapy are dizziness, drowsiness, ataxia and nausea. They can be largely avoided by starting with a low dose and increasing it slowly. Around 3% of patients treated with carbamazepine develop a generalised erythematous rash. Serious dermatological reactions can rarely occur (e.g. toxic epidermal necrolysis). Hyponatraemia can also be a problem.

Carbamazepine can induce a chronic low white blood cell (WBC) count. Many patients treated with carbamazepine have a WBC count at the lower end of the normal range, which rises on discontinuing treatment. One patient in 20,000 develops agranulocytosis and/or aplastic anaemia[19]. Raised ALP and GGT are, potentially, a sign of a hypersensitivity reaction to carbamazepine (a GGT of up to twice normal is common and should not cause concern). Normally, it would be recommended that therapy should be withdrawn, as this can progress to a multi-system hypersensitivity reaction (mainly manifesting itself as various skin reactions and a low WBC count, along with raised ALP and GGT), which can in turn lead to hepatitis. Fatalities have been reported. There is no clear timescale for these events, so it must not be assumed that raised LFTs for 6 months with no other clinical complications will not produce problems in the future. FBC and LFTs should be monitored in patients on long-term therapy.

Interactions with other drugs[20–22]

Carbamazepine is a potent inducer of hepatic cytochrome P450 enzymes and is metabolised by CYP3A4. Plasma levels of most **antidepressants**, most **antipsychotics**, **benzodiazepines**, some **cholinesterase inhibitors**, **methadone**, **thyroxine**, **theophylline**, **oestrogens**[23] and other steroids may be reduced by carbamazepine, resulting in treatment failure. Drugs that inhibit CYP3A4 will increase carbamazepine plasma levels and may precipitate toxicity. Examples include cimetidine, diltiazem, verapamil, dextropropoxyphene, erythromycin and SSRIs.

Pharmacodynamic interactions also occur. The anticonvulsant activity of carbamazepine is reduced by drugs that lower the seizure threshold (e.g. antipsychotics and antidepressants), the potential for carbamazepine to cause neutropenia may be increased by other drugs that have the potential to depress the bone marrow (e.g. clozapine), and the risk of hyponatraemia may be increased by other drugs that can deplete sodium (e.g. diuretics). Neurotoxicity has been reported with lithium and carbamazepine combinations[24]. This is rare. There are many complex interactions with other anticonvulsant drugs. The latest edition of the *BNF* should be checked before prescribing anticonvulsant polypharmacy (see also page 263).

As carbamazepine is structurally similar to the TCAs, in theory it should not be given within 14 days of discontinuing a MAOI. Most side-effects of carbamazepine are dose-related (peak plasma level-related), and increase in frequency and severity when the plasma level is >12 mg/l (this varies substantially from patient to patient). Side-effects can be minimised by using the slow-release preparation.

References

1. Vasudev K, Goswami U, Kohli K. Carbamazepine and valproate monotherapy: feasibility, relative safety and efficacy, and therapeutic drug monitoring in manic disorder. *Psychopharmacology* 2000; **150**: 15–23.
2. Chou JC-Y. Recent advances in treatment of acute mania. *J Clin Psychopharm* 1991; **11**: 3–21.
3. Keck PE, McElroy SL, Strakowski SM. Anticonvulsants and antipsychotics in the treatment of bipolar disorder. *J Clin Psychiatry* 1998; **59**(Suppl. 6): 74–81.
4. Small JG, Klapper MH, Milstein V. Carbamazepine compared with lithium in the treatment of mania. *Arch Gen Psychiatry* 1991; **48**: 915–921.
5. Klein E, Bental E, Lerer B. Carbamazepine and haloperidol vs placebo and haloperidol in excited psychoses. *Arch Gen Psychiatry* 1984; **48**: 915–921.
6. Dilsaver SC, Swann SC, Chen YW *et al.* Treatment of bipolar depression with carbamazepine: results of an open study. *Biol Psychiatry* 1996; **40**: 935–937.
7. Cullen M, Mitchell P, Brodaty H. Carbamazepine for treatment-resistant melancholia. *J Clin Psychiatry* 1991; **52**: 472–476.
8. Kramlinger KG, Post RM. The addition of lithium to carbamazepine. antidepressant efficacy in treatment resistant depression. *Arch Gen Psychiatry* 1989; **46**: 794–800.
9. Davis JM, Janicak PG, Hogan DM. Mood stabilisers in the prevention of recurrent affective disorders: a meta-analysis. *Acta Psychiatr Scand* 1999; **100**: 406–417.
10. Post RM, Leverich GS, Rosoff AS. Carbamazepine prophylaxis in refractory affective disorders: a focus on long-term follow-up. *J Clin Psychopharm* 1990; **10**: 318–327.
11. Erwin G, Harlong M, Moleman P *et al.* Prophylactic efficacy of lithium versus carbamazepine in treatment-naive bipolar patients. *J Clin Psychiatry* 2003; **64**: 144–151.
12. Joyce PR. Carbamazepine in rapid cycling bipolar affective disorder. *Int Clin Psychopharmacol* 1988; **3**: 123–129.
13. Okuma T. Effects of carbamazepine and lithium on affective disorders. *Neuropsychobiology* 1993; **27**: 138–145.
14. Brieden T, Ujeyl M, Naber D. Psychopharmacological treatment of aggression in schizophrenic patients. *Pharmacopsychiatry* 2002; **35**: 83–89.
15. Malcolm R, Myrick H, Roberts J. The effects of carbamazepine and lorazepam on single versus multiple previous alcohol withdrawals in an outpatient randomised trial. *J Gen Intern Med* 2002; **17**: 349–355.
16. Taylor D, Duncan D. Doses of carbamazepine and valproate in bipolar affective disorder. *Psychiatr Bull* 1997; **21**: 221–223.
17. Simhandl C, Denk E, Thau K. The comparative efficacy of carbamazepine low and high serum level and lithium carbonate in the prophylaxis of affective disorders. *J Affect Disorders* 1993; **28**: 221–231.
18. Taylor DM, Starkey K, Ginaiy S. Prescribing and monitoring of carbamazepine and valproate – a case note review. *Psychiatr Bull* 2000; **24**: 174–177.
19. Kaufman DW, Kelly JP, Jurgelon JM. Drugs in the aetiology of agranulocytosis and aplastic anaemia. *Eur J Haematol* 1996; **60**(Suppl.): 23–30.
20. Spina E, Perucca E. Clinical significance of pharmacokinetic interactions between antiepileptic and psychotropic drugs. *Epilepsia* 2002; **43**: 37–44.
21. Patsalos PN, Froscher W, Pisani F *et al.* The importance of drug interactions in epilepsy therapy. *Epilepsia* 2002; **43**: 365–385.
22. Ketler TA, Post RM, Worthington K. Principles of clinically important drug interactions with carbamazepine. I. *J Clin Psychopharm* 1991; **11**: 198–203.
23. Crawford P. Interactions between antiepileptic drugs and hormonal contraception. *CNS Drugs* 2002; **16**: 263–272.
24. Shula S, Godwin CD, Long LEB. Lithium–carbamazepine neurotoxicity and risk factors. *Am J Psychiatry* 1984; **141**: 1604–1606.

Bipolar disorder

Table   Mood stabilisers – brief details

Drug	Dose	Precautions
Lithium	Start on low (400 mg/day) dose Plasma levels to be monitored every 5–7 days until level is 0.6–1.0 mmol/l Once level is stable, check levels every 3–6 months or if drug interaction is suspected All samples must be taken 12 hours postdose	**Renal function** U&Es before commencing lithium. Excreted through kidney exclusively and potentially nephrotoxic. Change in body salt concentration can affect levels Significant proportion develop **hypothyroidism**: TFT before starting and at 6-monthly intervals. Treat with thyroxine Patients on long-term treatment should have calcium checked annually
Carbamazepine	Usual starting dose 200 mg b.d., slowly increased until dose 600–1000 mg/day is achieved. MR preparation possibly better tolerated Target range 8–12 mg/l Sample at trough Induces own metabolism: monitor every 2–4 weeks until stable and then every 3–6 months	Early **leucopenia** usually transient and benign but later falls in white cells may be serious. Warn patient about fever, infections, etc. Need baseline and regular FBCs every 2 weeks for first 2 months, and then every 3–6 months Carbamazepine **toxicity**: severe diplopia, nausea, ataxia, sedation
Valproate	Commence on 500 mg MR daily (Epilim) or 250 mg t.d.s. (Depakote), then increase until plasma levels reach 50–100 mg/l Trough samples required MR preparation may be given once daily, Depakote twice or three times daily	Check renal and hepatic function at baseline, then 6-monthly Full blood count at baseline, then 6-monthly
Lamotrigine	Dose as mood-stabiliser not certain, likely to be similar to that used in epilepsy (50–200 mg/day) As dose depends on concomitant medication, see manufacturer's information	Monitor patient for **rash** – more likely to occur in children, with concomitant valproate or if dose started too high or increased too quickly. Most rashes occur within 8 weeks of starting therapy
Topiramate	Dose not yet clear, but suggest starting at 25 mg a day and increasing weekly by 25 mg to a maximum of 200 mg/day Slow rate of increase if adverse effects troublesome	Monitor for signs **of visual disturbance** (stop topiramate immediately and refer) and **cognitive decline** (slow rate of dose increase)

Contraindications	Side-effects	Drug interactions
Pregnancy (see page 276–282) **Breast-feeding**: avoid (see page 276–282) **Renal impairment** (may be given if close monitoring practicable) Thyroidopathies Sick sinus syndrome	Thirst, polyuria GI upset Tremor (may treat with propranolol) Diabetes insipidus – may inhibit ADH (must maintain fluid intake) Acne Muscular weakness Cardiac arrhythmia Weight gain common (?related to thirst and intake of high-calorie drinks) Hypothyroidism Hyperthyroidism	**Antipsychotics** – all antipsychotics may increase lithium's neurotoxicity but this is rarely observed in practice **Diltiazem/verapamil** may also rarely be linked to neurotoxicity **Diuretics** (thiazides): increase lithium concentration **ACE inhibitors**: toxicity **NSAIDs** all cause toxicity except aspirin and sulindac Low-dose ibuprofen usually safe **COX 2** inhibitors can also cause toxicity **Alcohol** increases peak lithium concentration **Xanthines** increase lithium excretion **NaCl** increases lithium excretion
Pregnancy (see page 276–282) Breast-feeding (see page 276–282)	Drowsiness, ataxia, diplopia, nausea Agranulocytosis – 1 in 20,000 Aplastic anaemia – 1 in 20,000 Transient leucopenia in about 10% in first 2 months Hypersensitivity – hepatitis SIADH Rashes may be serious Toxic epidermal necrolysis in 1 in 20,000; monitor carefully throughout treatment; ask patient to report immediately any rash accompanied by fever/malaise	**Antipsychotics**: may add to CNS effects (drowsiness, ataxia, etc.) **Lithium:** CNS effects and increased risk of side-effects of both drugs **Ca^{++} channel blockers**: CNS effects **MAOIs** need 2 weeks washout ?Toxicity with **flu vaccine** Enzyme inducer affects many other drugs, including **phenytoin** and oral contraceptives. Also decreases **tricyclic and antipsychotic** plasma levels. See page 263
Pregnancy (see page 276–282) Breast-feeding (see page 276–282) Hepatic disease	*Commonly:* Nausea, vomiting and mild sedation Moderate weight gain Hair loss *Rarely:* Ataxia and headache Thrombocytopenia and platelet dysfunction Pancytopenia Pancreatitis	Complex interactions with other **anticonvulsants**: need to consult neurologist (see also page 263) Potentiates activity of **aspirin** and **warfarin** May increase **MAOI** and **TCA** levels Increases **lamotrigine** levels
Pregnancy (see page 276–282) Hepatic impairment	Rash, ataxia, diplopia, headache, vomiting	**Valproate** increases levels of lamotrigine Lamotrigine may increase levels of the active **carbamazepine epoxide metabolite**
Pregnancy – consult drug information services Breast-feeding	Nausea, weight loss, abdominal pain More rarely, confusion, impaired concentration, memory impairment, emotional lability, ataxia	Additive CNS effects with other anticonvulsants May increase levels of phenytoin

121

Treatment of acute mania or hypomania

Drug choice in mania and hypomania is made difficult by the dearth of robust comparative data relating to drug combinations – the most common therapeutic intervention. Studies have shown clear efficacy for many single drugs compared with placebo but studies comparing single drugs with combinations have methodological problems. There are few studies comparing different combinations.

The tables below outline treatments and a treatment strategy for mania and hypomania. These recommendations are based on individual studies cited, two excellent reviews[1,2] and NICE guidance on olanzapine and valproate semisodium[3].

Step	Suggested treatment	References
Step 1	**De novo mania or hypomania (no prior diagnosis of bipolar disorder)**	1–12
	Start antipsychotic (e.g. olanzapine, risperidone, quetiapine, conventionals)	
	Hypomania in a patient not receiving mood stabilisers	
	Start valproate* (1st choice) Or lithium* Or carbamazepine*	
	Mania or mixed episodes	
	Start or optimise mood stabiliser** and Start antipsychotic	
	All patients withdraw antidepressants	
Step 2	**Add benzodiazepine**	1, 2, 13–15
	Suggest:	
	lorazepam up to 4 mg/day or clonazepam up to 2 mg/day	
	Note – many centres use higher doses of benzodiazepines in mania.	
Step 3	Consider other antimanic agents and strategies – see table below.	

*Suggested starting doses:

- lithium 400 mg MR daily
- carbamazepine 200 mg MR twice daily
- valproate   Epilim Chrono 500 mg daily
              or
              Depakote 250 mg three times daily

Oral 'loading' with 20–30 mg/kg per day valproate semisodium is also possible and may have a rapid onset of action[16–18]. Intravenous 'loading' has also been attempted[19].

** Use of plasma concentration monitoring to optimise dose is strongly recommended[1,2,20].

Note that lithium may be less effective in mixed states[21] or where there is substance misuse[22].

Other treatments

Alphabetical order – no preference implied by order in the table

Consult specialist and primary literature before using any treatment listed below.

Treatment	Comments
Aripiprazole[23,24] 15–30 mg/day	Strong support for antimanic effect from several placebo-controlled trials. May be considered at Step 1. Not licensed for mania in UK.
Clozapine[25,26]	Established treatment option for refractory mania.
Gabapentin[27–29] (up to 2.4 G/day)	Probably only effective by virtue of an anxiolytic effect. Rarely used.
Lamotrigine[30,31] (up to 200 mg/day)	Possibly effective but better efficacy in bipolar depression.
Levetiracetam[32,33] (up to 4000 mg/day)	Possibly effective but controlled studies required.
Oxcarbazepine[34–36] (around 1000 mg/day)	Possibly effective but controlled studies required.
Phenytoin[37] (300–400 mg/day)	Rarely used. Limited data.
Ritanserin[38] (10 mg/day)	Supported by a single randomised, controlled trial. Well tolerated. May protect against EPSEs.
Topiramate[39–42] (up to 300 mg/day)	Possibly effective, even in refractory mania. Causes weight loss.
Ziprasidone[43]	Supported by a randomised, placebo-controlled study.

References

1. Goodwin GM, Young AH. The British Association for Psychopharmacology guidelines for treatment of bipolar disorder: a summary. *J Psychopharmacol* 2003; **17**: 3–6.
2. American Psychiatric Association. Practice guideline for the treatment of patients with bipolar disorder. *Am J Psychiatry* 2002; **159**(Suppl.): 1–50.
3. National Institute for Clinical Excellence. Olanzapine and valproate semisodium in the treatment of acute mania associated with bipolar disorder I disorder. Technology Appraisal 66, 2003.
4. Sachs GS. Decision tree for the treatment of bipolar disorder. *J Clin Psychiatry* 2003; **64**: 35–40.
5. Tohen M, Goldberg JF, Gonzalez-Pinto Arrillaga AM *et al.* A 12-week, double-blind comparison of olanzapine vs haloperidol in the treatment of acute mania. *Arch Gen Psychiatry* 2003; **60**: 1218–1226.
6. Baldessarini RJ, Hennen J, Wilson M *et al.* Olanzapine versus placebo in acute mania treatment responses in subgroups. *J Clin Psychopharm* 2003; **23**: 370–376.
7. Applebaum J, Levine J, Belmaker RH. Intravenous fosphenytoin in acute mania. *J Clin Psychiatry* 2003; **64**: 408–409.
8. Sachs G, Chengappa KNR, Suppes T *et al.* Quetiapine with lithium or divalproex for the treatment of bipolar mania: a randomized, double-blind, placebo-controlled study. *Bipolar Disord* 2004; **6**: 213–223.
9. Yatham LN, Paulsson B, Mullen J *et al.* Quetiapine versus placebo in combination with lithium or divalproex for the treatment of bipolar mania. *J Clin Psychopharm* 2004; **24**: 599–606.
10. Yatham LN, Binder C, Kusumakar V *et al.* Risperidone plus lithium versus risperidone plus valproate in acute and continuation treatment of mania. *Int Clin Psychopharmacol* 2004; **19**: 103–109.
11. Bowden CL, Myers JE, Grossman F, Xie Y. Risperidone in combination with mood stabilizers: a 10-week continuation phase study in bipolar 1 disorder. *J Clin Psychiatry* 2004; **65**: 707–714.
12. Hirschfeld RMA, Keck PE Jr, Kramer M *et al.* Rapid antimanic effect of risperidone monotherapy: a 3-week multicenter, double-blind, placebo-controlled trial. *Am J Psychiatry* 2004; **161**: 1057–1065.
13. Sachs GS, Rosenbaum JF, Jones J. Adjunctive clonazepam for maintenance treatment of bipolar affective disorder. *J Clin Psychopharm* 1990; **10**: 42–47.

Bipolar disorder

14. Modell JG, Lenox RH, Weiner S. Inpatient clinical trial of lorazepam for the management of manic agitation. *J Clin Psychopharm* 1985; **5**: 109–113.
15. Curtin F, Schulz P. Clonazepam and lorazepam in acute mania: a Bayesian meta-analysis. *J Affect Disorders* 2004; **78**: 201–208.
16. McElroy SL, Keck PE, Stanton SP *et al.* A randomized comparison of divalproex oral loading versus haloperidol in the initial treatment of acute psychotic mania. *J Clin Psychiatry* 1996; **57**: 142–146.
17. Hirschfeld RMA, Allen MH, McEvoy JP *et al.* Safety and tolerability of oral loading divalproex sodium in acutely manic bipolar patients. *J Clin Psychiatry* 1999; **60**: 815–818.
18. Hirschfeld RMA, Baker JD, Wozniak P *et al.* The safety and early efficacy of oral-loaded divalproex versus standard-titration divalproex, lithium, olanzapine, and placebo in the treatment of acute mania associated with bipolar disorder. *J Clin Psychiatry* 2003; **64**: 841–846.
19. Jagadhessan K, Duggal HS, Candra Gupta S *et al.* Acute antimanic efficacy and safety of intravenous valproate loading therapy: an open-label study. *Neuropsychobiology* 2003; **47**: 90–93.
20. Taylor DM, Duncan D. Doses of carbamazepine and valproate in bipolar affective disorder. *Psychiatr Bull* 1997; **21**: 221–223.
21. Swann AC, Secunda SK, Katz MM *et al.* Lithium treatment of mania: clinical characteristics, specificity of symptom change, and outcome. *Psychiatry Res* 1986; **18**: 127–141.
22. Goldberg JF, Garnò JL, Leon AC *et al.* A history of substance abuse complicates remission from acute mania in bipolar disorder. *J Clin Psychiatry* 1999; **60**: 733–740.
23. Lyseng-Williamson KA, Perry CM. Aripiprazole in acute mania associated with bipolar 1 disorder. *CNS Drugs* 2004; **18**: 367–376.
24. Keck PE, Marcus R, Tourkodimiris S *et al.* A placebo-controlled, double-blind study of the efficacy and safety of aripiprazole in patients with acute bipolar mania. *Am J Psychiatry* 2003; **160**: 1651–1658.
25. Mahmood T, Devlin M, Silverstone T. Clozapine in the management of bipolar and schizoaffective manic episodes resistant to standard treatment. *Aust NZ J Psychiatry* 1997; **31**: 424–426.
26. Green AI, Tohen M, Patel JK *et al.* Clozapine in the treatment of refractory psychotic mania. *Am J Psychiatry* 2000; **157**: 982–986.
27. Macdonald KJ, Young LT. Newer antiepileptic drugs in bipolar disorder. *CNS Drugs* 2002; **16**: 549–562.
28. Cabras PL, Hardoy MJ, Hardoy MC *et al.* Clinical experience with gabapentin in patients with bipolar or schizoaffective disorder: results of an open-label study. *J Clin Psychiatry* 1999; **60**: 245–248.
29. Pande AC, Crockatt JG, Janney CA *et al.* Gabapentin in bipolar disorder: a placebo-controlled trial of adjunctive therapy. *Bipolar Disord* 2000; **2**(3 Pt 2): 249–255.
30. Calabrese JR, Bowden CL, McElroy SL *et al.* Spectrum of activity of lamotrigine in treatment-refractory bipolar disorder. *Am J Psychiatry* 1999; **156**: 1019–1023.
31. Bowden CL, Calabrese JR, Sachs G *et al.* A placebo-controlled 18 month trial of lamotrigine and lithium maintenance treatment in recently manic or hypomanic patients with bipolar 1 disorder. *Arch Gen Psychiatry* 2003; **60**: 392–400.
32. Grunze H, Langosch J, Born C *et al.* Levetiracetam in the treatment of acute mania: an open add-on study with an on-off-on design. *J Clin Psychiatry* 2003; **64**: 781–784.
33. Goldberg JF, Burdick KE. Levetiracetam for acute mania (Letter). *Am J Psychiat* 2002; **159**: 148.
34. Benedetti A, Lattanzi L, Pini S *et al.* Oxcarbazepine as add-on treatment in patients with bipolar manic, mixed or depressive episode. *J Affect Disorders* 2004; **79**: 273–277.
35. Lande RG. Oxcarbazepine: efficacy, safety, and tolerability in the treatment of mania. *Int J Psychiatry Prac Clin* 2004; **8**: 37–40.
36. Ghaemi SN, Berv DA, Klugman J *et al.* Oxcarbazepine treatment of bipolar disorder. *J Clin Psychiatry* 2003; **64**: 943–945.
37. Mishory A, Yaroslavsky Y, Bersudsky Y *et al.* Phenytoin as an antimanic anticonvulsant: a controlled study. *Am J Psychiatry* 2000; **157**: 463–465.
38. Akhondzadeh S, Mohajari H, Mohammadi MR *et al.* Ritanserin as an adjunct to lithium and haloperidol for the treatment of medication-naive patients with acute mania: a double blind and placebo controlled trial. *BMC Psychiatry* 2003; **3**: 1–7.
39. Grunze HCR, Normann C, Langosch J *et al.* Antimanic efficacy of topiramate in 11 patients in an open trial with an on-off-on design. *J Clin Psychiatry* 2001; **62**: 464–468.
40. Lakshmi NY, Kuusmakar V, Calabrese JR *et al.* Third generation anticonvulsants in bipolar disorder: a review of efficacy and summary of clinical recommendations. *J Clin Psychiatry* 2002; **63**: 275–283.
41. Vieta E, Goikolea JM, Pinto AG *et al.* 1-year follw up of patients treated with risperidone and topiramate for a manic episode. *J Clin Psychiatry* 2003; **64**: 834–839.
42. Vieta E, Torrent C, Garcia-Ribas G *et al.* Use of topiramate in treatment-resistant bipolar spectrum disorders. *J Clin Psychopharm* 2002; **22**: 431–435.
43. Keck PE Jr, Versiani M, Potkin S *et al.* Ziprasidone in the treatment of acute bipolar mania: a three-week, placebo-controlled, double-blind, randomized trial. *Am J Psychiatry* 2003; **160**: 741–748.

Further reading

Joffe RT, Macqueen GM, Marriott M *et al.* Induction of mania and cycle acceleration in bipolar disorder: effect of different classes of antidepressant. *Acta Psychiatr Scand* 2002; **105**: 427–430.

Table   Drugs for acute mania – relative costs (January 2005)

Drug	Cost for 30 days' treatment	Comments
Lithium (Priadel) 800 mg/day	£2.95	Add cost of plasma level monitoring
Carbamazepine (Tegretol Retard) 800 mg/day	£11.08	Self-induction complicates acute treatment
Sodium valproate (Epilim Chrono) 1500 mg/day	£18.19	Not licensed for mania, but may be given once daily
Valproate semisodium (Depakote) 1500 mg/day	£72.19	Licensed for mania, but given two or three times daily
Haloperidol (Serenace) 10 mg/day	£8.81	Most widely used typical antipsychotic
Olanzapine (Zyprexa) 15 mg/day	£127.69	Most widely used atypical
Quetiapine (Seroquel) 600 mg/day	£170.00	
Risperidone (Risperidal) 4 mg/day	£68.69	Non-sedative but effective

Bipolar disorder

Antipsychotics in bipolar disorder

Typical antipsychotics have long been used in mania and several studies support their use in a variety of hypomanic and manic presentations[1–3]. Their effectiveness seems to be enhanced by the addition of a mood stabiliser[4,5]. In the longer-term treatment of bipolar disorder, typicals are widely used (presumably as prophylaxis)[6] but robust supporting data are absent[7]. The observation that typical antipsychotics may induce depression and tardive dyskinesia in bipolar patients militates against their long-term use[7–9].

Among atypical antipsychotics, olanzapine, risperidone and quetiapine have been most robustly evaluated and are licensed in the UK for the treatment of mania. Olanzapine is probably most widely used. It is more effective than placebo in mania[10,11], and at least as effective as valproate semi-sodium[12] and lithium[13]. As with typical drugs, olanzapine may be most effective when used in combination with a mood-stabiliser[14,15]. Data suggest olanzapine may offer benefits in longer-term treatment[16,17] and it is formally licensed as prophylaxis.

Clozapine seems to be effective in refractory bipolar conditions, including refractory mania[18–20]. Risperidone has shown efficacy in mania[21], particularly in combination with a mood-stabiliser[2,22]. Data relating to quetiapine[23–25] are compelling but those relating to amisulpride[26] are scarce.

References

1. Prien R, Point P, Caffey E et al. Comparison of lithium carbonate and chlorpromazine in the treatment of mania. *Arch Gen Psychiatry* 1972; **26**: 146–153.
2. Sachs G, Grossman F, Nassir G et al. Combination of a mood stabilizer with risperidone or haloperidol for treatment of acute mania: a double-blind, placebo-controlled comparison of efficacy and safety. *Am J Psychiatry* 2002; **159**: 1146–1154.
3. McElroy S, Keck P, Stanton S et al. A randomized comparison of divalproex oral loading versus haloperidol in the initial treatment of acute psychotic mania. *J Clin Psychiatry* 1996; 57: 142–146.
4. Chou J, Czobor P, Owen C et al. Acute mania: haloperidol dose and augmentation with lithium or lorazepam. *J Clin Psychopharm* 1999; **19**: 500–505.
5. Small JG, Kellams JJ, Milstein V et al. A placebo-controlled study of lithium combined with neuroleptics in chronic schizophrenia patients. *Am J Psychiatry* 1975; **132**: 1315–1317.
6. Soares J, Barwell M, Mallinger A et al. Adjunctive antipsychotic use in bipolar patients: an open 6-month prospective study following an acute episode. *J Affect Disorders* 1998; **56**: 1–8.
7. Keck P, McElroy S, Strakowski S. Anticonvulsants and antipsychotics in the treatment of bipolar disorder. *J Clin Psychiatry* 1998; **59**(Suppl. 6): 74–81.
8. Tohen M, Zarate C. Antipsychotic agents and bipolar disorder. *J Clin Psychiatry* 1998; **59**(Suppl. 1): 38–49.
9. Zarate CA, Tohen M. Double-blind comparison of the continued use of antipsychotic treatment versus its discontinuation in remitted manic patients. *Am J Psychiatry* 2004; **161**: 169–171.
10. Tohen M, Sanger T, Mcelroy S et al. Olanzapine versus placebo in the treatment of acute mania. *Am J Psychiatry* 1999; **156**: 702–709.
11. Tohen M, Jacobs T, Grundy S et al. Efficacy of olanzapine in acute bipolar mania. *Arch Gen Psychiatry* 2000; 57: 841–849.
12. Tohen M, Barker R, Altshuler L et al. Olanzapine versus divalproex in the treatment of acute mania. *Am J Psychiatry* 2002; **159**: 1011–1017.
13. Berk M, Ichim I, Brook S. Olanzapine compared to lithium in mania: a double-blind randomised controlled trial. *Int Clin Psychopharm* 1999; **13**: 339–343.
14. Tohen M, Chengappa R, Suppes T et al. Efficacy of olanzapine in combination with valproate or lithium in the treatment of mania in patients partially nonresponsive to valproate or lithium monotherapy. *Arch Gen Psychiatry* 2002; **69**: 62–69.
15. Tohen M, Chengappa KNR, Suppes T et al. Relapse prevention in bipolar 1 disorder: 18-month comparison of olanzapine plus mood stabiliser vs mood stabiliser alone. *Br J Psychiatry* 2004; **184**: 337–345.
16. Sanger T, Grundy S, Gibson J et al. Long-term olanzapine therapy in the treatment of bipolar I disorder: an open-label continuation phase study. *J Clin Psychiatry* 2001; **62**: 273–280.
17. Vieta E, Reinares M, Corbella B et al. Olanzapine as long-term adjunctive therapy in treatment-resistant bipolar disorder. *J Clin Psychopharm* 2001; **21**: 469–473.
18. Calabrese J, Kimmel S, Woyshville MJ et al. Clozapine for treatment-refractory mania. *Am J Psychiatry* 1996; **153**: 759–764.
19. Green A, Tohen M, Patel J et al. Clozapine in the treatment of refractory psychotic mania. *Am J Psychiatry* 2000; **157**: 982–986.

20. Calabrese J, Kimmel S, Woyshville MJ *et al.* Clozapine in treatment-refractory mood disorders. *J Clin Psychiatry* 1994; **55**: 91–93.
21. Segal J, Berk M, Brook S. Risperidone compared with both lithium and haloperidol in mania: a double-blind randomised controlled trial. *Clin Neuropharmacol* 1998; **21**: 176–180.
22. Vieta E, Herraiz M, Parramon G *et al.* Risperidone in the treatment of mania: efficacy and safety results from a large multicentre, open study in Spain. *J Affect Disorders* 2002; **72**: 15–19.
23. Ghaemi N, Katzow J. The use of quetiapine for treatment-resistant bipolar disorder: a case series. *Ann Clin Psychiatry* 1999; **11**: 137–140.
24. Sachs G, Mullen JA, Devine NA *et al.* Quetiapine versus placebo as adjunct to mood stabilizer for the treatment of acute bipolar mania. Presented at the 15th Congress of the European College of Neuropsychopharmacology, 5–9 October 2002, Barcelona, Spain.
25. Altamura AC, Salvadori D, Madaro D *et al.* Efficacy and tolerability of quetiapine in the treatment of bipolar disorder: preliminary evidence from a 12-month open label study. *J Affect Disorders* 2003; **76**: 267–271.
26. Pariante C, Orru M, Carpinello B *et al.* Multiple sclerosis and major depression resistant to treatment. Case of a patient with antidepressive therapy induced mood disorder associated with manic features (Italian). *Clin Ther* 1995; **146**: 449–452.

Bipolar disorder

Bipolar depression

Bipolar depression is a common and debilitating disorder which differs from unipolar disorder in severity, timecourse, recurrence and response to drug treatment. Episodes of bipolar depression are, compared with unipolar depression, more rapid in onset, more severe, shorter and more likely to involve reverse neurovegetative symptoms such as hyperphagia and hypersomnia[1]. Around 15% of people with bipolar disorder commit suicide[2], a statistic which aptly reflects the severity and frequency of depressive episodes. Bipolar depression entails greater socio-economic burden than both mania and unipolar depression[3].

The drug treatment of bipolar depression is somewhat controversial for two reasons. First, there is a dearth of well-conducted, randomised, controlled trials reported in the literature and second, the condition entails consideration of lifelong outcome rather than discrete episode response[4]. We have some knowledge of the therapeutic effects of drugs in depressive episodes but more limited awareness of the therapeutic or deleterious effects of drugs in the longer term. The tables below give some broad guidance on treatment options in bipolar depression.

Table　Established treatments	
Drug/regime	**Comments**
Lithium[1,5–8]	Lithium is probably effective in treating bipolar depression but supporting data are confounded by cross-over designs incorporating abrupt switching to placebo. There is some evidence that lithium prevents depressive relapse but its effects on manic relapse are considered more robust. Fairly strong support for lithium in reducing suicidality in bipolar disorder.
Lithium and antidepressant[9–16]	Antidepressants are widely used in bipolar depression, particularly for breakthrough episodes occurring in those on mood stabilisers. They appear to be effective, although there is a risk of cycle acceleration and/or switching. Tricyclics and MAOIs are usually avoided. SSRIs are generally recommended. Venlafaxine and bupropion (amfebutamone) have also been used. There is limited evidence that antidepressants are effective only when lithium plasma levels are below 0.8 mmol/l. Continuing antidepressant treatment after resolution of symptoms may protect against depressive relapse, although this is controversial.
Lamotrigine[1,6,17–20]	Lamotrigine appears to be effective both as a treatment for bipolar depression and as prophylaxis against further episodes. It does not induce switching or rapid cycling. Note that, at the time of writing, published and unpublished data combined are insufficient to support the formal licensing of lamotrigine in bipolar depression. Treatment is complicated by the risk of rash, which is associated with speed of dose titration. The necessity for titration may limit clinical utility. A further complication is the question of dose: 50 mg/day has efficacy, but 200 mg/day is probably better. In the USA doses of up to 1200 mg/day have been used (mean around 250 mg/day).
Olanzapine and fluoxetine[6,10,21]	This combination ('zyp-zac') is more effective than both placebo and olanzapine alone in treating bipolar depression. The dose is 6 and 25 mg or 12 and 50 mg/day. Early data suggest prophylactic effectiveness for the combination.

Table Alternative treatments – refer to primary literature before using

Drug/regime	Comments
Quetiapine[10,22–24]	A randomised, controlled trial has demonstrated clear efficacy for doses of 300 mg and 600 mg daily (as monotherapy) in bipolar I and bipolar II depression.
	As expected, quetiapine appears not to be associated with switching to mania; longer-term data are awaited.
Pramipexole[25,26]	Pramipexole is a dopamine agonist which is widely used in Parkinson's disease. Two small placebo-controlled trials suggest useful efficacy in bipolar depression. Effective dose averages around 1.7 mg/day. Both studies used pramipexole as an adjunct to existing mood-stabiliser treatment. Neither study detected an increased risk of switching to mania/hypomania (a theoretical consideration) but data are insufficient to exclude this possibility. Probably best reserved for specialist centres.
Valproate[1,6,27,28]	Limited evidence of efficacy as monotherapy but recommended in some guidelines. Probably protects against depressive relapse but database is small.
Carbamazepine[1,6,28,29]	Occasionally recommended but database is poor and effect modest. May have useful activity when added to other mood-stabilisers.
Antidepressants[30–36]	'Unopposed' antidepressants (i.e. without mood-stabiliser protection) are generally avoided in bipolar depression because of the risk of switching. There is also evidence that they are relatively less effective in bipolar depression than in unipolar depression. Nonetheless short-term use of fluoxetine, venlafaxine and moclobemide seems reasonably effective and safe even as monotherapy. Overall, however, unopposed antidepressant treatment should probably be avoided, especially in bipolar I disorder.

Table Other possible treatments – seek specialist advice before using

Drug/regime	Comments
Gabapentin[1,37,38]	Open studies suggest modest effect when added to mood-stabilisers or antipsychotics. Doses average around 1750 mg/day. Anxiolytic effect may account for apparent effect in bipolar depression.
Inositol[39]	Small, randomised, pilot study suggests that 12 g/day inositol is effective in bipolar depression.
Riluzole[40]	Riluzole shares some pharmacological characteristics with lamotrigine. Database is limited to a single case report supporting use in bipolar depression.
Thyroxine[41]	Limited evidence of efficacy as augmentation. Doses average around 300 µg/day.
Mifepristone[42]	Some evidence of mood-elevating properties in bipolar depression. May also improve cognitive function. Dose is 600 mg/day.

Bipolar disorder

References

1. Malhi GS, Mitchell PB, Salim S. Bipolar depression management options. *CNS Drugs* 2003; 17: 9–25.
2. Haddad PM, Dursun SM. Pharmacological management of bipolar depression. *Acta Psychiatr Scand* 2002; 105: 401–403.
3. Hirschfeld RMA. Bipolar depression: the real challenge. *Eur Neuropsychopharm* 2004; 14: S83–S88.

4. Baldassano CF, Ballas CA, O'Reardon JP. Rethinking the treatment paradigm for bipolar depression: the importance of long-term management. *CNS Spectrum* 2004; **9**(Suppl. 9): 11–18.

5. Geddes JR, Burgess S, Hawton K *et al*. Long-term lithium therapy for bipolar disorder: systematic review and meta-analysis of randomized controlled trials. *Am J Psychiatry* 2004; **161**: 217–222.

6. Yatham NL, Calabrese JR, Kusumakar V. Bipolar depression: criteria for treatment selection, definition of refractoriness, and treatment options. *Bipolar Disord* 2003; **5**: 85–97.

7. Calabrese JR, Bowden CL, Sachs G *et al*. A placebo-controlled 18-month trial of lamotrigine and lithium maintenance treatment in recently depressed patients with bipolar I disorder. *J Clin Psychiatry* 2003; **64**: 1013–1024.

8. Prein RF, Klett CJ, Caffey EM Jr. Lithium carbonate and imipramine in prevention of affective episodes. A comparison in recurrent affective illness. *Arch Gen Psychiatry* 1973; **3**: 420–425.

9. Montgomery SA, Schatzberg AF, Guelfi JD *et al*. Pharmacotherapy of depression and mixed states in bipolar disorder. *J Affect Disorders* 2000; **59**: S39–S56.

10. Calabrese JR, Kaspar S, Johnson G *et al*. International Consensus Group on Bipolar I Depression Treatment Guidelines. *J Clin Psychiatry* 2004; **65**: 4.

11. Nemeroff CB, Evans DL, Gyulai L *et al*. Double-blind, placebo-controlled comparison of imipramine and paroxetine in the treatment of bipolar depression. *Am J Psychiatry* 2001; **6**: 906–912.

12. Vieta E, Martinez-Aran A, Goikolea JM *et al*. A randomized trial comparing paroxetine and venlafaxine in the treatment of bipolar depressed patients taking mood stabilisers. *J Clin Psychiatry* 2002; **63**: 508–512.

13. Young LT, Joffe RT, Robb JC *et al*. Double-blind comparison of addition of a second mood stabiliser versus an antidepressant to an initial mood stabiliser for treatment of patients with bipolar depression. *Am J Psychiatry* 2000; **157**: 124–126.

14. Fawcett JA. Lithium combinations in acute and maintenance treatment of unipolar and bipolar depression. *J Clin Psychiatry* 2003; **64**: 32–37.

15. Altshuler L, Kiriakos L, Calcagno J *et al*. The impact of antidepressant discontinuation versus antidepressant continuation on 1-year risk for relapse of bipolar depression: a retrospective chart review. *J Clin Psychiatry* 2001; **62**: 612–616.

16. Erfurth A, Michael N, Stadtland C *et al*. Bupropion as add-on strategy in difficult-to-treat bipolar depressive patients. *Neuropsychobiology* 2002; **45**: 33–36.

17. Baldassano CF, Datto SM, Littman L *et al*. What drugs are best for bipolar depression? *Ann Clin Psychiatry* 2003; **15**: 225–232.

18. Calabrese JR, Bowden CL, Sachs GS *et al*. A double-blind placebo-controlled study of lamotrigine monotherapy in outpatients with bipolar I depression. *J Clin Psychiatry* 1999; **60**: 79–88.

19. Bowden CL, Mitchell P, Suppes T. Lamotrigine in the treatment of bipolar depression. *Eur Neuropsychopharm* 1999; **4**: S113–S117.

20. Marangell LB, Martinez JM, Ketter TA *et al*. Lamotrigine treatment of bipolar disorder: data from the first 500 patients in STEP-BD. *Bipolar Disord* 2004; **6**: 139–143.

21. Tohen M, Vieta E, Calabrese J *et al*. Efficacy of olanzapine and olanzapine-fluoxetine combination in the treatment of bipolar I depression. *Arch Gen Psychiatry* 2003; **60**: 1079–1088.

22. Calabrese J, Macfadden W, McCoy R *et al*. Double-blind, placebo-controlled study of quetiapine in bipolar depression. Presented at the 157th Annual Meeting of the American Psychiatric Association, 2004.

23. Macfadden W, Calabrese J, McCoy R *et al*. Double-blind, placebo-controlled study of quetiapine in bipolar I depression. Presented at the XXIVth Collegium Internationale Neuro-Psychopharmacologicum (CINP) Congress, 2004.

24. Macfadden W, Calabrese J, McCoy R *et al*. Antianxiety effects analysis of quetiapine in bipolar depression. Presented at the 157th Annual Meeting of the American Psychiatric Association, 2004.

25. Goldberg JF, Burdick KE, Endick CJ. Preliminary randomized, double-blind, placebo-controlled trial of pramipexole added to mood stabilisers for treatment-resistant bipolar depression. *Am J Psychiatry* 2004; **161**: 564–566.

26. Zarate CA Jr, Payne JL, Singh J *et al*. Pramipexole for bipolar II depression: a placebo-controlled proof of concept study. *Biol Psychiatry* 2004; **56**: 54–60.

27. Sachs GS, Altshuler L, Keeter TA *et al*. Divalproex versus placebo for the treatment of bipolar depression. Presented at the Americal College of Neuropsychopharmacology Conference, Puerto Rico, 2001.

28. Goodwin GM. Evidence-based guidelines for treating bipolar disorder: recommendations from the British Association for Psychopharmacology. *J Psychopharmacol* 2003; **17**: 149–173.

29. Dilsaver SC, Swann C, Chen YW *et al*. Treatment of bipolar depression with carbamazepine: results of an open study. *Biol Psychiatry* 1996; **40**: 935–937.

30. Amsterdam JD, Shults J, Brunswick DJ *et al*. Short-term fluoxetine monotherapy for bipolar type II or bipolar NOS major depression – low manic switch rate. *Bipolar Disord* 2004; **6**: 75–81.

31. Amsterdam JD, Garcia-Espana F, Fawcett J *et al*. Efficacy and safety of fluoxetine in treating bipolar II major depressive episode. *J Clin Psychopharm* 1998; **18**: 435–440.

32. Amsterdam J. Efficacy and safety of venlafaxine in the treatment of bipolar II major depressive episode. *J Clin Psychopharm* 1998; **18**: 414–417.

33. Amsterdam JD, Garcia-Espana F. Venlafaxine monotherapy in women with bipolar II and unipolar major depression. *J Affect Discorders* 2000; **59**: 225–229.

34. Silverstone T. Moclobemide vs. imipramine in bipolar depression: a multicentre double-blind clinical trial. *Acta Psychiatr Scand* 2001; **104**: 104–109.

35. Nassir Ghaemi S, Rosenquist JK, Ko JY *et al*. Antidepressant treatment in bipolar versus unipolar depression. *Am J Psychiatry* 2004; **161**: 163–165.

36. Post RM, Leverich GS, Nolen WA *et al.* A re-evaluation of the role of antidepressants in the treatment of bipolar depression: data from the Stanley Foundation Bipolar Network. *Bipolar Disord* 2003; 5: 396–406.
37. Wang PW, Santosa C, Schumacher M *et al.* Gabapentin augmentation therapy in bipolar depression. *Bipolar Disord* 2002; 4: 296–301.
38. Ashton CH, Young AH. Gaba-ergic drugs: exit stage left; enter stage night. *J Psychopharmacol* 2003; 17: 174–178.
39. Chengappa KR, Levine J, Gershon S *et al.* Inositol as an add-on treatment for bipolar depression. *Bipolar Disord* 2000; 2: 47.
40. Singh J, Zarate CA, Krystal AD. Case report: successful riluzole augmentation therapy in treatment-resistant bipolar depression following the development of rash with lamotrigine. *Psychopharmacology* 2004; 173: 227–228.
41. Bauer M. Thyroid hormone augmentation with levothyroxine in bipolar depression. *Bipolar Disord* 2002; 4: 109–110.
42. Young AH, Gallagher P, Watson S *et al.* Improvements in neurocognitive function and mood following adjunctive treatment with mifepristone (RU-486) in bipolar disorder. *Neuropsychopharmacology* 2004; 29: 1538–1545.

Further reading

Silverstone PH, Silverstone T. A review of acute treatments for bipolar depression. *Int Clin Psychopharmacol* 2004; 19: 113–124.

Rapid-cycling bipolar affective disorder

Rapid-cycling is usually defined as bipolar disorder in which four or more episodes of (hypo) mania or depression occur in a 12-month period. It is generally held to be less responsive to drug treatment than non-rapid-cycling bipolar illness[1,2] and entails considerable depressive morbidity and suicide risk[3]. The following table outlines a treatment strategy for rapid cycling based on rather limited data and very few direct comparisons of drugs[4]. In practice, response to treatment is sometimes idiosyncratic: individuals sometimes show significant response only to one or two drugs. Spontaneous or treatment-related remissions occur in around a third of rapid-cyclers[5].

Step	Suggested treatment	References
Step 1	Withdraw antidepressants.	6–8
Step 2	Evaluate possible precipitants (e.g. alcohol, thyroid dysfunction, external stressors).	2, 8
Step 3	Optimise mood stabiliser treatment (see page 122) Consider combining mood-stabilisers. Lithium may be relatively less effective.	9, 10
Step 4	Consider other treatment options: (alphabetical order) Clozapine (usual doses) Lamotrigine (up to 225 mg/day) Levetiracetam (up to 2000 mg/day) Nimodipine (180 mg/day) Olanzapine (usual doses) Quetiapine (300–600 mg/day) Risperidone (up to 6 mg/day) Thyroxine (150–400 µg/day) Choice of drug determined by patient factors – no comparative efficacy data to guide choice.	11–21

References

1. Calabrese JR, Shelton MD, Rapport DJ *et al.* Current research on rapid cycling bipolar disorder and its treatment. *J Affect Disorders* 2001; **67**: 241–255.
2. Kupta RW, Luckenbaugh DA, Post RM *et al.* Rapid and non-rapid cycling bipolar disorder: a meta-analysis of clinical studies. *J Clin Psychiatry* 2003; **64**: 1483–1494.
3. Coryell W, Soloman D, Turvey C *et al.* The long-term course of rapid-cycling bipolar disorder. *Arch Gen Psychiatry* 2003; **60**: 914–920.
4. Tondo L, Hennen J, Baldessarini RJ. Rapid-cycling bipolar disorder: effects of long-term treatments. *Acta Psychiatr Scand* 2003; **108**: 4–14.
5. Koukopoulos A, Sani G, Koukopoulos AE *et al.* Duration and stability of the rapid-cycling course: a long-term personal follow-up of 109 patients. *J Affect Disorders* 2003; **73**: 75–85.
6. Wehr TA, Goodwin FK. Can antidepressants cause mania and worsen the course of affective illness? *Am J Psychiatry* 1987; **144**: 1403–1411.
7. Altshuler LL, Post RM, Leverich GS. Antidepressant-induced mania and cycle acceleration: a controversy revisited. *Am J Psychiatry* 1995; **152**: 1130–1138.
8. American Psychiatric Association. Practice guideline for the treatment of patients with bipolar disorder. *Am J Psychiatry* 2002; **159**(Suppl.): s51–s50.
9. Calabrese JR, Woyshville MJ. A medication algorithm for treatment of bipolar rapid cycling? *Clin Psychiatry* 1995; **56**(Suppl. 3): 11–18.
10. Taylor DM, Duncan D. Treatment options for rapid-cycling bipolar affective disorder. *Psychiatr Bull* 1996; **20**: 601–603.

11. Sanger TM, Tohen M, Vieta E *et al.* Olanzapine in the acute treatment of bipolar I disorder with a history of rapid cycling. *J Affect Disorders* 2003; **73**: 155–161.
12. Calabrese JR, Meltzer HY, Markovitz PJ. Clozapine prophylaxis in rapid cycling bipolar disorder. *J Clin Psychopharm* 1991; **11**: 396–397.
13. Vieta E, Parramon G, Padrell E *et al.* Quetiapine in the treatment of rapid cycling bipolar disorder. *Bipolar Disord* 2002; **4**: 335–340.
14. Goodnick PJ. Nimodipine treatment of rapid cycling bipolar disorder. *J Clin Psychiatry* 1995; **56**: 330.
15. Pazzagila PJ, Post RM, Ketter TA *et al.* Preliminary controlled trial of nimodipine in ultra-rapid cycling affective dysregulation. *Psychiatry Res* 1993; **49**: 257–272.
16. Bauer MS, Whybrow PC. Rapid cycling bipolar affective disorder. *Arch Gen Psychiatry* 1990; **47**: 435–440.
17. Fatemi SH, Rapport DJ, Calabrese JR *et al.* Lamotrigine in rapid-cycling bipolar disorder. *J Clin Psychiatry* 1997; **58**: 522–527.
18. Calabrese JR, Suppes T, Bowden CL *et al.* A double-blind, placebo-controlled, prophylaxis study of lamotrigine in rapid-cycling bipolar disorder. *J Clin Psychiatry* 2000; **61**: 841–850.
19. Braunig P, Kruger S. Levetiracetam in the treatment of rapid cycling bipolar disorder. *J Clin Psychopharm* 2003; **17**: 239–241.
20. Vieta E, Gasto C, Colom F *et al.* Treatment of refractory rapid cycling bipolar disorder with risperidone. *J Clin Psychopharm* 1998; **18**: 172–174.
21. Jacobsen FM. Risperidone in the treatment of affective illness and obsessive-compulsive disorder *J Clin Psychiatry* 1995; **56**: 423–429.

Prophylaxis in bipolar disorder

The evidence base is weak. Most evidence supports the efficacy of lithium[1,2]. Carbamazepine is somewhat less effective[2] and the long-term efficacy of valproate is uncertain[3-5]. Typical antipsychotics have traditionally been used and are perceived to be effective although the objective evidence base is, again, weak. Emerging evidence supports the efficacy of some atypical antipsychotics. Whether atypicals are more effective than typicals or are truly associated with a reduced overall side-effect burden remains untested.

A significant proportion of patients with bipolar illness fail to respond adequately to a single mood-stabiliser and combinations of mood-stabilisers[6] or a mood-stabiliser and an antipsychotic[7] may improve outcome. This needs to be balanced against the side-effect burden associated with polypharmacy. The patient's views about 'acceptable risk' of recurrence versus 'acceptable side-effect burden' are paramount.

References

1. Geddes JR, Burgess S, Hawton K. Long-term lithium therapy for bipolar disorder: systematic review and meta-analysis of randomised controlled trials. *Am J Psychiatry* 2004; **161**: 217–222.
2. Erwin G, Harlong M, Moleman P *et al.* Prophylactic efficacy of lithium versus carbamazepine in treatment-naïve bipolar patients. *J Clin Psychiatry* 2003; **64**: 144–151.
3. Bowden CL, Calabrese JR, McElroy SL *et al.* A randomised, placebo-controlled 12-month trial of divalproex and lithium in the treatment of outpatients with bipolar 1 disorder. *Arch Gen Psychiatry* 2000; **57**: 481–489.
4. Tohen M, Ketter TA, Zarate CA *et al.* Olanzapine versus divalproex sodium for the treatment of acute mania and maintenance of remission: a 47 week study. *Am J Psychiatry* 2003; **160**: 1263–1271.
5. Macritchie KA, Geddes J, Scott J *et al.* Valproic acid, valproate and divalproex in the maintenance treatment of bipolar disorder. Cochrane Database of Systematic Reviews 2004. www.cochrane.org.uk
6. Freeman MP, Stoll AL. Mood stabiliser combinations: a review of safety and efficacy. *Am J Psychiatry* 1998; **155**: 12–21.
7. Tohen M, Chengappa KNR, Suppes T *et al.* Relapse prevention in bipolar 1 disorder : 18-month comparison of olanzapine plus mood stabiliser v mood stabiliser alone. *Br J Psychiatry* 2004; **184**: 337–345.

Further reading

American Psychiatric Association. Practice guidelines for the treatment of patients with bipolar disorder. *Am J Psychiatry* 2002; **159**(Suppl.): 1–50.
Goodwin GM, Young AH. The British Association for Psychopharmacology guidelines for treatment of bipolar disorder: a summary. *J Psychopharmacol* 2003; **17**: 3–6.
Sachs GS. Decision tree for the treatment of bipolar disorder. *J Clin Psychiatry* 2003; **64**: 35–40.

chapter 4

Depression and anxiety

Antidepressant drugs – tricyclics*

Tricyclic	Licensed indication	Licensed doses (elderly doses not included)	Main adverse effects	Major interactions	Approx. half-life (h)	Cost (£)
Amitriptyline	Depression Nocturnal enuresis in children	30–200 mg/day 7–10 yr: 10–20 mg 11–16 yr: 25–50 mg at night for max. 3 months	Sedation, often with hangover; postural hypotension; tachycardia/arrhythmia; dry mouth, blurred vision, constipation, urinary retention	SSRIs (except citalopram), phenothiazines, cimetidine – ↑ plasma levels of TCAs Alcohol Antimuscarinics Antipsychotics (esp. pimozide/thioridazine) MAOIs	9–25 18–96 Active metabolite (nortriptyline)	0.04/50 mg
Clomipramine	Depression Phobic and obsessional states Adjunctive treatment of cataplexy associated with narcolepsy	10–250 mg/day 10–150 mg/day 10–75 mg/day	As for amitriptyline	As for amitriptyline	19–37 54–77 Active metabolite (desmethyl-clomipramine)	0.09/50 mg
Dosulepin (dothiepin)	Depression	75–225 mg/day	As for amitriptyline	As for amitriptyline	11–40 22–60 Active metabolite (desmethyldosulepin)	0.10/75 mg
Doxepin	Depression	10–300 mg/day (up to 100 mg as a single dose)	As for amitriptyline	As for amitriptyline	8–25 28–52 Active metabolite (desmethyldoxepin)	0.05/50 mg

	Indication	Dose	Side effects	Notes	Half-life (hours)	
Imipramine	Depression	10–200 mg/day (up to 100 mg as a single dose; up to 300 mg in hospital patients)	As for amitriptyline but less sedative	As for amitriptyline	4–18 12–24 Active metabolite (desipramine)	0.04/25 mg
	Nocturnal enuresis in children	7 yr: 25 mg 8–11 yr: 25–50 mg >11 yr: 50–75 mg at night for max. 3 months				
Lofepramine	Depression	140–210 mg/day	As for amitriptyline but less sedative/anticholinergic/cardiotoxic Constipation common	As for amitriptyline	1.5–6 12–24 Active metabolite (desipramine)	0.18/70 mg
Nortriptyline	Depression	30–150 mg/day	As for amitriptyline but less sedative/anticholinergic/hypotensive Constipation may be problematic	As for amitriptyline	18–96	0.25/25 mg
	Nocturnal enuresis in children	7 yr: 10 mg 8–11 yrs: 10–20 mg >11 yr: 25–35 mg at night for max. 3 months				
Trimipramine	Depression	30–300 mg/day	As for amitriptyline but more sedative	As for amitriptyline Safer with MAOIs than other tricyclics	7–23	0.28/50 mg

* For full details refer to the manufacturer's information

Antidepressant drugs – SSRIs*

SSRI	Licensed indication	Licensed doses (elderly doses not included)	Main adverse effects	Major interactions	Approx. half-life (h)	Cost (£)
Citalopram	Depression – treatment of the initial phase and as maintenance therapy against potential relapse or recurrence	20–60 mg/day Use lowest dose – evidence for higher doses poor	Nausea, vomiting, dyspepsia, abdominal pain, diarrhoea, rash, sweating, agitation, anxiety, headache, insomnia, tremor, sexual dysfunction (male and female), hyponatraemia, cutaneous bleeding disorders Discontinuation symptoms may occur. See pages 176 et seq	Not a potent inhibitor of most cytochrome enzymes MAOIs – avoid Avoid – St John's wort Caution with alcohol (although no interaction seen)/NSAIDs/tryptophan/ warfarin	33 Has weak active metabolites	0.53/20 mg (generic available – price may vary) Drops 0.72/16 mg/ 8 drops (= 20 mg tablet)
	Panic disorder ± agoraphobia	10 mg for 1 week, increasing up to 60 mg/day				
Escitalopram	Depression Panic disorder ± agoraphobia Social anxiety disorder	10–20 mg/day 5 mg/day for 1 week, increasing up to 20 mg/day 20 mg/day	As for citalopram	As for citalopram	~30 Has weak active metabolites	0.53/10 mg
Fluoxetine	Depression ± anxiety	20 mg/day	As for citalopram but insomnia and agitation more common Rash may occur more frequently May alter insulin requirements	Inhibits CYP2D6, CYP3A4. Increases plasma levels of some antipsychotics/ some benzos/carbamazepine/ ciclosporin/phenytoin/tricyclics MAOIs – never Avoid: selegiline/St John's wort Caution – alcohol (although no interaction seen)/NSAIDs/ tryptophan/warfarin	2–3 days	0.09/20 mg (generic – price may vary)
	OCD	20–60 mg/day			4–16 days Active metabolite (norfluoxetine)	Liquid 0.84/20 mg/5 ml
	Bulimia nervosa	60 mg/day Higher doses possible – see SPC				
Fluvoxamine	Depression	100–300 mg/day b.d. if >100 mg	As for citalopram but nausea more common	Inhibits CYP1A2/2C9/3A4 Increases plasma levels of some benzos/carbamazepine/ciclosporin/ methadone/olanzapine/phenytoin/ propranolol/ theophylline/some tricyclics/warfarin MAOIs – never Caution: alcohol/lithium/ NSAIDs/St John's wort/ tryptophan/warfarin	17–22	0.60/100 mg
	OCD	100–300 mg/day b.d. if >100 mg				

Paroxetine	Depression ± anxiety OCD Panic disorder ± agoraphobia Social phobia PTSD Generalised anxiety disorder	20–50 mg/day Use lowest dose – evidence for higher doses poor 20–60 mg/day 10–50 mg/day 20–50 mg/day 20–50 mg/day 20 mg/day	As for citalopram but antimuscarinic effects and sedation more common Extrapyramidal symptoms more common, but rare Discontinuation symptoms common – withdraw slowly	Potent inhibitor of CYP2D6 Increases plasma level of some antipsychotics/tricyclics MAOIs – never Avoid: St John's wort Caution: alcohol/lithium/NSAIDs/tryptophan/warfarin	~ 24 (non-linear kinetics)	0.49/20 mg (generic – price may vary) Liquid 1.38/20 mg/10 ml
Sertraline	Depression ± anxiety and prevention of relapse or recurrence of depression ± anxiety OCD (under specialist supervision in children) PTSD in women	50–200 mg/day Use 50–100 mg – evidence for higher doses poor 50–200 mg/day (adults) 6–12 yr: 25–50 mg/day, may be increased in steps of 50 mg at intervals of one week 13–17 yr: 50–200 mg/day 25–50 mg/day	As for citalopram	Inhibits CYP2D6 (more likely to occur at doses ≥100 mg/day). Increases plasma levels of some antipsychotics/tricyclics. Avoid: St John's wort Caution: alcohol (although no interaction seen)/lithium/NSAIDs/tryptophan/warfarin	~ 26 Has a weak active metabolite	0.95/100 mg (0.58/50 mg)

* For full details refer to the manufacturer's information

139

Antidepressant drugs – MAOIs*

MAOI	Licensed indication	Licensed doses (elderly doses not included)	Main adverse effects	Major interactions	Approx. half-life (h)	Cost (£)
Isocarboxazid	Depression	30 mg/day in single or divided doses, increased after 4 weeks to max. 60 mg/day for 4–6 weeks 10–40 mg/day maintenance	Postural hypotension, dizziness, drowsiness, insomnia, headaches, oedema, anticholinergic adverse effects, nervousness, paraesthesia, weight gain, hepatotoxicity, leucopenia, hypertensive crisis	Tyramine in food, sympathomimetics, alcohol, opioids, antidepressants, levodopa, $5HT_1$ agonists	36	0.53/10 mg
Phenelzine	Depression	15 mg t.d.s. – q.i.d. (hospital patients: max. 30 mg t.d.s.) Consider reducing to lowest possible maintenance dose	As for isocarboxazid but more postural hypotension, less hepatotoxicity	As for isocarboxazid Probably safest of MAOIs and is the one that should be used if combinations are considered	1.5	0.20/15 mg
Tranylcypromine	Depression	10 mg b.d. Doses >30 mg/day under close supervision only Usual maintenance: 10 mg/day Last dose no later than 3 pm	As for isocarboxazid but insomnia, nervousness, hypertensive crisis more common than with other MAOIs; hepatotoxicity less common Mild dependence as amphetamine-like structure	As for isocarboxazid but interactions more severe Never use in combination therapy with other antidepressants	2.5	0.18/10 mg

					2–4	0.31/150 mg
Moclobemide (Reversible inhibitor of MAO-A)	Depression Social phobia	150–600 mg/day b.d. after food 300–600 mg/day b.d. after food Last dose before 3 pm	Sleep disturbances, nausea, agitation, confusion Hypertension reported – may be related to tyramine ingestion	Tyramine interactions rare and mild but possible if high doses (>600 mg/day) used or if large quantities of tyramine ingested CNS excitation/depression with dextromethorphan/pethidine Avoid: clomipramine/levodopa/selegiline/sympathomimetics/SSRIs Caution with fentanyl/morphine/tricyclics Cimetidine – use half-dose of moclobemide		

* For full details refer to the manufacturer's information

Antidepressant drugs – others*

Antidepressant	Licensed indication	Licensed doses (elderly doses not included)	Main adverse effects	Major interactions	Approx. half-life (h)	Cost (£)
Duloxetine	Depression (and other non-psychiatric indications)	60–120 mg/day Limited data to support advantage of doses above 60 mg/day	Nausea, insomnia, dizziness, dry mouth, somnolence, constipation, anorexia. Very small increases in heart rate and blood pressure. Probably clinically insignificant	Metabolised by CYP1A2 and CYP2D6. Inhibitor of CYP2D6 Caution with drugs acting on either enzyme MAOIs – avoid Caution: alcohol (although no interaction seen)	12 (metabolites inactive)	0.99/60 mg
Mianserin	Depression	30–90 mg daily	Sedation, rash; rarely: blood dyscrasia, jaundice, arthralgia No anticholinergic effects Sexual dysfunction uncommon Low cardiotoxicity	Other sedatives, alcohol MAOIs: avoid Effect on hepatic enzymes unclear, so caution is required	10–20 2-desmethyl-mianserin is major metabolite (?activity)	0.14/30 mg
Mirtazapine	Depression	15–45 mg/day	Increased appetite, weight gain, drowsiness, oedema, dizziness, headache, ?blood dyscrasia Nausea/sexual dysfunction relatively uncommon	Minimal effect on CYP2D6/1A2/3A Caution: alcohol/sedatives	20–40 25 Active metabolite (demethyl-mirtazapine)	0.64/30 mg Dispersible tablets (generic available – price may vary)
Reboxetine	Depression – acute and maintenance	4–6 mg b.d.	Insomnia, sweating, dizziness, dry mouth, constipation, tachycardia, urinary hesitancy Erectile dysfunction may occur rarely	Metabolised by CYP3A4 – avoid drugs inhibiting this enzyme (e.g. erythromycin ketoconazole). Minimal effect on CYP2D6/3A4 MAOIs: avoid No interaction with alcohol	13	0.32/4 mg

Trazodone	Depression ± anxiety	150–300 mg/day (up to 600 mg/day in hospitalised patients) b.d. dosing above 300 mg/day	Sedation, dizziness, headache, nausea, vomiting, tremor, postural hypotension, tachycardia, priapism	Caution: sedatives/alcohol/other antidepressants/digoxin/phenytoin MAOIs: avoid	5–13 (biphasic) 4–9 Active metabolite (mCPP)	0.44/100 mg Liquid 0.71/100 mg/ 10 ml
	Anxiety	75–300 mg/day	Not anticholinergic less cardiotoxic than tricyclics			
Venlafaxine	Depression ± anxiety and prevention of relapse or recurrence of depression	75–375 mg/day (b.d.) with food 75–225 mg XL/day (o.c.) with food	Nausea, insomnia, dry mouth, somnolence, dizziness, sweating, nervousness, headache, sexual dysfunction	Metabolised by CYP2D6/3A4 – caution with drugs known to inhibit both isozymes Minimal effects on CYP2D6 No effects on CYP1A2/2C9/3A4 MAOIs: avoid	5 11 Active metabolite (O-desmethyl-venlafaxine)	0.70/75 mg 0.84/75 mg XL
	Generalised anxiety disorder (XL prep only)	75 mg XL/day (discontinue if no response after 8 weeks)	Elevation of blood pressure at higher doses. UK MHRA recommend: venlafaxine is initiated only by specialists; avoid use in heart disease; ECG monitoring Discontinuation symptoms common – withdraw slowly	Caution: alcohol (although no interaction seen)/cimetidine/clozapine/warfarin		

* For full details refer to the manufacturer's information

Treatment of affective illness

Depression

Basic principles of prescribing in depression

- Discuss with the patient choice of drug and utility/availability of other, non-pharmacological treatments.

- Discuss with the patient likely outcomes, such as gradual relief from depressive symptoms over several weeks.

- Prescribe a dose of antidepressant (after titration, if necessary) that is likely to be effective.

- For a single episode, continue treatment for at least 4–6 months after resolution of symptoms (multiple episodes may require longer).

- Withdraw antidepressants gradually; always inform patients of the risk and nature of discontinuation symptoms.

Official guidance on the treatment of depression

NICE guidelines[1] – a summary
- Antidepressants are not recommended in mild depression – watchful waiting, problem-solving and exercise are more effective.
- When an antidepressant is prescribed, a generic SSRI is recommended.
- All patients should be informed about the withdrawal effects of antidepressants.
- For severe or resistant depression a combination of antidepressant and CBT is recommended.
- Patients with two prior episodes and functional impairment should be treated for at least 2 years.

MHRA/CSM Expert Working Group on SSRIs[2] – a summary
- Use the lowest possible dose.
- Monitor closely in early stages for restlessness, agitation and suicidality. This is particularly important in young people (<30 years).
- Doses should be tapered gradually on stopping.
- Venlafaxine should be initiated only by specialists. Avoid in heart disease. ECG monitoring is recommended.

References

1. National Institute of Clinical Excellence. Depression: management of depression in primary and secondary care. Clinical Guideline 23, December 2004.
2. Committee on Safety of Medicines. December 2004. www.mhra.gov.uk.

Depression & anxiety

Drug treatment of depression

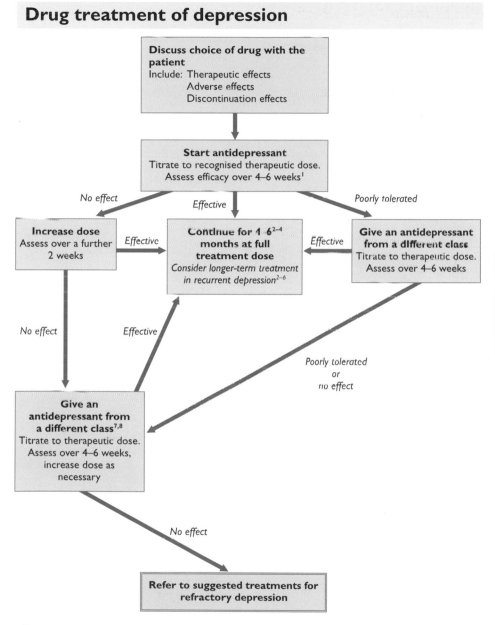

Discuss choice of drug with the patient
Include: Therapeutic effects
Adverse effects
Discontinuation effects

Start antidepressant
Titrate to recognised therapeutic dose.
Assess efficacy over 4–6 weeks[1]

No effect *Effective* *Poorly tolerated*

Increase dose
Assess over a further 2 weeks

Effective

Continue for 4–6[2–4] months at full treatment dose
Consider longer-term treatment in recurrent depression[2–6]

Effective

Give an antidepressant from a different class
Titrate to therapeutic dose.
Assess over 4–6 weeks

No effect *Effective*

Poorly tolerated or no effect

Give an antidepressant from a different class[7,8]
Titrate to therapeutic dose.
Assess over 4–6 weeks, increase dose as necessary

No effect

Refer to suggested treatments for refractory depression

Depression & anxiety

Notes

- Tools such as the Montgomery–Asberg Depression Rating Scale and the Hamilton Depression Rating Scale are recommended to assess drug effect.
- Switching between drug classes in cases of poor tolerability is not well supported by published studies but has a strong theoretical basis. In cases of non-response, there is some evidence that switching within a drug class can be effective[8,9], but switching between classes is, in practice, the most common option (see page 171).

References

1. Snow V, Lascher S, Mottur-Pilson C *et al.* Pharmacologic treatment of acute major depression and dysthymia. *Ann Intern Med* 2000; **132**: 738–742.
2. Anderson IM, Nutt DJ, Deakin JFW. Evidence-based guidelines for treating depressive disorders with antidepressants: a revision of the 1993 British Association for Psychopharmacology guidelines. *J Psychopharmacol* 2000; **14**: 3–19.
3. Crismon ML, Trivedi M, Pigott TA *et al.* The Texas Medication Algorithm Project: Report of the Texas Consensus Conference Panel on Medication Treatment of Major Depressive Disorder. *J Clin Psychiatry* 1999; **60**: 142–156.
4. American Psychiatric Association. Practice guideline for major depressive disorder in adults. *Am J Psychiatry* 1993; **150**: 1–26.
5. Kocsis JH, Friedman RA, Markowitz JC *et al.* Maintenance therapy for chronic depression. *Arch Gen Psychiatry* 1996; **53**: 769–774.
6. Dekker J, de Jonghe F, Tuynman H. The use of anti-depressants after recovery from depression. *Eur J Psychiat* 2000; **14**: 207–212.
7. Nelson JC. Treatment of antidepressant nonresponders: augmentation or switch? *J Clin Psychiatry* 1998; **59**: 35–41.
8. Joffe RT. Substitution therapy in patients with major depression. *CNS Drugs* 1999; **11**: 175–180.
9. Thase ME, Feighner JP, Lydiard RB. Citalopram treatment of fluoxetine nonresponders. *J Clin Psychiatry* 2001; **62**: 683–687.

Further reading

Barbui C, Hotopf M. Amitriptyline v. the rest: still the leading antidepressant after 40 years of randomised controlled trials. *Br J Psychiatry* 2001; **178**: 129–144.
Smith D, Dempster C, Glanville J, *et al.* Efficacy and tolerability of venlafaxine compared with selective serotonin reuptake inhibitors and other antidepressants: a meta-analysis. *Br J Psychiatry* 2002; **180**: 396–404.

Recognised minimum effective doses – antidepressants

Tricyclics

Tricyclics	Unclear; at least 75–100 mg/day[1], possibly 125 mg/day[2]
Lofepramine	140 mg/day[3]

SSRIs

Citalopram	20 mg/day[4]
Escitalopram	10 mg/day[5]
Fluoxetine	20 mg/day[6]
Fluvoxamine	50 mg/day[7]
Paroxetine	20 mg/day[8]
Sertraline	50 mg/day[9]

Others

Duloxetine	60 mg/day[10,11]
Mirtazapine	30 mg/day[12]
Moclobemide	300 mg/day[13]
Reboxetine	8 mg/day[14]
Trazodone	150 mg/day[15]
Venlafaxine	75 mg/day[16]

Depression & anxiety

References

1. Farukawa TA, McGuire H, Barbui C. Meta-analysis of effects and side effects of low dosage tricyclic antidepressants in depression: systematic review. *BMJ* 2002; **325**: 991–995.
2. Donoghue J, Taylor DM. Suboptimal use of antidepressants in the treatment of depression. *CNS Drugs* 2000; **13**: 365–383.
3. Lancaster SG, Gonzalez JP. Lofepramine – a review of its pharmacodynamic and pharmaco-kinetic properties, and therapeutic efficacy in depressive illness. *Drugs* 1989; **37**: 123–140.
4. Montgomery SA, Pedersen V, Tanghoj P *et al.* The optimal dosing regimen for citalopram – a meta-analysis of nine placebo-controlled studies. *Int Clin Pyschopharm* 1994; **9**(Suppl. 1): 35–40.
5. Burke WJ, Gergel I, Bose A. Fixed-dose trial of the single isomer SSRI escitalopram in depressed outpatients. *J Clin Psychiatry* 2002; **63**: 331–336.
6. Altamura AC, Montgomery SA, Wernicke JF. The evidence for 20 mg a day of fluoxetine as the optimal dose in the treatment of depression. *Br J Psychiatry* 1998; **153**(Suppl. 3): 109–112.
7. Walczak DD, Apter JT, Halikas JA. The oral dose–effect relationship for fluvoxamine: a fixed-dose comparison against placebo in depressed outpatients. *Ann Clin Psychiatry* 1996; **8**: 139–151.
8. Dunner DL, Dunbar GC. Optimal dose regimen for paroxetine. *J Clin Psychiatry* 1992; **53**(Suppl. 2): 21–26.
9. Moon CA, Jago W, Wood K *et al.* A double-blind comparison of sertraline and clomipramine in the treatment of major depressive disorder and associated anxiety in general practice. *J Psychopharmacol* 1994; **8**: 171–176.
10. Goldstein DJ, Lu Y, Detke MJ *et al.* Duloxetine in the treatment of depression: a double-blind placebo-controlled comparison with paroxetine. *J Clin Psychopharm* 2004; **24**: 389–399.
11. Detke MJ, Lu Y, Goldstein DJ *et al.* Duloxetine, 60 mg once daily, for major depressive disorder: a randomized double-blind placebo-controlled trial. *J Clin Psychiatry* 2002; **63**: 308–315.
12. Van-Moffaert M, De Wilde J, Vereecken A *et al.* Mirtazapine is more effective than trazodone: a double-blind controlled study in hospitalized patients with major depression. *Int Clin Psychopharmacol* 1995; **10**: 3–9.
13. Priest RG, Schmid-Burgk W. Moclobemide in the treatment of depression. *Review of Contemporary Pharmacotherapy* 1994; **5**: 35–43.
14. Schatzberg AF. Clinical efficacy of reboxetine in major depression. *J Clin Psychiatry* 2000; **61**(Suppl. 10): 31–38.
15. Brogden RN, Heel RC, Speight TM *et al.* Trazodone: a review of its pharmacological properties and therapeutic use in depression and anxiety. *Drugs* 1981; **21**: 401–429.
16. Feighner JP, Entsuah AR, McPherson MK. Efficacy of once-daily venlafaxine extended release (XR) for symptoms of anxiety in depressed outpatients. *J Affect Disorders* 1998; **47**: 55–62.

Antidepressant prophylaxis

First episode

A single episode of depression should be treated for 4–6 months after recovery (i.e. a total of 9 months in all)[1,2]. If antidepressant therapy is stopped immediately on recovery, 50% of patients experience a return of their depressive symptoms[1].

Recurrent depression

Of those patients who have one episode of major depression, 50–85% will go on to have a second episode, and 80–90% of those who have a second episode, will go on to have a third[3]. Many factors are known to increase the risk of recurrence, including a family history of depression, recurrent dysthymia, concurrent non-affective psychiatric illness, chronic medical illness and social factors (e.g. lack of confiding relationships and psychosocial stressors). Some prescription drugs may precipitate depression[4]. Up to 15% of people with depression take their own life[3].

The figure below outlines the risk of recurrence for multiple-episode patients: those recruited to the study had already experienced at least three episodes of depression, with 3 years or less between episodes[5,6].

A meta-analysis of antidepressant continuation studies[7] concluded that continuing treatment with antidepressants reduces the odds of depressive relapse by around two-thirds, which is approximately equal to halving the absolute risk. This benefit persisted at 36 months and seemed to be similar across heterogeneous patient groups (first episode, multiple episode and chronic), although none of the studies included first-episode patients only. Specific studies in first-episode patients are required to confirm that treatment beyond 6–9 months confers additional benefit in this patient group.

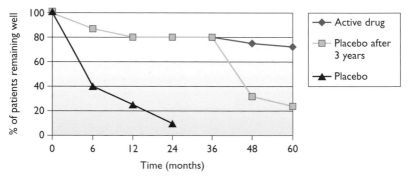

Dose for prophylaxis

Adults should receive the same dose as used for acute treatment. There is very limited evidence that lower doses are effective[8,9]. There is some evidence to support the use of lower doses in elderly patients: dosulepin 75 mg/day offers effective prophylaxis[8]. There is no evidence to support the use of lower than standard doses of SSRIs[10].

Relapse rates after ECT are similar to those after stopping antidepressants[11]. Antidepressant prophylaxis will be required, ideally with a different drug from the one that failed to get the patient well in the first instance, although good data in this area are lacking. There is some support for the use of a combination of lithium and nortriptyline[12].

Key points that patients should know

- A single episode of depression should be treated for 6 months after recovery.
- The risk of recurrence of depressive illness is high and increases with each episode.
- Those who have had multiple episodes may require treatment for many years.
- The chances of staying well are greatly increased by taking antidepressants.
- Antidepressants are:
  - effective
  - not addictive
  - not known to lose their efficacy over time
  - not known to cause new long-term side-effects.
- Medication needs to be continued at the treatment dose. If side-effects are intolerable, it may be possible to find a more suitable alternative.
- If patients decide to stop their medication, this must not be done suddenly, as this may lead to unpleasant discontinuation effects (see page 171). The medication needs to be reduced slowly under the supervision of a doctor.

References

1. Loonen AJ, Peer PG, Zwanikken GJ. Continuation and maintenance therapy with antidepressive agents: meta-analysis of research. *Pharm Weekly Sci* 1991; **13**: 167–175.
2. Reimherr FW, Amsterdam JD, Quitkin FM. Optimal length of continuation therapy in depression: a prospective assessment during long-term fluoxetine treatment. *Am J Psychiatry* 1998; **155**: 1247–1253.
3. Forshall S, Nutt D. Maintenance pharmacotherapy of unipolar depression. *Psychiatr Bull* 1999; **23**: 370–373.
4. Patten SB, Love EJ. Drug-induced depression. *Psychother Psychoso* 1997; **66**: 63–73.
5. Frank E, Kupfer DJ, Perel JM *et al.* Three-year outcomes for maintenance therapies in recurrent depression. *Arch Gen Psychiatry* 1990; **47**: 1093–1099.
6. Kupfer DJ, Frank E, Perel JM *et al.* Five-year outcome for maintenance therapies in recurrent depression. *Arch Gen Psychiatry* 1992; **49**: 769–773.
7. Geddes JR, Carney SM, Davies C *et al.* Relapse prevention with antidepressant drug treatment in depressive disorders: a systematic review. *Lancet* 2003; **361**: 653–661.
8. Frank E, Kupfer DJ, Perel JM. Comparison of full dose versus half dose pharmacotherapy in the maintenance treatment of recurrent depression. *J Affect Disorders* 1993; **27**: 139–145.
9. Old Age Depression Interest Group. How long should the elderly take antidepressants? A double-blind placebo controlled study of continuation/prophylaxis therapy with dothiepin. *Br J Psychiatry* 1993; **162**: 175–182.
10. Franchini L, Gasperini M, Perez J *et al.* Dose-response efficacy of paroxetine in preventing depressive recurrences: a randomised double-blind study. *J Clin Psychiatry* 1998; **59**: 229–232.
11. Nobler MS, Sackeim HA. Refractory depression and electroconvulsive therapy. In: Nolen WA, Zohar J, Roose SP *et al.* (eds.) *Refractory Depression: current strategies and future directions.* Chichester: John Wiley & Sons Ltd, 1994, pp. 69–81.
12. Sackeim HA, Haskett RF, Mulsant BH *et al.* Continuation therapy in the prevention of relapse following ECT: a randomized controlled trial. *JAMA* 2001; **285**: 1299–1307.

Further reading

Jackson GA, Maciver I. Psychiatrist's attitudes to maintenance drug treatment in depression. *Psychiatr Bull* 1999; **23**: 74–77.

Depression & anxiety

Treatment of refractory depression – first choice

Table First choice: commonly used treatments generally well supported by published literature

Treatment	Advantages	Disadvantages	Refs
Add **lithium** Aim for plasma level of 0.4–1.0 mmol/l	• Well established • Effective in around half of cases • Well supported in the literature • Recommended by NICE	• Sometimes poorly tolerated at higher plasma levels • Potentially toxic (NICE recommend ECG) • Usually needs specialist referral • Plasma monitoring is essential	1–3
ECT	• Well established • Effective • Well supported in the literature	• Poor reputation in public domain • Necessitates general anaesthetic • Needs specialist referral • Usually reserved for last-line treatment • Usually combined with other treatments	4,5
Venlafaxine (high dose) (>200 mg/day)	• Usually well tolerated • Can be initiated in primary care • Recommended by NICE	• Limited support in literature • Nausea and vomiting more common • Discontinuation reactions common • Blood pressure monitoring essential • ECG required	6–8
Add **tri-iodothyronine** (20–50 µg/day)	• Usually well tolerated • Some literature support	• TFT monitoring required • Usually needs specialist referral • Trials mainly support tricyclic augmentation • Some negative studies • Becoming less popular	9,10
Add **tryptophan** 2–3 g t.d.s.	• Usually well tolerated • Well researched, but few data in refractory depression	• Theoretical risk of eosinophilia–myalgia syndrome • Data relate mainly to combination with tricyclics/MAOIs • Risk of serotonin syndrome • Becoming less popular	10–12
SSRI + mianserin or mirtazapine	• Recommended by NICE • Usually well tolerated • Reasonable literature support • Becoming more widely used	• Risk of serotonin syndrome (inform patient) • Risk of blood dyscrasia with mianserin	13–15

Note: Data relating to augmentation strategies in refractory depression are poor by evidence-based standards[16,17]. Recommendations are therefore partly based on clinical experience and expert consensus.

Always consider non-drug approaches (e.g. CBT).

References

1. Fava M, Rosenbaum JF, McGrath PJ *et al.* Lithium and tricyclic augmentation of fluoxetine treatment. *Am J Psychiatry* 1994; **151**: 1372–1374.
2. Dinan TG. Lithium augmentation in sertraline-resistant depression: a preliminary dose-response study. *Acta Psychiatr Scand* 1993; **88**: 300–301.
3. Bauer M, Döpfmer S. Lithium augmentation in treatment-resistant depression: meta-analysis of placebo-controlled studies. *J Clin Psychopharm* 1999; **19**: 427–434.
4. Folkerts HW, Michael N, Tölle R *et al.* Electroconvulsive therapy vs paroxetine in treatment-resistant depression – a randomized study. *Acta Psychiatr Scand* 1997; **96**: 334–342.
5. Gonzalez-Pinto A, Gutierrez M, Gonzalez N *et al.* Efficacy and safety of venlafaxine-ECT combination in treatment-resistant depression. *J Neuropsych Clin Neurosci* 2002; **14**: 206–209.
6. Poiriere MF, Boyer P. Venlafaxine and paroxetine in treatment-resistant depression. *Br J Psychiatry* 1999; **175**: 12–16.
7. Nierenberg AA, Feighner JP, Rudolph R *et al.* Venlafaxine for treatment-resistant unipolar depression. *J Clin Psychopharm* 1994; **14**: 419–423.
8. Smith D, Dempster C, Glanville J *et al.* Efficacy and tolerability of venlafaxine compared with selective serotonin reuptake inhibitors and other antidepressants: a meta-analysis. *Br J Psychiatry* 2002; **180**: 396–404.
9. Joffe RT, Singer W. A comparison of tri-iodothyronine and thyroxine in the potentiation of tricyclic antidepressants. *Psychiatry Res* 1990; **32**: 241–251.
10. Anderson IM. Drug treatment of depression: reflections on the evidence. *Advan Psych Treat* 2003; **9**: 11–20.
11. Smith S. Tryptophan in the treatment of resistant depression – a review. *Pharm J* 1998; **261**: 819–821.
12. Cowen PJ. New drugs, old problems revisiting pharmacological management of treatment-resistant depression. *Advan Psych Treat* 2005; **11**: 19–27.
13. Carpenter LL, Yasmin S, Price LH. A double-blind placebo controlled study of antidepressant augmentation with mirtazapine. *Biol Psychiatry* 2002; **51**: 183–188.
14. Carpenter LL, Jocic Z, Hall JM *et al.* Mirtazapine augmentation in the treatment of refractory depression. *J Clin Psychiatry* 1999; **60**: 45–49.
15. Ferreri M, Lavergne F, Berlin I *et al.* Benefits from mianserin augmentation of fluoxetine in patients with major depression non-responders to fluoxetine alone. *Acta Psychiatr Scand* 2001; **103**: 66–72.
16. Lam R, Wan D, Cohen N *et al.* Combining antidepressants for treatment-resistant depression: a review. *J Clin Psychiatry* 2002; **63**: 685–693.
17. Stimpson N, Agrawal N, Lewis G. Randomised controlled trials investigating pharmacological and psychological interventions for treatment-refractory depression. Systematic review. *Br J Psychiatry* 2002; **181**: 284–294.

Treatment of refractory depression – second choice

Table Second choice: less commonly used, variably supported by published evaluations (alphabetical order – no preference implied by order)

Treatment	Advantages	Disadvantages	References
Add lamotrigine (aim for 200 mg/day but lower doses may be effective)	• Reasonably well researched • Quite widely used • Probably more robust data for bipolar depression	• Slow titration • Risk of rash • Appropriate dosing unclear	1–5
Add pindolol (5 mg t.d.s. or 7.5 mg once daily)	• Well tolerated • Can be initiated in primary care • Reasonably well researched (but combined with SSRIs, trazodone, venlafaxine only)	• Data mainly relate to acceleration of response • Refractory data contradictory – some negative studies • Appropriate dosing unclear – higher doses may be more effective	6–10
Combine olanzapine and fluoxetine (12.5 mg + 50 mg daily)	• Well researched (but few *published* studies) • Usually well tolerated	• Expensive • Risk of weight gain • Limited clinical experience in UK	11–14
Combine MAOI and TCA (e.g. trimipramine + phenelzine)	• Widely used in 1960s and 1970s • Inexpensive • Still fairly widely used	• Potential for severe interaction • Needs specialist referral • Becoming less popular	15, 16

Depression & anxiety

References

1. Calabrese JR, Bowden CL, Sachs GS. A double-blind placebo-controlled study of lamotrigine monotherapy in outpatients with bipolar I depression. *J Clin Psychiatry* 1999; **60**: 79–88.
2. Maltese TM. Adjunctive lamotrigine treatment for major depression (Letter). *Am J Psychiatry* 1999; **156**: 1833.
3. Normann C, Hummel B, Scharer L *et al*. Lamotrigine as adjunct to paroxetine in acute depression: a placebo-controlled, double-blind study. *J Clin Psychiatry* 2002; **63**: 337–344.
4. Barbee J, Jamhour N. Lamotrigine as an augmentation agent in treatment-resistant depression. *J Clin Psychiatry* 2002; **63**: 737–741.
5. Barbosa L, Berk M, Vorster M. A double-blind, randomized, placebo-controlled trial of augmentation with lamotrigine or placebo in patients concomitantly treated with fluoxetine for resistant major depressive episodes. *J Clin Psychiatry* 2003; **64**: 403–407.
6. Rabiner E, Bhagwagar Z, Gunn R *et al*. Pindolol augmentation of selective serotonin reuptake inhibitors: PET evidence that the dose used in clinical trials is too low. *Am J Psychiatry* 2001; **158**: 2080–2082.
7. McAskill R, Mir S, Taylor D. Pindolol augmentation of antidepressant therapy. *Br J Psychiatry* 1998; **173**: 203–208.
8. Räsänen P, Hakko H, Tuhonen J. Pindolol and major affective disorders: a three-year follow-up study of 30,483 patients. *J Clin Psychopharm* 1999; **19**: 297–302.
9. Perry EB Jr, Berman RM, Sanacora G *et al*. Pindolol augmentation in depressed patients resistant to selective serotonin reuptake inhibitors: a double-blind, randomized, controlled trial. *J Clin Psychiatry* 2004; **65**: 238–243.
10. Sokolski KN, Conney JC, Brown BJ *et al*. Once-daily high-dose pindolol for SSRI-refractory depression. *Psychiatry Res* 2004; **125**: 81–86.
11. Dube S, Andersen S, Paul S *et al*. Meta-analysis of olanzapine/fluoxetine use in treatment-resistant depression. Presented at 15th European College of Neuropsychopharmacology, 5–9 October 2002, Barcelona, Spain.
12. Corya SA, Andersen SW, Detke HC *et al*. Long-term antidepressant efficacy and safety of olanzapine/fluoxetine combination: a 76-week open-label study. *J Clin Psychiatry* 2003; **64**: 1349–1356.
13. Corya S, Andersen S, Paul S *et al*. Safety meta-analysis of olanzapine/fluoxetine combination versus fluoxetine. Presented at 15th European College of Neuropsychopharmacology, 5–9 October 2002, Barcelona, Spain.
14. Shelton RC, Tollefson GD, Tohen M *et al*. A novel augmentation strategy for treating resistant major depression. *Am J Psychiatry* 2001; **158**: 131–134.
15. White K, Simpson G. The combined use of MAOIs and tricyclics. *J Clin Psychiatry* 1984; **45**: 67–69.
16. Kennedy N, Paykel ES. Treatment and response in refractory depression: results from a specialist affective disorders service. *J Affect Disorders* 2004; **81**: 49–53.

Treatment of refractory depression – other reported treatments

Table Other reported treatments (alphabetical order – no preference implied).

Prescribers *must* familiarise themselves with the primary literature before using these strategies.

Treatment	Comments	References
Add amantadine (up to 300 mg/day).	Limited data.	1
Add bupropion (amfebutamone) 300 mg/day.	Reasonably well supported.	2–4
Add carbergoline 2 mg/day.	Very limited data.	5
Add clonazepam 0.5–1.0 mg/day.	Use of benzodiapines is widespread but not well supported.	6
Add metyrapone 1 g/day.	Data relate to non-refractory illness.	7
Add reboxetine 2–8 mg/day.	Reasonably well supported.	8–10
Add risperidone 0.5–1.0 mg/day.	Limited data but becoming more widely used.	11, 12
Add yohimbine Up to 30 mg/day.	Data relate to non-refractory illness.	13
Add ziprasidone Up to 160 mg/day.	Reasonably well supported.	14
Buspirone Up to 60 mg/day.	Reasonably well supported. Usually added to antidepressant treatment.	15
Dexamethasone 3–4 mg/day.	Use for 4 days only. Limited data.	16, 17
Ketoconazole 400–800 mg/day.	Rarely used. Risk of hepatotoxity.	18
Modafanil 100–400 mg/day.	Data mainly relate to non-refractory illness. Usually added to antidepressant treatment.	19–21
Nortriptyline ± lithium.	Re-emergent treatment option.	22, 23
Oestrogens (various regimens).	Limited data.	24
Omega–3-triglycerides EPA 1–2 g/day.	Developing database. Usually added to antidepressant treatment.	25–27
Pramipexole 100–200 mg/day.	Few data in refractory unipolar depression.	28

Depression & anxiety

Table Other reported treatments – continued

Treatment	Comments	References
Riluzole 100–200 mg/day.	Very limited data.	29
S-adenosyl-L-methionine 400 mg/day IM; 1600 mg/day oral	Limited data in refractory depression.	30, 31
SSRI + TCA.	Formerly widely used.	32
rTMS.	Very limited data.	33
TCA – high dose.	Formerly widely used.	34
Testosterone gel.	Effective in those with low testosterone levels.	35
Vagus nerve stimulation.	Developing database but uncertain efficacy.	36
Venlafaxine – high dose. (up to 600 mg/day).	Cardiac monitoring essential.	37
Venlafaxine + IV clomipramine.	Cardiac monitoring essential.	38

References

1. Stryjer R, Strous RD, Shaked G *et al.* Amantadine as augmentation therapy in the management of treatment-resistant depression. *Int Clin Psychopharmacol* 2003; **18**: 93–96.
2. Fatemi SH, Emamian ES, Kist DA. Venlafaxine and bupropion combination therapy in a case of treatment-resistant depression. *Ann Pharmacother* 1999; **33**: 701–703.
3. Pierre JM, Gitlin MJ. Buprorion-tranylcypromine combination for treatment-refractory depression. *J Clin Psychiatry* 2000; **61**: 449–450.
4. Lam RW, Hossie H, Solomans K *et al.* Citalopram and bupropion-SR: combining versus switching in patients with treatment-resistant depression. *J Clin Psychiatry* 2004; **65**: 337–340.
5. Takahashi H, Yoshida K, Higuchi H *et al.* Addition of a dopamine agonist, cabergoline, to a serotonin-noradrenalin reuptake inhibitor, milnacipran, as a therapeutic option in the treatment of refractory depression: two case reports. *Clin Neuropharmacol* 2003; **26**: 230–232.
6. Smith WT, Londborg PD, Glaudin V *et al.* Short-term augmentation of fluoxetine with clonazepam in the treatment of depression: a double-blind study. *Am J Psychiatry* 1998; **155**: 1339–1345.
7. Jahn H, Schick M, Kiefer F *et al.* Metyrapone as additive treatment in major depression. *Arch Gen Psychiatry* 2004; **61**: 1235–1244.
8. Dursun S, Devarajan S, Kutcher S. The 'Dalhousie serotonin cocktail' for treatment-resistant major depressive disorder. *J Psychopharmacol* 2001; **15**: 136–138.
9. Devarajan S, Dursun S. Citalopram plus reboxetine in treatment-resistant depression. *Can J Psychiatry* 2000; **45**: 489–490.
10. Rubio G, San L, Lopez-Munoz F *et al.* Reboxetine adjunct for partial or nonresponders to antidepressant treatment. *J Affect Disorders* 2004; **81**: 67–72.
11. Ostroff RB, Nelson JC. Risperidone augmentation of selective serotonin reuptake inhibitors in major depression. *J Clin Psychiatry* 1999; **60**: 256–259.
12. Stoll AL, Haura G. Tranylcypromine plus risperidone for treatment refractory major depression (Letter). *J Clin Psychopharm* 2000; **20**: 495–497.
13. Sanacora G, Berman RM, Cappiello A *et al.* Addition of the α2-antagonist yohimbine to fluoxetine: effects on rate of antidepressant response. *Neuropsychopharmacology* 2004; **29**: 1166–1171.
14. Papkostas GI, Petersen TJ, Nierenberg AA *et al.* Ziprasidone augmentation of selective serotonin reuptake inhibitors (SSRIs) for SSRI-resistant major depressive disorder. *J Clin Psychiatry* 2004; **65**: 217–221.
15. Appelberg B, Syvalahti E, Koskinen T. Patients with severe depression may benefit from buspirone augmentation of selective serotonin reuptake inhibitors: results from a placebo-controlled, randomized, double-blind, placebo, wash-in study. *J Clin Psychiatry* 2001; **62**: 448–452.
16. Dinan TG, Lavelle E, Cooney J *et al.* Dexamethasone augmentation in treatment-resistant depression. *Acta Psychiatr Scand* 1997; **95**: 58–61.

17. Bodani M, Sheehan B, Philpot M. The use of dexamethasone in elderly patients with antidepressant-resistant depressive illness. *J Psychopharmacol* 1999; **13**: 196–197.
18. Wolkowitz OM, Reus VI, Chan T *et al*. Antiglucocorticoid treatment of depression: double-blind ketoconazole. *Biol Psychiatry* 1999; **45**: 1070–1074.
19. DeBattista C, Lembke A, Solvason HB *et al*. A prospective trial of modafinil as an adjunctive treatment of major depression. *J Clin Psychopharm* 2004; **24**: 87–90.
20. Ninan PT, Hassman HA, Glass SJ *et al*. Adjunctive modafinil at initiation of treatment with a selective serotonin reuptake inhibitor enhances the degree and onset of therapeutic effects in patients with major depressive disorder and fatigue. *J Clin Psychiatry* 2004; **65**: 414–420.
21. Menza MA, Kaufman KR, Castellanos A. Modafinil augmentation of antidepressant treatment in depression. *J Clin Psychiatry* 2000; **61**. 378–381.
22. Nierenberg AA, Papakostas GI, Petersen T *et al*. Nortriptyline for treatment-resistant depression. *J Clin Psychiatry* 2003; **64**: 35–39.
23. Nierenberg AA, Papakostas GI, Petersen T *et al*. Lithium augmentation of nortriptyline for subjects resistant to multiple antidepressants. *J Clin Psychopharm* 2003; **23**: 92–95.
24. Stahl SM. Basic psychopharmacology of antidepressants. II. Oestrogen as an adjunct to antidepressant treatment. *J Clin Psychiatry* 1998; **59**(Suppl. 4): 15–24.
25. Peet M, Horrobin D. A dose ranging study of the effects of ethyl-eicosapentanoate in patients with ongoing depression despite apparently adequate treatment with standard drugs. *Arch Gen Psychiatry* 2002; **59**. 913–919.
26. Su KP, Huang SY, Chiu CC *et al*. Omega-3 fatty acids in major depressive disorder: a preliminary double-blind, placebo-controlled trial. *Eur Neuropsychopharm* 2003; **13**: 267–271.
27. Nemets B, Stahl Z, Belmaker RH. Addition of omega-3 fatty acid to maintenance medication treatment for recurrent unipolar depressive disorder. *Am J Psychiatry* 2002; **159**: 477–479.
28. Whiskey E, Taylor D. Pramipexole in unipolar and bipolar depression. *Psychiatr Bull* 2004; **28**: 438–440.
29. Zarate CA, Payne JL, Quiroz J *et al*. An open-label trial of riluzole in patients with treatment-resistant major depression. *Am J Psychiatry* 2004; **161**: 171–174.
30. Pancheri P, Scapicchio P, Delle Chiaie R. A double-blind, randomized parallel-group, efficacy and safety study of intramuscular S-adenosyl-L-methionine, 1,4-butanedisulphonate (SAMe) versus imipramine in patients with major depressive disorder. *Int J Neuropsychopharm* 2002; **5**. 287–294.
31. Alpert JE, Papakostas G, Mischoulon D *et al*. S-adenosyl-L-methionine (SAMe) as an adjunct for resistant major depressive disorder. An open trial following partial or nonresponse to selective serotonin reuptake inhibitors or venlafaxine. *J Clin Psychopharm* 2004; **24**: 661–664.
32. Taylor D. Selective serotonin reuptake inhibitors and tricyclic antidepressants in combination: interactions and therapeutic uses. *Br J Psychiatry* 1995; **167**: 575–580.
33. Huang CC, Su TP. An open trial of daily left prefrontal cortex repetitive transcranial magnetic stimulation for treating medication-resistant depression. *Eur Psychiatry* 2004; **19**: 523–524.
34. Malhi GS, Bridges PK. Management of resistant depression. *Int J Psychiatry Clin Pract* 1997; **1**: 269–276.
35. Pope HG Jr, Cohane GH, Kanayama G *et al*. Testosterone gel supplementation for men with refractory depression: a randomized, placebo-controlled trial. *Am J Psychiatry* 2003; **160**: 105–111.
36. Matthews K, Eljamel MS. Vagus nerve stimulation and refractory depression. Please can you switch me on doctor? *Br J Psychiatry* 2003; **183**: 181–183.
37. Harrison CL, Ferrier N, Young AH. Tolerability of high-dose venlafaxine in depressed patients. *J Psychopharm* 2004; **18**: 200–204.
38. Fountoulakis KN, Iacovides A, St Kaprinis G. Combined oral venlafaxine and intravenous clomipramine-A: successful temporary response in a patient with extremely refractory depression. *Can J Psychiatry* 2004; **49**: 73–74.

Depression & anxiety

Psychotic depression

The response to tricyclic antidepressants alone in patients with psychotic major depression (PMD) is poorer than in patients with non-psychotic major depression; one meta-analysis found rates to be 35% and 67%, respectively[1]. It is now well established by many studies that the response of PMD to a combination of an antipsychotic and a TCA is superior to either alone[2,3], although this is not entirely undisputed[4]. Amoxapine is a TCA that also has an antipsychotic-like pharmacological profile. While advocated by some as a single agent for PMD, this is based on one underpowered trial suggesting equal efficacy to a tricyclic/antipsychotic combination[5].

PMD is one of the indications for ECT; ECT is at least as effective as combined antidepressant/ antipsychotic therapy[2,6] and may be more effective in psychotic than non-psychotic depression[7]. However, the usual caveats to ECT use apply, including contraindications, side-effects and the tendency to relapse.

There are fewer studies of newer antidepressants and atypical antipsychotics, either alone or in combination, specifically for PMD, although open studies suggest they are also efficacious[8]. A recent large RCT showed response rates of 64% for combined olanzapine and fluoxetine compared to 35% for olanzapine alone and 28% for placebo[9]. There was no fluoxetine alone group.

Long-term outcome is generally poorer for PMD than for simple depression[10].

Novel approaches being developed include those based on antiglucocorticoid strategies; one small open study found rapid effects of the glucocorticoid receptor antagonist mifepristone[11], although these findings have been criticised[12].

There is no specific indication for other therapies or augmentation strategies in PMD over and above that for resistant depression or psychosis seen elsewhere.

References

1. Chan CH, Janicak PG, Davis JM et al. Response of psychotic and nonpsychotic depressed patients to tricyclic antidepressants. J Clin Psychiatry 1987; 48: 197–200.
2. Kroessler DK. Relative efficacy rates for therapies of delusional depression. Conv Ther 1985; 1: 173–182.
3. Spiker DG, Weiss JC, Dealy RS et al. The pharmacological treatment of delusional depression. Am J Psychiatry 1985; 142: 430–436.
4. Mulsant BH, Sweet RA, Rosen J et al. The double-blind randomized comparison of nortriptyline plus perphenazine versus nortriptyline plus placebo in the treatment of psychotic depression in late life. J Clin Psychiatry 2001; 62: 597–604.
5. Anton RF, Burch EA. A comparison study of amoxapine vs amitriptyline plus perphenazine in the treatment of psychotic depression. Am J Psychiatry 1990; 147: 1203–1218.
6. Parker G, Roy K, Hadzi-Pavlovic D et al. Psychotic (delusional) depression: a meta-analysis of physical treatments. J Affect Disorders 1992; 24: 17–24.
7. Petrides G, Fink M, Husain MM et al. ECT remission rates in psychotic versus nonpsychotic depressed patients: a report from CORE. J ECT 2001; 17: 244–253.
8. Wheeler Vega JA, Mortimer AM, Tyson PJ. Somatic treatment of psychotic depression: review and recommendations for practice. J Clin Psychopharm 2000; 20: 504–519.
9. Rothschild AJ, Williamson DJ, Tohen MF et al. A double-blind, randomized study of olanzapine and olanzapine/fluoxetine combination for major depression with psychotic features. J Clin Pyschopharm 2004; 24: 365–373.
10. Flint A, Rifat S. Two-year outcome of psychotic depression in late life. Am J Psychiatry 1998; 155: 178–183.
11. Belanoff JK, Rothschild AJ, Cassidy F et al. An open label trial of C-1073 (mifepristone) for psychotic major depression. Biol Psychiatry 2002; 52: 386–392.
12. Rubin RT. Dr. Rubin replies (Letter). Am J Psychiatry 2004; 161: 1722.

Further reading

Bell MA, Rothschild AJ. Psychotic depression: state-of-the-art algorithm improves odds for remission. *Current Psychiatry Online.* At www.currentpsychiatry.com.

Electroconvulsive therapy (ECT) and psychotropics

The table below summarises the effect of various psychotropics on seizure duration during ECT. Note that there are few well-controlled studies in this area and so recommendations should be viewed with this in mind.

Drug	Effect on ECT seizure duration	Comments[1-10]
Benzodiazepines	Reduced	All may raise seizure threshold and so should be avoided where possible. Many are long-acting and may need to be discontinued some days before ECT. Benzodiazepines may also complicate anaesthesia
		If sedation is required, consider hydroxyzine. If very long term and essential, continue and use higher stimulus
SSRIs	Minimal effect; small increase possible	Generally considered safe to use during ECT. Beware complex pharmacokinetic interactions with anaesthetic agents
Venlafaxine	Minimal effect	Limited data suggest no effect on seizure duration but possibility of increased risk of asystole with doses above 300 mg/day. ECG advised
TCAs	Possibly increased	Few data relevant to ECT but many TCAs lower seizure threshold. TCAs are associated with arrhythmia following ECT and should be avoided in elderly patients and those with cardiac disease. In others, it is preferable to continue TCA treatment during ECT. Close monitoring is essential. Beware hypotension
MAOIs	Minimal effect	Data relating to ECT very limited but long history of ECT use during MAOI therapy
		MAOIs probably do not affect seizure duration but interactions with sympathomimetics occasionally used in anaesthesia are possible and may lead to hypertensive crisis
		MAOIs may be continued during ECT but the anaesthetist must be informed. Beware hypotension
Lithium	Possibly increased	Conflicting data on lithium and ECT. The combination may be more likely to lead to delirium and confusion, and some authorities suggest discontinuing lithium 48 hours before ECT. In the UK, ECT is often used during lithium therapy but starting with a low stimulus and with very close monitoring. The combination is generally well tolerated
		Note that lithium potentiates the effects of non-depolarising neuromuscular blockers such as suxamethonium
Antipsychotics	Possibly increased	Few published data but widely used. Phenothiazines and clozapine are perhaps most likely to prolong seizures, and some suggest withdrawal before ECT. However, safe concurrent use has been reported. ECT and antipsychotics appear generally to be a safe combination
Anticonvulsants	Reduced	If used as a mood-stabiliser, continue but be prepared to use higher energy stimulus. If used for epilepsy, their effect is to normalise seizure threshold. Interactions are possible. Valproate may prolong the effect of thiopental; carbamazepine may inhibit neuromuscular blockade
Barbiturates	Reduced	All barbiturates reduce seizure duration in ECT but are widely used as sedative anaesthetic agents
		Thiopental and methohexital may be associated with cardiac arrhythmia

For drugs known to lower seizure threshold, treatment is best begun with a low-energy stimulus (50 mC). Staff should be alerted to the possibility of prolonged seizures and IV diazepam should be available. With drugs known to elevate seizure threshold, higher stimuli may, of course, be required. Methods are available to lower seizure threshold or prolong seizures[11], but discussion of these is beyond the scope of this book.

ECT frequently causes confusion and disorientation; more rarely, it causes delirium. Close observation is essential. Very limited data support the use of thiamine (200 mg daily) in reducing post-ECT confusion[12]. Ibuprofen may be used to prevent headache[13].

References

1. Bazire S. *Psychotropic Drug Directory*. Salisbury: Fivepin Publishing, 2003.
2. Curran S, Freeman CP. ECT and drugs. In: Freeman CP (ed.) *The ECT Handbook – the Second Report of the Royal College of Psychiatrists' Special Committee on ECT*. Dorchester: Henry Ling Ltd, Dorset Press, 1995.
3. Jarvis MR, Goewert AJ, Zorumski CF. Novel antidepressants and maintenance electroconvulsive therapy. *Ann Clin Psychiatry* 1993; 4: 275–284.
4. Kellner CH, Nixon DW, Bernstein HJ. ECT – drug interactions: a review. *Psychopharmacol Bull* 1991; 27: 595–609.
5. Maidment I. The interaction between psychiatric medicines and ECT. *Hosp Pharm* 1997; 4: 102–105.
6. Welch CA. Electroconvulsive therapy. In: Ciraulo DA, Shader RI, Greenblatt DJ *et al.* (eds). *Drug Interactions in Psychiatry*, 2nd edn. Baltimore, MD: Williams & Wilkins, 1995.
7. Gonzalez-Pinto A, Gutierrez M, Gonzalez N *et al.* Efficacy and safety of venlafaxine–ECT combination in treatment-resistant depression. *J Neuropsych Clin Neurosci* 2002; 14: 206–209.
8. Naguib M, Koorn R. Interactions between psychotropics, anaesthetics and electroconvulsive therapy. *CNS Drugs* 2002; 16: 230–247.
9. Jha AK, Stein GS, Fenwick P. Negative interaction between lithium and electroconvulsive therapy – a case-control study. *Br J Psychiatry* 1996; 168: 241–243.
10. Dolenc TJ, Habl SS, Barnes RD *et al.* Electroconvulsive therapy in patients taking monoamine oxidase inhibitors. *J ECT* 2004; 20: 258–261.
11. Datta C, Rai AK, Ilivicky HJ *et al.* Augmentation of seizure induction in electroconvulsive therapy: a clinical reappraisal. *J ECT* 2002; 18: 118–125.
12. Linton CR, Reynolds MTP, Warner NJ. Using thiamine to reduce post-ECT confusion. *Int J Geriatr Psychiat* 2002; 17: 189–192.
13. Leung M, Hollander Y, Brown GR. Pretreatment with ibuprofen to prevent electroconvulsive therapy-induced headache. *J Clin Psychiatry* 2003; 64: 551–553.

Further reading

National Institute for Clinical Excellence. Guidance on the use of electroconvulsive therapy. Technology Appraisal 59, April 2003.
Patra KK, Coffey CE. Implications of herbal alternative medicine for electroconvulsive therapy. *J ECT* 2004; 20: 186–194.

Depression & anxiety

Antidepressant-induced hyponatraemia

Most antidepressants have been associated with hyponatraemia. The mechanism of this adverse effect is probably the syndrome of inappropriate secretion of antidiuretic hormone (SIADH). Hyponatraemia is a rare but potentially serious adverse effect of antidepressants that demands careful monitoring, particularly in those patients at greatest risk (see table below).

Table   Risk factors[1–4]
Old age
Female sex
Low body weight
Some drug treatments *(e.g. diuretics, NSAIDs, carbamazepine, cancer chemotherapy)*
Reduced renal function *(especially acute and chronic renal failure)*
Medical co-morbidity (e.g. *hypothyroidism, diabetes, COPD, hypertension, head injury, CVA, various cancers*)
Warm weather (summer)

Antidepressants

No antidepressant has been shown *not* to be associated with hyponatraemia and most have a reported association[5]. It has been suggested that serotonergic drugs are relatively more likely to cause hyponatraemia[6,7], although this is disputed[8]. There are certainly literature reports of hyponatraemia occurring with noradrenergic drugs[9,10].

Monitoring

All patients taking antidepressants should be observed for signs of hyponatraemia (dizziness, nausea, lethargy, confusion, cramps, seizures). Serum sodium should be determined (at baseline and 2 and 4 weeks, and then 3-monthly[11]) for those at high risk of drug-induced hyponatraemia. The high-risk factors are as follows:

- extreme old age (>80 years)
- history of hyponatraemia
- co-therapy with other drugs known to be associated with hyponatraemia (as above)
- reduced renal function (GFR < 50 ml/min)
- medical co-morbidity (as above).

Note that hyponatraemia is common in elderly patients so monitoring is essential[12,13].

Treatment[14]

Withdraw antidepressant immediately (note risk of discontinuation effects which may complicate clinical picture):

- If serum sodium is >125 mmol/l – monitor sodium daily until normal.
- If serum sodium is <125 mmol/l – refer to specialist medical care.

Restarting treatment

- Consider ECT.
- Prescribe a drug from a different class. Consider noradrenergic drugs such as reboxetine and lofepramine. Begin with a low dose, increasing slowly, and monitor closely. If hyponatraemia recurs and continued antidepressant use is essential, consider water restriction and/or careful use of demeclocycline (see *BNF*).

Other psychotropics

Carbamazepine has a well-known association with SIADH. Note also that antipsychotic use has been linked to hyponatraemia[15-17] (see page 104).

References

1. Spigset O, Hedenmalm K. Hyponatraemia in relation to treatment with antidepressants: a survey of reports in the World Health Organization data base for spontaneous reporting of adverse drug reactions. *Pharmacotherapy* 1997; 17: 348–352.
2. Madhusoodanan S, Bogunovic OJ, Moise D *et al.* Hyponatraemia associated with psychotropic medications: a review of the literature and spontaneous reports. *Adverse Drug React Toxicological Rev* 2002; 21: 17–29.
3. Wilkinson TJ, Begg EJ, Winter AC *et al.* Risk factors with hyponatraemia with SSRIs assessed. *Br J Clin Pharmacol* 1999; 47: 211–217.
4. McAskill R, Taylor D. Psychotropics and hyponatraemia. *Psychiatr Bull* 1997; 21: 33–35.
5. Thomas A, Verbalis JG. Hyponatraemia and the syndrome of inappropriate antidiuretic hormone secretion associated with drug therapy in psychiatric patients. *CNS Drugs* 1995; 5: 357–369.
6. Movig KLL, Leufkens HGM, Lenderink AW *et al.* Serotonergic antidepressants associated with an increased risk for hyponatraemia in the elderly. *Eur J Clin Pharmacol* 2002; 58: 143–148.
7. Movig KLL, Leufkens HGM, Lenderink AW *et al.* Association between antidepressant drug use and hyponatraemia: a case-control study. *Br J Clin Pharmacol* 2002; 53: 363–369.
8. Kirby D, Ames D. Hyponatraemia and selective serotonin re-uptake inhibitors in elderly patients. *Int J Geriatr Psychiat* 2001; 16: 484–493.
9. Ranieri P, Franzoni S, Trabucchi M. Reboxetine and hyponatremia. *New Engl J Med.* 2000; 342: 215–216.
10. Liskin B, Walsh BT, Roose SP *et al.* Imipramine-induced inappropriate ADH secretion. *J Clin Psychopharm* 1984; 4: 146–147.
11. Arinzon ZH, Yehoshua AL, Fidelman ZG. Delayed recurrent SIADH associated with SSRIs. *Ann Pharmacother* 2002; 36: 1175–1177.
12. Fabian TJ, Amico JA, Kroboth PD *et al.* Paroxetine-induced hyponatremia in older adults. *Arch Intern Med* 2004; 164: 327–332.
13. Fabian TJ, Amico JA, Kroboth PD *et al.* Paroxetine-induced hyponatremia in the elderly due to the syndrome of inappropriate secretion of antidiuretic hormone (SIADH). *J Geriat Psychiat Neurol* 2003; 16: 160–164.
14. Sharma H, Pompei P. Antidepressant-induced hyponatraemia in the aged. *Drugs Aging* 1996; 8: 430–435.
15. Ohsawa H, Kishimoto T, Motoharu H *et al.* An epidemiological study on hyponatremia in psychiatric patients in mental hospitals in Nara Prefecture. *J J Psychiat Neurol* 1992; 46: 883–889.
16. Leadbetter RA, Shutty MS. Differential effects of neuroleptics and clozapine on polydipsia and intermittent hyponatraemia. *J Clin Psychiatry* 1994; 55: 110–113.
17. Collins A, Anderson J. SIADH induced by two atypical antipsychotics. *Int J Geriat Psychiat* 2000; 15: 282–285.

Further reading

Anon. Management of antipsychotic drug-induced SIADH. *Drug Therapy Perspectives* 1985; 6: 12–16.
Wee R, Lim WK. Selective serotonin re-uptake inhibitors (SSRIs) and hyponatraemia in the elderly. *Int J Geriat Psychiat* 2004; 19: 590–591.

Depression & anxiety

Post-stroke depression

Post-stroke depression is a common problem seen in at least 30–40% of survivors of intracerebral haemorrhage[1,2]. Depression probably slows functional rehabilitation[3], but antidepressants may be beneficial through relieving depressive symptoms and allowing faster rehabilitation[4].

Prophylaxis

The high incidence of depression after stroke makes prophylaxis worthy of consideration. Nortriptyline, fluoxetine and sertraline may prevent post-stroke depression[5,6], but data are very limited. Mianserin seems ineffective[7] but mirtazapine may protect against depressive episodes and treat them[8]. Amitriptyline appears to prevent central post-stroke pain[9].

Treatment

Treatment is complicated by medical co-morbidity and by the potential for interaction with other co-prescribed drugs (especially warfarin). Contraindication to antidepressant treatment seems to be substantially more likely with tricyclics than with SSRIs[10]. Fluoxetine[11], citalopram[12] and nortriptyline[13] are probably the most studied and seem to be effective. SSRIs and nortriptyline are widely recommended for post-stroke depression. Despite early fears, SSRIs seem not to increase risk of stroke[14], although some doubt remains[15].

Post-stroke depression – recommended drugs

SSRIs*
Nortriptyline

* If patient is also taking warfarin, suggest citalopram[16].

References

1. Gainotti G, Antonucci G, Marra C et al. Relation between depression after stroke, antidepressant therapy, and functional recovery. *J Neurol Neurosurg Psychiatry* 2001; **71**: 258–261.
2. Hayee MA, Akhtar N, Haque A et al. Depression after stroke – analysis of 297 stroke patients. *Bangladesh Med Res Council Bull* 2001; **27**: 96–102.
3. Paolucci S, Antonucci G, Grasso MG et al. Post-stroke depression, antidepressant treatment and rehabilitation results: a case-control study. *Cerebrovasc Dis* 2001; **12**: 264–271.
4. Gainotti G, Marra C. Determinants and consequences of post-stroke depression. *Curr Opin Neurol* 2002; **15**: 85–89.
5. Narushima K, Kosier JT, Robinson RG. Preventing poststroke depression: a 12-week double-blind randomized treatment trial and 21-month follow-up. *J Nerv Ment Dis* 2002; **190**: 296–303.
6. Rasmussen A, Lunde M, Poulsen DL et al. A double-blind, placebo-controlled study of sertraline in the prevention of depression in stroke patients. *Psychosomatics* 2003; **44**: 216–221.
7. Palomaki H, Kaste M, Berg A et al. Prevention of poststroke depression: 1 year randomised placebo controlled double blind trial of mianserin with 6 month follow up after therapy. *J Neurol Neurosurg Psychiatry* 1999; **66**: 490–494.
8. Niedermaier N, Bohrer E, Schulte K et al. Prevention and treatment of poststroke depression with mirtazapine in patients with acute stroke. *J Clin Psychiatry* 2004; **65**: 1619–1623.
9. Lampl C, Yazdi K, Röper C. Amitriptyline in the prophylaxis of central poststroke pain: preliminary results of 39 patients in a placebo-controlled, long-term study. *Stroke* 2002; **33**: 3030–3032.
10. Cole MG, Elie LM, McCusker J et al. Feasibility and effectiveness of treatments for post-stroke depression in elderly inpatients: systematic review. *J Geriatr Psychiat Neurol* 2001; **14**: 37–41.

11. Wiart L, Petit H, Joseph PA *et al.* Fluoxetine in early poststroke depression: a double-blind placebo-controlled study. *Stroke* 2000; **31**: 1829–1832.
12. Andersen G, Vestergaard K, Lauritzen L. Effective treatment of poststroke depression with the selective serotonin reuptake inhibitor citalopram. *Stroke* 1994; **25**: 1099–1104.
13. Robinson R, Schultz SK, Castillo C *et al.* Nortriptyline versus fluoxetine in the treatment of depression and in short-term recovery after stroke: a placebo-controlled, double blind study. *Am J Psychiatry* 2000; **157**: 351–359.
14. Bak S, Tsiropoulos I, Kjaersgaard JO *et al.* Selective serotonin reuptake inhibitors and the risk of stroke: a population-based case-control study. *Stroke* 2002; **33**: 1465–1473.
15. Ramasubbu R. SSRI treatment-associated stroke: causality assessment in two cases. *Ann Pharmacother* 2004; **38**: 1197–1201.
16. Sayal KS, Duncan-McConnell DA, McConnell HW *et al.* Psychotropic interactions with warfarin. *Acta Psychiatr Scand* 2000; **102**: 250–255.

Treatment of depression in the elderly

The prevalence of most physical illnesses increases with age. Many physical problems such as cardio-vascular disease, chronic pain and Parkinson's disease are associated with a high risk of depressive illness[1]. The morbidity and mortality associated with depression are increased, as the elderly are more physically frail and therefore more likely to suffer serious consequences from self-neglect (e.g. life-threatening dehydration or hypothermia) and immobility (e.g. venous stasis). Almost 20% of completed suicides occur in the elderly[2].

The elderly may take longer to respond to antidepressants than younger adults[3] and may require to be treated for longer periods overall. Flint and Rifat[4] found that, of a cohort of elderly people who had recovered from a first episode of depression and had received antidepressants for 2 years, 60% relapsed within 2 years if antidepressant treatment was withdrawn. Lower doses of antidepressants may be effective as prophylaxis. Dothiepin (dosulepin) 75 mg/day has been shown to be effective in this regard[5]. There is no evidence to suggest that the response to antidepressants is reduced in the physically ill[6], although outcome in the elderly in general is often suboptimal[7,8].

There is no ideal antidepressant. All are associated with problems (see table on page 164). Choice is determined by the individual clinical circumstances of each patient, particularly physical co-morbidity and concomitant medication (both prescribed and 'over the counter').

References

1. Katona C, Livingston G. Impact of screening old people with physical illness for depression. *Lancet* 2000; **356**: 91–92.
2. Cattell H, Jolley DJ. One hundred cases of suicide in elderly people. *Br J Psychiatry* 1995; **166**: 451–457.
3. Paykel ES, Raman R, Cooper Z *et al.* Residual symptoms after partial remission: an important outcome in depression. *Psychol Med* 1995; **25**: 1171–1180.
4. Flint AJ, Rifat SL. Recurrence of first-episode geriatric depression after discontinuation of maintenance antidepressants. *Am J Psychiatry* 1999; **156**: 943–945.
5. Old Age Depression Special Interest Group. How long should the elderly take antidepressants? A double blind placebo controlled study of continuation/prophylaxis therapy with dothiepin. *Br J Psychiatry* 1993; **162**: 175–182.
6. Evans M, Hammond M, Wilson K *et al.* Placebo-controlled treatment trial of depression in elderly physically ill patients. *Int J Geriatr Psychiat* 1997; **12**: 817–824.
7. Heeren TJ, Derksen P, Heycop TH *et al.* Treatment, outcome and predictors of response in elderly depressed in-patients. *Br J Psychiatry* 1997; **170**: 436–440.
8. Tuma TA. Outcome of hospital-treated depression at 4.5 years: an elderly and a younger adult cohort compared. *Br J Psychiatry* 2000; **178**: 224–228.

Further reading

Movig KL, Leufkens HG, Lenderink AW. Serotonergic antidepressants associated with an increased risk of hyponatraemia in the elderly. *Eur J Clin Pharmacol* 2002; **58**: 143–148.

National Service Framework for Older People. London: Department of Health (a whole supplement dedicated to the use of medicines in older people), 2001.

Pacher P, Ungvari Z. Selective serotonin reuptake inhibitor antidepressants increase the risk of falls and hip fractures in elderly people by inhibiting cardiovascular ion channels. *Med Hypotheses* 2001; **57**: 469–471.

Spina E, Scordo MG. Clinically significant drug interactions with antidepressants in the elderly. *Drugs Aging* 2002; **19**: 299–320.

Van Walraven C, Mamdani MM, Wells PS *et al.* Inhibition of serotonin re-uptake by antidepressants and upper gastrointestinal bleeding in elderly patients: retrospective cohort study. *BMJ* 2001; **323**: 655–658.

Wilson K, Mottram P, Sivanranthan A *et al.* Antidepressants versus placebo for depressed elderly (Cochrane review). In: *Cochrane Database of Systematic Reviews*. Issue 2, 2002; Update Software.

Depression & anxiety

Table Antidepressants and the elderly

	Anticholinergic side-effect (urinary retention, dry mouth, blurred vision, constipation)	Postural hypotension	Sedation
Older tricyclics	Variable: moderate with nortriptyline, imipramine and dosulepin (dothiepin). Marked with others	All can cause postural hypotension Dosage titration is required	Variable: from minimal with imipramine to profound with trimipramine
Lofepramine	Moderate, although constipation/sweating can be severe	Can be a problem but generally better tolerated than the older tricyclics	Minimal
SSRIs	Dry mouth can be a problem with paroxetine	Much less of a problem, but an increased risk of falls is documented with SSRIs	Can be a problem with paroxetine Unlikely with the other SSRIs
Others	Minimal with mirtazapine and venlafaxine. Can be rarely a problem with reboxetine Duloxetine – few effects	Hypotension not a problem with venlafaxine but it can increase BP at higher doses No effect with duloxetine	Mirtazapine, mianserin and trazodone are sedative Duloxetine – neutral effects

Weight gain	Safety in overdose	Other side-effects	Drug interactions
All tricyclics can cause weight gain	Dothiepin and amitriptyline are the most toxic (seizures and cardiac arrhythmia)	Seizures, anticholinergic-induced cognitive impairment	Mainly pharmacodynamic: increased sedation with benzodiazepines, increased hypotension with diuretics, increased constipation with other anticholinergic drugs, etc.
Few data, but lack of spontaneous reports may indicate less potential than the older tricyclics	Relatively safe	Raised LFTs	
Paroxetine and possibly citalopram may cause weight gain Others are weight neutral	Safe with the possible exception of citalopram (one minor metabolite is possibly cardiotoxic)	GI effects and headaches, hyponatraemia, increased risk of GI bleeds in the elderly, orofacial dyskinesia with paroxetine	Fluvoxamine, fluoxetine and paroxetine are potent inhibitors of several hepatic cytochrome enzymes (see page 183). Sertraline is safer and citalopram is the safest
Greatest problem is with mirtazapine	All are relatively safe	Insomnia and hypokalaemia with reboxetine	Duloxetine inhibits CYP2D6 Moclobemide and venlafaxine inhibit CYP450 enzymes Check for potential interactions Reboxetine is safe

Cardiac effects of antidepressants

Drug	Heart rate	Blood pressure	QTc
Tricyclics[1,2]	Increase in heart rate	Postural hypotension	Prolongation of QTc interval
Lofepramine[1,3]	Modest increase in heart rate	Less decrease in postural blood pressure compared with other TCAs	Can possibly prolong QTc interval at higher doses *(desipramine is main metabolite)*
MAOIs[1]	Decrease in heart rate	Postural hypotension. Risk of hypertensive crisis	Unclear but may shorten QTc interval
Fluoxetine[4–6]	Small decrease in mean heart rate	Minimal effect on blood pressure	No effect on QTc interval
Paroxetine[7,8]	Small decrease in mean heart rate	Minimal effect on blood pressure	No effect on QTc interval
Sertraline[9,10]	Minimal effect on heart rate	Minimal effect on blood pressure	No effect on QTc interval
Citalopram[11]	Small decrease in heart rate	Slight drop in systolic blood pressure	No effect on QTc interval in normal doses
Fluvoxamine[12]	Minimal effect on heart rate	Small drops in systolic blood pressure	No significant effect on QTc
Venlafaxine[13,14]	Marginally increased	Some increase in postural blood pressure. At higher doses increase in blood pressure	Possible prolongation in overdose – data unclear
Duloxetine[15–17]	Slight increase	No significant effect	No effect on QTc
Mirtazapine[18]	Minimal change in heart rate	Minimal effect on blood pressure	No effect on QTc interval
Reboxetine[19,20]	Significant increase in heart rate	Marginal increase in both systolic and diastolic blood pressure. Postural decrease at higher doses	Unclear
Moclobemide[21,22]	Marginal decrease in heart rate	Minimal effect on blood pressure. Isolated cases of hypertensive episodes	No effect on QTc interval
Trazodone[1]	Decrease in heart rate more common, although increase can also occur	Can cause significant postural hypotension	Can prolong QTc interval

Notes: SSRIs are generally recommended in cardiac disease but beware cytochrome-mediated interactions with co-administered cardiac drugs. SSRIs may protect against myocardial infarction[23], and untreated depression worsens prognosis in cardiovascular disease[24]. Treatment of depression with SSRIs should not therefore be

Arrhythmia	Conduction disturbance	Licensed restrictions post-MI	Comments
Class I anti-arrhythmic activity	Slows down cardiac conduction	CI in patients with recent MI	TCAs affect cardiac contractility. Some TCAs linked to ischaemic heart disease. Association with sudden cardiac death
May occur at higher doses	Benign effect on cardiac conduction	CI in patients with recent MI	Less cardiotoxic than other TCAs. Reasons unclear
May cause arrhythmia and decrease LVF	No clear effect on cardiac conduction	Use with caution in patients with cardiovascular disease	
Few cases reported in literature	None	Caution. Clinical experience is limited	Safe post MI
None	None	General caution in cardiac patients	Safe post MI
None	None	None – probably drug of choice	Safe post MI
None	None	Caution, although no ECG changes	Minor metabolite which may ↑ QTc interval
None	None	Caution	Limited changes in ECG have been observed
Some reports of cardiac arrhythmia	Rare reports of conduction abnormalities	Caution. Has not been evaluated in post-MI patients	Evidence for arrhythmogenic potential is very slim and disputed
None	None	Caution in patients with recent MI	Limited clinical experience
None	None	Caution in patients with recent MI	
Rhythm abnormalities may occur	Atrial and ventricular ectopic beats, especially in the elderly	Caution in patient with cardiac disease	
None	None	None	
Several case reports of arrhythmia	May have a minimal effect on cardiac conduction	Care in patients with severe cardiac disease	May be arrhythmogenic in patients with pre-existing cardiac disease

withheld post-MI. Protective effects of treatment of depression post-MI appear to relate to antidepressant administration: CBT may be ineffective in this respect[25]. Note that the mild anti-coagulant effect of SSRIs may have adverse consequences too: upper GI bleeding is more common in those taking SSRIs[26].

References

1. Warrington SJ, Padgham C, Lader M. The cardiovascular effects of antidepressants. *Psychol Med* 1989; Suppl. 16 (monograph).
2. Hippisley-Cox J, Pringle M, Hammersley V *et al.* Antidepressants as a risk factor for ischaemic heart disease in primary care. *BMJ* 2001; 323: 666–669.
3. Stern H, Konetschny J, Herrmann L *et al.* Cardiovascular effects of single doses of the antidepressants amitriptyline and lofepramine in healthy subjects. *Pharmacopsychiatry* 1985; 18: 272–277.
4. Fisch C. Effect of fluoxetine on the electrocardiogram. *J Clin Psychiatry* 1985; 46: 42–44.
5. Ellison ME, Milofsky JE, Ely E. Fluoxetine-induced bradycardia and syncope in two patients. *J Clin Psychiatry* 1990; 51: 385–386.
6. Roose SP, Glassman AH, Attia E *et al.* Cardiovascular effects of fluoxetine in depressed patients with heart disease. *Am J Psychiatry* 1998; 155: 660–665.
7. Kuhs H, Rudolf GA. Cardiovascular effects of paroxetine. *Psychopharmacology* 1990; 102: 379–382.
8. Roose SP, Laghrissi-Thode F, Kennedy JS *et al.* Comparison of paroxetine and nortriptyline in depressed patients with ischemic heart disease. *J Am Med Assoc* 1998; 279: 287–291.
9. Shapiro PA, Lespérance F, Frasure-Smith N *et al.* An open-label preliminary trial of sertraline for treatment of major depression after acute myocardial infarction (the SADHAT trial). *Am Heart J* 1999; 137: 1100–1106.
10. Glassman AH, O'Connor CM, Califf RM *et al.* Sertraline treatment of major depression in patients with acute MI or unstable angina. *J Am Med Assoc* 2002; 288: 701–709.
11. Rasmussen SL, Overø KF, Tanghøj P. Cardiac safety of citalopram: prospective trials and retrospective analyses. *J Clin Psychopharmacol* 1999; 19: 407–415.
12. Strik JJ, Honig A, Lousberg R *et al.* Cardiac side effects of two selective serotonin reuptake inhibitors in middle-aged and elderly patients. *Int Clin Psychopharmacol* 1998; 13: 263–267.
13. ABPI. Venlafaxine SPC. *Compendium of Data Sheets and Summaries of Product Characteristics,* 1999.
14. Khawaja IS, Feinstein RE. Cardiovascular effects of selective serotonin reuptake inhibitors and other novel antidepressants. *Heart Disease* 2003; 5: 153–160.
15. Sharma A, Goldberg MJ, Cerimele BJ. Pharmacokinetics and safety of duloxetine, a dual-serotonin and norepinephrine reuptake inhibitor. *J Clin Pharmacol* 2000; 40: 161–167.
16. Schatzberg AF. Efficacy and tolerability of duloxetine, a novel dual reuptake inhibitor in the treatment of major depressive disorder. *J Clin Psychiatry* 2003; 64: 30–37.
17. Detke MJ, Lu Y, Goldstein DJ *et al.* Duloxetine, 60 mg once daily, for major depressive disorder: a randomised double-blind placebo-controlled trial. *J Clin Psychiatry* 2002; 63: 308–315.
18. Montgomery SA. Safety of mirtazapine: a review. *Int Clin Psychopharmacol* 1995; 10(Suppl. 4): 37–45.
19. Mucci M. Reboxetine: a review of antidepressant tolerability. *J Psychopharmacol* 1997; 11(Suppl. 4): S33–S37.
20. Holm KJ, Spencer CM. Reboxetine: a review of its use in depression. *CNS Drugs* 1999; 12: 65–83.
21. Moll E, Neumann N, Schmid-Burgk W *et al.* Safety and efficacy during long-term treatment with moclobemide. *Clin Neuropharmacol* 1994; 17(Suppl. 1): S74–S87.
22. Hilton S, Jaber B, Ruch R. Moclobemide safety: monitoring a newly developed product in the 1990s. *J Clin Psychopharmacol* 1995; 15(Suppl. 2): 76S–83S.
23. Sauer WH, Berlin JA, Kimmel SE. Selective serotonin inhibitors and myocardial infarction. *Circulation* 2001; 104: 1894–1898.
24. Davies SJC, Jackson PR, Potokar J *et al.* Treatment of anxiety and depressive disorders in patients with cardiovascular disease. *BMJ* 2004; 328: 939–943.
25. ENRICHD Investigators. Effects of treating depression and low perceived social support on clinical events after myocardial infarction. The enhancing recovery in coronary heart disease patients (ENRICHD) randomized trial. *J Am Med Assoc* 2003; 289: 3106–3116.
26. Dalton SO, Johansen C, Mellemkjaer L. Use of selective serotonin reuptake inhibitors and risk of upper gastrointestinal tract bleeding: a population-based study. *Arch Intern Med* 2003; 163: 59–64.

Further reading

Alvarez W, Pickworth KK. Safety of antidepressant drugs in the patient with cardiac disease. *Pharmacotherapy* 2003; 23: 754–771.
Roose SP. Treatment of depression in patients with heart disease. *Biol Psychiatry* 2003; 54: 262–268.
Von Kanel R. Platelet hyperactivity in clinical depression and the beneficial effect of antidepressant drug treatment: how strong is the evidence? *Acta Psychiatr Scand* 2004; 110: 163–177.

Antidepressants and sexual dysfunction

Primary sexual disorders are common, although reliable normative data are lacking[1]. Reported prevalence rates vary depending on the method of data collection (low numbers with spontaneous reports, increasing with confidential questionnaires and further still with direct questioning)[1,2]. Physical illness, psychiatric illness, substance misuse and prescribed drug treatment can all cause sexual dysfunction[1,2]. Baseline sexual functioning should be determined, if possible (questionnaires may be useful), because sexual function can affect quality of life and compliance (sexual dysfunction is one of the major causes of treatment dropout[3]). Complaints of sexual dysfunction may also indicate progression or inadequate treatment of underlying medical or psychiatric conditions. It may also be the result of drug treatment and intervention may greatly improve quality of life[4]. The normal human sexual response is described on page 99.

Effects of depression

Both depression and the drugs used to treat it can cause disorders of desire, arousal and orgasm. The precise nature of the sexual dysfunction may indicate whether depression or treatment is the more likely cause. For example, 40–50% of people with depression report diminished libido and problems regarding sexual arousal in the month before diagnosis, compared with only 15–20% who experience orgasm problems prior to taking an antidepressant[5].

Effects of antidepressant drugs

Antidepressants can cause sedation, hormonal changes, disturbance of cholinergic/adrenergic balance, peripheral alpha-adrenergic antagonism, inhibition of nitric oxide and increased serotonin neurotransmission, all of which can result in sexual dysfunction[6]. Sexual dysfunction has been reported as a side-effect of all antidepressants, although rates vary (see table below). Individual susceptibility also varies and all effects are reversible.

Not all of the sexual side-effects of antidepressants are undesirable[1]: serotonergic antidepressants are effective in the treatment of premature ejaculation and may also be beneficial in paraphilias.

Table Sexual adverse effects of antidepressant drugs

Drug	Approximate prevalence	Type of problem
Tricyclics[7–10]	30%	Decreased libido, erectile dysfunction, delayed orgasm, impaired ejaculation. Prevalence of delayed orgasm with clomipramine may be double that with other TCAs. Painful ejaculation reported rarely
Trazodone[3,11–13]	Unknown	Impaired ejaculation and both increases and decreases in libido reported. Used in some cases to promote erection. Priapism occurs in approximately 0.01%
MAOIs[3,14]	40%	Similar to TCAs, although prevalence may be higher[1]. Moclobemide much less likely to cause problems than older MAOIs (4% v 40%)
SSRIs[3,15–18]	60–70%	Decreased libido and delayed orgasm. Paroxetine is associated with more erectile dysfunction and decreased vaginal lubrication than the other SSRIs. High prevalence with SSRIs may be due to selective reporting. Difficult to determine relative prevalence but there is evidence that ejaculatory delay is worse with paroxetine than citalopram[19] Penile anaesthesia has been reported rarely with fluoxetine
Venlafaxine[3]	70%	Decreased libido and delayed orgasm common. Erectile dysfunction less common
Mirtazapine[3,16]	25%	Decreased libido and delayed orgasm possible. Erectile dysfunction less common
Reboxetine[20]	5–10%	Various abnormalities of orgasmic function

Treatment

Spontaneous remission occurs in approximately 10% of cases and partial remission in a further 11%[3]. If this does not happen, the dose may be reduced or the antidepressant discontinued where appropriate.

Drug 'holidays' or delayed dosing may be used[21]. This approach is problematic as the patient may relapse or experience antidepressant discontinuation symptoms. More logical is a switch to a different drug that is less likely to cause the specific sexual problem experienced (see table above). Note that amfebutamone (buproprion – not licensed for depression in UK) may have the lowest risk of sexual dysfunction[22] among newer antidepressants. Data relating to duloxetine are limited at the time of writing.

Adjunctive or 'antidote' drugs may also be used (see page 101 for further information).

References

1. Baldwin DS, Thomas SC, Birtwistle J. Effects of antidepressant drugs on sexual function. *Int J Psychiatry Clin Pract* 1997; **1**: 47–58.
2. Pollack MH, Reiter S, Hammerness P. Genitourinary and sexual adverse effects of psychotropic medication. *Int J Psychiat Med* 1992; **22**: 305–327.
3. Montejo AL, Llorca G, Izquierdo JA *et al*. Incidence of sexual dysfunction associated with antidepressant agents: a prospective multicentre study of 1022 outpatients. *J Clin Psychiatry* 2001; **62**(Suppl. 3): 10–20.
4. Segraves RT. Effects of psychotropic drugs on human erection and ejaculation. *Arch Gen Psychiatry* 1989; **46**: 275–284.
5. Kennedy SH, Dickens SE, Eisfeld BS *et al*. Sexual dysfunction before antidepressant therapy in major depression. *J Affect Disorders* 1999; **56**: 201–208.
6. Clayton AH. Recognition and assessment of sexual dysfunction associated with depression. *J Clin Psychiatry* 2001; **62**: 5–9.
7. Harrison WM, Rabkin JG, Ehrhardt AA *et al*. Effects of antidepressant medication on sexual function: a controlled study. *J Clin Psychopharmacol* 1986; **6**: 144–149.
8. Beaumont G. Sexual side effects of clomipramine. *J Int Med Res* 1977; **51**: 37–44.
9. Rickels K, Robinson DS, Schweizer E *et al*. Nefazodone: aspects of efficacy. *J Clin Psychiatry* 1995; **56**(Suppl. 6): 43–46.
10. Sovner R. Anorgasmia associated with imipramine but not desipramine: case report. *J Clin Psychiatry* 1983; **44**: 345–346.
11. Garbell N. Increased libido in women receiving trazodone. *Am J Psychiatry* 1986; **143**: 781–782.
12. Sullivan G. Increased libido in three men treated with trazodone. *J Clin Psychiatry* 1988; **49**: 202–203.
13. Thompson JW, Ware MR, Blashfield RK. Psychotropic medication and priapism: a comprehensive review. *J Clin Psychiatry* 1990; **51**: 430–433.
14. Lesko LM, Stotland NL, Segraves RT. Three cases of female anorgasmia associated with MAOIs. *Am J Psychiatry* 1982; **139**: 1353–1354.
15. Herman JB, Brotman AW, Pollack MH *et al*. Fluoxetine induced sexual dysfunction. *J Clin Psychiatry* 1990; **51**: 25–27.
16. Gelenberg AJ, Laukes C, McGahuey C *et al*. Mirtazepine substitution in SSRI-induced sexual dysfunction. *J Clin Psychiatry* 2000; **61**: 356–360.
17. Jacobsen FM. Fluoxetine-induced sexual dysfunction and an open trial of yohimbine. *J Clin Psychiatry* 1992; **53**: 119–122.
18. Lauerma H. Successful treatment of citalopram-induced anorgasmia by cyproheptadine. *Acta Psychiatr Scand* 1996; **93**: 69–70.
19. Waldinger MD, Zwinderman AH, Olivier B. SSRIs and ejaculation: a double-blind, randomized, fixed-dose study with paroxetine and citalopram. *J Clin Psychopharmacol* 2001; **21**: 556–560.
20. Haberfellner EM. Sexual dysfunction caused by reboxetine. *Pharmacopsychiat* 2002; **35**: 77–78.
21. Rothschild AJ. Selective serotonin reuptake inhibitor-induced sexual dysfunction: efficacy of a drug holiday. *Am J Psychiatry* 1995; **152**: 1514–1516.
22. Clayton AH, Pradko JF, Croft HA *et al*. Prevalence of sexual dysfunction among newer antidepressants. *J Clin Psychiatry* 2002; **63**: 357–366.

Further reading

Fava M, Rankin M. Sexual functioning and SSRIs. *J Clin Psychiatry* 2002; **63**(Suppl. 5): 13–16.

Antidepressants – swapping and stopping

General guidelines

- All antidepressants have the potential to cause withdrawal phenomena. When taken continuously *for 6 weeks or longer,* antidepressants should not be stopped abruptly unless a serious adverse event has occurred (e.g. cardiac arrhythmia with a tricyclic). (See page 176.)
- When changing from one antidepressant to another, abrupt withdrawal should usually be avoided. Cross-tapering is preferred, in which the dose of the ineffective or poorly tolerated drug is slowly reduced while the new drug is slowly introduced.

Example		Week 1	Week 2	Week 3	Week 4
Withdrawing dosulepin	150 mg OD	100 mg OD	50 mg OD	25 mg OD	Nil
Introducing citalopram	Nil	10 mg OD	10 mg OD	20 mg OD	20 mg OD

- The speed of cross-tapering is best judged by monitoring patient tolerability. No clear guidelines are available, so caution is required.
- Note that the co-administration of some antidepressants, even when cross-tapering, is absolutely contraindicated. In other cases, theoretical risks or lack of experience preclude recommending cross-tapering.
- In some cases cross-tapering may not be considered necessary. An example is when switching from one SSRI to another: their effects are so similar that administration of the second drug is likely to ameliorate withdrawal effects of the first. However, there is little firm evidence of this occurring.
- Potential dangers of simultaneously administering two antidepressants include pharmacodynamic interactions (serotonin syndrome[1–4], hypotension, drowsiness) and pharmacokinetic interactions (e.g. elevation of tricyclic plasma levels by some SSRIs).

Serotonin syndrome – symptoms[1,2]	
Increasing severity ↓	Restlessness Diaphoresis Tremor Shivering Myoclonus Confusion Convulsions Death

- The advice given in the following table should be treated with caution and patients should be very carefully monitored when switching.

References

1. Sternbach H. The serotonin syndrome. *Am J Psychiatry* 1999; **148**: 705–713.
2. Mir S, Taylor D. Serotonin syndrome. *Psychiatr Bull* 1999; **23**: 742–747.
3. Pan JJ. Serotonin syndrome induced by low-dose venlafaxine. *Ann Pharmacother* 2003; **37**: 209–211.
4. Houlihan DJ. Serotonin syndrome resulting from coadministration of tramadol, venlafaxine, and mirtazapine. *Ann Pharmacother* 2004; **38**: 411–413.

Depression & anxiety

Table   Antidepressants – swapping and stopping[*]

To From	MAOIs- hydrazines	Tranyl- cypromine[a]	Tricyclics	Citalopram/ escitalopram	Fluoxetine	Paroxetine
MAOIs- hydrazines	Withdraw and wait for 2 weeks	Withdraw and wait for 2 weeks	Withdraw and wait for 2 weeks	Withdraw and wait for 2 weeks	Withdraw and wait for 2 weeks	Withdraw and wait for 2 weeks
Tranyl- Cypromine	Withdraw and wait for 2 weeks	–	Withdraw and wait for 2 weeks	Withdraw and wait for 2 weeks	Withdraw and wait for 2 weeks	Withdraw and wait for 2 weeks
Tricyclics	Withdraw and wait for 1 week	Withdraw and wait for 1 week	Cross-taper cautiously	Halve dose and add citalopram then slow withdrawal[c]	Halve dose and add fluoxetine then slow withdrawal[c]	Halve dose and add paroxetine then slow withdrawal[c]
Citalopram/ escitalopram	Withdraw and wait for 1 week	Withdraw and wait for 1 week	Cross-taper cautiously[c]	–	Withdraw then start fluoxetine at 10 mg/day	Withdraw and start paroxetine at 10 mg/day
Paroxetine	Withdraw and wait for 2 weeks	Withdraw and wait for 1 week	Cross-taper cautiously with very low dose of tricylic[c]	Withdraw and start citalopram	Withdraw then start fluoxetine	–
Fluoxetine[d]	Withdraw and wait 5–6 weeks	Withdraw and wait 5–6 weeks	Stop fluoxetine Wait 4–7 days Start tricyclic at very low dose and increase very slowly	Stop fluoxetine Wait 4–7 days Start citalopram at 10 mg/day and increase slowly	–	Stop fluoxetine Wait 4–7 days, then start paroxetine 10 mg/day

[*] Note: Advice given in this table is partly derived from manufacturers' information and partly theoretical. Caution is required in every instance

Sertraline	Trazodone	Moclobemide	Reboxetine	Venlafaxine	Mirtazapine	Duloxetine
Withdraw and wait for 2 weeks	Withdraw and wait for 2 weeks	Withdraw and wait for 2 weeks[b]	Withdraw and wait for 2 weeks	Withdraw and wait for 2 weeks	Withdraw and wait for 2 weeks	Withdraw and wait for 2 weeks
Withdraw and wait for 2 weeks	Withdraw and wait for 2 weeks	Withdraw and wait for 2 weeks[b]	Withdraw and wait for 2 weeks	Withdraw and wait for 2 weeks	Withdraw and wait for 2 weeks	Withdraw and wait for 2 weeks
Halve dose and add sertraline then slow withdrawal[c]	Halve dose and add trazodone, then slow withdrawal	Withdraw and wait at least 1 week	Cross-taper cautiously	Cross-taper cautiously, starting with venlafaxine 37.5 mg/day	Cross-taper cautiously	Cross-taper cautiously, start at 60 mg alt die increase slowly
Withdraw and start sertraline at 25 mg/day	Withdraw before starting titration of trazodone	Withdraw and wait at least 2 weeks	Cross-taper cautiously	Withdraw citalopram Start venlafaxine 37.5 mg/day and increase very slowly	Cross-taper cautiously	Withdraw – start at 60 mg alt die Increase slowly
Withdraw and start sertraline at 25 mg/day	Withdraw before starting titration of trazodone	Withdraw and wait at least 2 weeks	Cross-taper cautiously	Withdraw paroxetine Start venlafaxine 37.5 mg/day and increase very slowly	Cross-taper cautiously	Withdraw, start at 60 mg alt die Increase slowly
Stop fluoxetine Wait 4–7 days, then start sertraline 25 mg/day	Stop fluoxetine Wait 4–7 days then start low-dose trazodone	Withdraw and wait at least 5 weeks	Withdraw Start reboxetine at 2 mg b.d. and increase cautiously	Withdraw Wait 4–7 days Start venlafaxine at 37.5 mg/day Increase very slowly	Withdraw, wait 4–7 days and start mirtazapine cautiously	Withdraw, wait 4–7 days and start at 60 mg alt die Increase slowly

Table Antidepressants – swapping and stopping[*] – (cont.)

To From	MAOIs- hydrazines	Tranyl- cypromine[a]	Tricyclics	Citalopram/ escitalopram	Fluoxetine	Paroxetine
Sertraline	Withdraw and wait for 2 weeks[b]	Withdraw and wait for 2 weeks	Cross-taper cautiously with very low dose of tricyclic[c]	Withdraw then start citalopram	Withdraw then start fluoxetine	Withdraw then start paroxetine
Trazodone	Withdraw and wait at least 1 week	Withdraw and wait at least 1 week	Cross-taper cautiously with very low dose of tricyclic	Withdraw then start citalopram	Withdraw then start fluoxetine	Withdraw then start paroxetine
Moclobemide	Withdraw and wait 24 hours	Withdraw and wait 24 hours	Withdraw and wait 24 hours	Withdraw and wait 24 hours	Withdraw and wait 24 hours	Withdraw and wait 24 hours
Reboxetine	Withdraw and wait at least 1 week	Withdraw and wait at least 1 week	Cross-taper cautiously	Cross-taper cautiously	Cross-taper cautiously	Cross-taper cautiously
Venlafaxine	Withdraw and wait at least 1 week	Withdraw and wait at least 1 week	Cross-taper cautiously with very low dose of tricyclic[c]	Cross-taper cautiously Start with 10 mg/day	Cross-taper cautiously Start with 20 mg every other day	Cross-taper cautiously Start with 10 mg/day
Mirtazapine	Withdraw and wait for 1 week	Withdraw and wait for 1 week	Withdraw then start tricyclic	Withdraw then start citalopram	Withdraw then start fluoxetine	Withdraw then start paroxetine
Duloxetine	Withdraw and wait 1 week	Withdraw and wait 1 week	Cross-taper cautiously with very low dose of tricylic	Withdraw then start citalopram	Withdraw then start fluoxetine	Withdraw then start paroxetine
Stopping[e]	Reduce over 4 weeks	Reduce over 4 weeks	Reduce over 4 weeks	Reduce over 4 weeks	At 20 mg/day, just stop At 40 mg/day, reduce over 2 weeks	Reduce over 4 weeks or longer, if necessary[f]

Notes

[a] SPC for tranylcypromine suggests at least 1-week gap between cessation of prior drug and starting tranylcypromine.

[b] Abrupt switching is possible but not recommended.

[c] Do not co-administer clomipramine and SSRIs or venlafaxine. Withdraw clomipramine before starting.

[d] Beware: interactions with fluoxetine may still occur for 5 weeks after stopping fluoxetine because of its long half-life.

[e] See general guidelines (page 176).

[f] Withdrawal effects seem to be more pronounced. Slow withdrawal over 1–3 months may be necessary.

Sertraline	Trazodone	Moclobemide	Reboxetine	Venlafaxine	Mirtazapine	Duloxetine
–	Withdraw before starting trazodone/nefazodone	Withdraw and wait at least 2 weeks	Cross-taper cautiously	Withdraw. Start venlafaxine at 37.5 mg/day	Cross-taper cautiously	Withdraw, start at 60 mg alt die Increase slowly
Withdraw then start sertraline	–	Withdraw and wait at least 1 week	Withdraw, start reboxetine at 2 mg b.d. and increase cautiously	Withdraw. Start venlafaxine at 37.5 mg/day	Cross-taper cautiously	Withdraw, start at 60 mg alt die Increase slowly
Withdraw and wait 24 hours	Withdraw and wait 24 hours	–	Withdraw and wait 24 hours	Withdraw and wait 24 hours	Withdraw and wait 24 hours	Withdraw and wait 24 hours
Cross-taper cautiously	Cross-taper cautiously	Withdraw and wait at least 1 week	–	Cross-taper cautiously	Cross-taper cautiously	Cross-taper cautiously
Cross-taper cautiously Start with 25 mg/day	Cross-taper cautiously	Withdraw and wait at least 1 week	Cross-taper cautiously	–	Cross-taper cautiously	Withdraw, start at 60 mg alt die Increase slowly
Withdraw then start sertraline	Withdraw then start trazodone	Withdraw and wait 1 week	Withdraw then start reboxetine	Withdraw then start venlafaxine	–	Withdraw, start at 60 mg alt die Increase slowly
Withdraw then start sertraline	Withdraw then start trazodone	Withdraw and wait 1 week	Cross-taper cautiously	Withdraw then start venlafaxine	Withdraw then start mirtazapine	–
Reduce over 4 weeks	Reduce over 4 weeks	Reduce over 4 weeks	Reduce over 4 weeks	Reduce over 4 weeks or longer, if necessary[f]	Reduce over 4 weeks	–

Antidepressant discontinuation symptoms

What are discontinuation symptoms?

The term 'discontinuation symptoms' is used to describe symptoms experienced on stopping prescribed drugs that are not drugs of dependence. There is an important semantic difference between 'discontinuation' and 'withdrawal' symptoms – the latter implies addiction; the former does not. While this distinction is important for precise medical terminology, it may be irrelevant to patient experience. Discontinuation symptoms may occur after stopping many drugs, including antidepressants, and can often be explained in the context of 'receptor rebound'[1] – e.g. an antidepressant with potent anticholinergic side-effects may be associated with diarrhoea on discontinuation.

Discontinuation symptoms may be entirely new or similar to some of the original symptoms of the illness, and so cannot be attributed to other causes. They are experienced by at least a third of patients[2].

The onset is usually within 5 days of stopping treatment (depending on the half-life of the anti depressant) or occasionally during taper or after missed doses[3,4] (short-half-life drugs only). Symptoms can vary in form and intensity and occur in any combination. They are usually mild and self-limiting, but can occasionally be severe and prolonged. The perception of symptom severity is probably made worse by the absence of forewarnings. Some symptoms are more likely with individual drugs.

Table Antidepressant discontinuation symptoms

	MAOIs	TCAs	SSRIs and related
Symptoms	**Common** Agitation, irritability, ataxia, movement disorders, insomnia, somnolence, vivid dreams, cognitive impairment, slowed speech, pressured speech **Occasionally** Hallucinations, paranoid delusions	**Common** Flu-like symptoms (chills, myalgia, excessive sweating, headache, nausea), insomnia, excessive dreaming **Occasionally** Movement disorders, mania, cardiac arrhythmia	**Common** Flu-like symptoms, 'shock-like' sensations, dizziness exacerbated by movement, insomnia, excessive (vivid) dreaming, irritability, crying spells **Occasionally** Movement disorders, problems with concentration and memory
Drugs most commonly associated with discontinuation symptoms	All Tranylcypromine is partly metabolised to amphetamine and is therefore associated with a true 'withdrawal syndrome'	Amitriptyline Imipramine	Paroxetine Venlafaxine

Clinical relevance[2]

The symptoms of a discontinuation reaction may be mistaken for a relapse of illness or the emergence of a new physical illness[5] leading to unnecessary investigations or reintroduction of the antidepressant. Symptoms may be severe enough to interfere with daily functioning, and those who have experienced discontinuation symptoms may reason (perhaps appropriately) that antidepressants are 'addictive' and not wish to accept treatment.

Who is most at risk?[1,2,5]

Although anyone can experience discontinuation symptoms, the risk is increased in those prescribed short-half-life drugs[3] (e.g. paroxetine, venlafaxine), particularly if they do not take them regularly. Two-thirds of patients prescribed antidepressants may skip a few doses from time to time[6]. The risk is also increased in those who have been taking antidepressants for 8 weeks or longer[7], those who have developed anxiety symptoms at the start of antidepressant therapy (particularly with SSRIs), those receiving other centrally acting medication (e.g. antihypertensives, antihistamines, antipsychotics), children and adolescents, and those who have experienced discontinuation symptoms before.

How to avoid[1,2,5]

Generally, antidepressant therapy should be discontinued over at least a 4-week period (this is not required with fluoxetine)[5]. The shorter the half life of the drug, the more important that this rule is followed. The end of the taper may need to be slower, as symptoms may not appear until the reduction in the total daily dosage of the antidepressant is (proportionately) substantial. Patients receiving MAOIs may need to be tapered over a longer period. Tranylcypromine may be particularly difficult to stop. At risk patients (see above) may need a slower taper.

Many people suffer symptoms despite slow withdrawal. For these patients the option of abrupt withdrawal should be discussed. Some may prefer to face a week or two of intense symptoms rather than months of less severe discontinuation syndrome.

How to treat[2,5]

There are few systematic studies in this area. Treatment is pragmatic. If symptoms are mild, reassure the patient that these symptoms are not uncommon after discontinuing an antidepressant and will pass in a few days. If symptoms are severe, reintroduce the original antidepressant (or another with a longer half-life from the same class) and taper gradually while monitoring for symptoms.

Some evidence supports the use of anticholinergic agents in tricyclic withdrawal[8] and fluoxetine for symptoms associated with stopping clomipramine[9] or venlafaxine[10] – fluoxetine, having a longer plasma half-life, seems to be associated with a lower incidence of discontinuation symptoms than other similar drugs[11].

Key points that patients should know

- Antidepressants are not addictive; a survey of 2000 people across the UK conducted in 1991 found that 78% thought that antidepressants were addictive[12]. It is important to dispel this myth. In order for a drug to be addictive it must also fulfil certain other criteria including tolerance, escalating use, etc. This should be discussed. Note, however, that this semantic and categorical distinction may be lost on many people.
- Patients should be informed that they may experience discontinuation symptoms (and the most likely symptoms associated with the drug that they are taking) when they stop their antidepressant.
- Antidepressants should not be stopped abruptly. The dose should be tapered down over at least 4 weeks. Fluoxetine is an exception to this rule[3].
- Discontinuation symptoms may occur after missed doses if the antidepressant prescribed has a short half-life.

References

1. Antidepressant discontinuation syndrome: update on serotonin reuptake inhibitors. *J Clin Psychiatry* 1997; **58**(Suppl. 7): 3–40.
2. Lejoyeux M, Ades J, Mourad I. Antidepressant withdrawal syndrome: recognition, prevention and management. *CNS Drugs* 1996; **5**: 278–292.
3. Rosenbaum JF, Fava M, Hoog SL *et al.* Selective serotonin reuptake inhibitor discontinuation syndrome: a randomised controlled trial. *Biol Psychiatry* 1998; **44**: 77–88.
4. Michelson D, Fava M, Amsterdam J *et al.* Interruption of selective serotonin reuptake inhibitor treatment. *Br J Psychiatry* 2000; **176**: 363–368.
5. Haddad PM. Antidepressant discontinuation syndromes. *Drug Safety* 2001; **24**: 183–197.
6. Meijer WEE, Bouvy ML, Heerdink ER. Spontaneous lapses in dosing during chronic treatment with selective serotonin reuptake inhibitors. *Br J Psychiatry* 2001; **179**: 519–522.
7. Kramer JC, Klein DF, Fink M. Withdrawal symptoms following discontinuation of imipramine therapy. *Am J Psychiatry* 1961; **118**: 549–550.
8. Dilsaver SC, Feinberg M, Greden JF. Antidepressant withdrawal symptoms treated with anticholinergic agents. *Am J Psychiatry* 1983; **140**: 249–251.
9. Benazzi F. Fluoxetine for clomipramine withdrawal symptoms. *Am J Psychiatry* 1999; **156**: 661–662.
10. Giakas WJ, Davis JM. Intractable withdrawal from venlafaxine treated with fluoxetine. *Psychiat Ann* 1997; **27**: 85–92.
11. Coupland NJ, Bell CJ, Potokar JP. Serotonin reuptake inhibitor withdrawal. *J Clin Psychopharmacol* 1996; **16**: 356–362.
12. Priest RG, Vize C, Roberts A *et al.* Lay people's attitudes to treatment of depression: results of opinion pole for Defeat Depression Campaign just before its launch. *BMJ* 1996; **313**: 858–859.

Depression & anxiety

St John's wort

St John's wort (SJW) is the popular name for the plant *Hypericum perforatum*. It contains a combination of at least 10 different components, including hypericins, flavonoids and xanthons[1]. Preparations of SJW are often unstandardised and this has complicated the interpretation of clinical trials.

The active ingredient and mechanism of action of SJW are unclear although many hypotheses have been proposed. At one time MAO inhibition was thought to be the most likely mechanism of action but more recent research has shown that this may account for only a small part of SJW's antidepressant effect[2]. Reuptake inhibition of both noradrenaline and serotonin has been demonstrated, as has the upregulation of serotonin receptors[3]. At this time no firm conclusions can be drawn.

SJW is not a licensed preparation in the UK but is available as a herbal or complementary therapy. (It is licensed in Germany for the treatment of depression.)

Evidence for SJW in the treatment of depression

A number of trials have been published that look at the efficacy of SJW in the treatment of depression. They have been extensively reviewed[1,4,5] and most authors conclude that SJW may be effective in the treatment of mild-to-moderate depression. This conclusion is suitably cautious in view of the following limitations of the studies:

- The active component of SJW for treating depression has not yet been determined. The trials used different preparations of SJW which were standardised according to their total content of hypericins. However, recent evidence suggests that hypericins alone do not treat depression[6]. It is illogical to recommend a treatment where the dosage stated is not that of the active ingredient.

- None of the trials has lasted longer than 8 weeks.

- SJW was often compared to subtherapeutic doses of standard antidepressants. Patients showed a surprisingly good response to low doses of TCAs used in the trials, a result which also brings into question the methodology of the studies. A more recent study found SJW to be as effective as imipramine 150 mg daily in the treatment of mild-to-moderate depression[7].

- SJW is often said to be much better tolerated than standard antidepressants. This is misleading, since only two trials have compared SJW to the newer antidepressants such as the SSRIs[8,9].

SJW may prove to be an effective and well-tolerated treatment for mild-to-moderate depression. NICE confirm that this is likely to be true[10]. It should not, however, be prescribed: we lack understanding of what constitutes a therapeutic dose of an unlicensed herbal treatment. Until more trials are conducted to address these points, we should continue to use antidepressants which are proven to be effective and whose long-term effects and possible interactions with other drugs have been determined.

Note also that SJW has been shown, in an underpowered study, to be ineffective in the treatment of severe depression[11].

Adverse effects

The most common side-effects of SJW are dry mouth, nausea, constipation, fatigue, dizziness, headache and restlessness[4,5,7,12]. In addition, SJW contains a red pigment that can cause photosensitivity reactions[13]. In common with other antidepressant drugs, SJW has been known to precipitate hypomania in people with bipolar affective disorder[14].

Drug interactions

It is thought that SJW is an inducer of the hepatic cytochrome P450 system[15]. Studies have shown that SJW significantly reduces plasma concentrations of digoxin and indinavir[16,17] (a drug used in the treatment of HIV). According to a number of case reports, SJW has lowered the plasma concentrations of theophylline, cyclosporin, warfarin and the combined oral contraceptive pill and has led to treatment failure[15]. There is a theoretical risk that SJW may interact with some anticonvulsant drugs[18]. Serotonin syndrome has been reported when SJW was taken together with sertraline, paroxetine, nefazodone and the triptans[18,19] (a group of serotonin agonists used to treat migraine). SJW should not be taken with any drugs that have a predominantly serotonergic action.

Key points that patients should know

- The evidence so far available suggests that SJW may be effective in the treatment of mild (not severe) depression, but we do not know enough about how much should be taken or what the side-effects are.

- The symptoms of depression can sometimes be caused by other physical or mental illness. It is important that these possible causes are investigated.

- SJW can interact with other medicines, resulting in serious side-effects. Some important drugs may be metabolised more rapidly and therefore become ineffective with serious consequences (e.g. increased viral load in HIV, reduced anticoagulant effect with warfarin leading to thrombosis).

- SJW is not suitable for some groups of people, including anyone who is severely depressed.

- It is always best to consult the doctor if any herbal or natural remedy is being taken or the patient is thinking of taking one.

Many people regard herbal remedies as 'natural' and therefore harmless[20]. They are not aware of the potential of such remedies for causing side-effects or interacting with other drugs. A small US study (n=22) found that people tend to take SJW because it is easy to obtain alternative medicines and also because they perceive herbal medicines as being purer and safer than prescription medicines. Few would discuss this medication with their conventional health-care provider[12]. Clinicians need to be proactive in asking patients if they use such treatments and try to dispel the myth that natural is the same as safe.

References

1. Linde K, Ramirez G, Mulrow CD *et al*. St John's wort for depression – an overview and meta-analysis of randomised controlled trials. *BMJ* 1996; **313**: 253–258.
2. Colt JM. In vitro receptor binding and enzyme inhibition by *Hypericum perforatum* extract. *Psychopharmacology* 1997; **30**(Suppl. 2): 108–112.
3. Muller WE, Rolli M, Schafer C *et al*. Effects of *Hypericum* extract (LI116) in biochemical models of antidepressant activity. *Psychopharmacology* 1997; **30**(Suppl. 2): 102–107.
4. Volz HP. Controlled clinical trials of *Hypericum* extracts in depressed patients – an overview. *Pharmacopsychiatry* 1997; **30**(Suppl. 2): 72–76.
5. Gaster B, Holroyd J. St Johns's wort for depression – a systematic review. *Arch Intern Med* 2000; **160**: 152–156.
6. Teufel-Mayer R, Gleitz J. Effects of long-term administration of *Hypericum* extracts on the affinity and density of the central serotonergic 5HT1a and 5HT2a receptors. *Pharmacopsychiatry* 1997; **30**(Suppl. 2): 113–116.
7. Woelk H. Comparison of St John's wort and imipramine for treating depression: randomised controlled trial. *BMJ* 2000; **321**: 356–359.
8. Brenner R, Azbel V, Madhusoodanan S *et al*. Comparison of an extract of *Hypericum* (LI160) and sertraline in the treatment of depression: a double blind randomised pilot study. *Clin Ther* 2000; **22**: 411–419.
9. Behnke K, Jensen JS, Graubaum HJ *et al*. *Hypericum perforatum* versus fluoxetine in the treatment of mild to moderate depression. *Advances in Therapy* 2002; **19**: 43–52.
10. National Institute for Clinical Excellence. Treatment guidelines for depression 2004. www.nice.org.uk.
11. Davidson JRT, Gadde KM, Fairbank JA *et al*. Effect of *Hypericum perforatum* (St John's wort) in major depressive disorder: a randomised controlled trial. *J Am Med Assoc* 2002; **287**: 1807–1814.
12. Wagner PJ, Jester D, LeClair B *et al*. Taking the edge off – why patients choose St John's wort. *J Fam Practice* 1999; **48**: 615–619.
13. Bore GM. Acute neuropathy after exposure to sun in a patient treated with St John's wort. *Lancet* 1998; **352**: 1121–1122.
14. Nierenburg AA, Burr T, Mathews J *et al*. Mania associated with St John's wort. *Bio Psychiat* 1999; **46**: 1707–1708.
15. Ernst E. Second thoughts about safety of St John's wort. *Lancet* 1999; **354**: 2014–2015.
16. Johne A, Brockmoller J, Bauer S *et al*. Pharmacokinetic interaction of digoxin with a herbal extract from St John's wort (*Hypericum perforatum*). *Clin Pharmacol Ther* 1999; **66**: 338–345.
17. Piscitelli SC, Burstein AH, Chaitt D *et al*. Indinavir concentrations and St John's wort. *Lancet* 2000; **355**: 547–548.
18. Anon. Reminder: St John's wort (*Hypericum perforatum*) interactions. *Current Problems in Pharmacovigilance* 2000; **26**: 6.
19. Lantz MS, Buchalter E, Giambanco V. St John's wort and antidepressant drug interactions in the elderly. *J Geriatr Psychiat Neurol* 1999; **12**: 7–10.
20. Barnes J, Mills SY, Abbot NC *et al*. Different standards for reporting ADRs to herbal remedies and conventional OTC medicines: face-to-face interviews with 515 users of herbal remedies. *Br J Clin Pharmacol* 1998; **45**: 496–500.

Further reading

Szegedi A, Kohnen R, Dienel A *et al*. Acute treatment of moderate to severe depression with hypericum extract WS 5570 (St John's Wort): randomised controlled double blind non-inferiority trial versus paroxetine. *BMJ*, doi: 10.1136/bmj.38356.655266.82.published 11 Feb 2005.

Werneke U, Horn O, Taylor D. How effective is St John's wort? The evidence revisited. *J Clin Psychiatry* 2004; **65**: 611–617.

Whiskey E, Werneke U, Taylor D. A systematic review and meta-analysis of *Hypericum perforatum* in depression: a comprehensive clinical review. *Int Clin Psychopharmacol* 2001; **16**: 239–252.

Drug interactions with antidepressants

Drugs can interact with each other in two different ways:

1. *Pharmacokinetic interactions* where one drug interferes with the absorption, distribution, metabolism or elimination of another drug. This may result in subtherapeutic effect or toxicity. The largest group of pharmacokinetic interactions involves drugs that inhibit or induce hepatic CYP450 enzymes (see the table opposite). Other enzyme systems include FMO[1] and UGT[2]. While both of these enzyme systems are involved in the metabolism of psychotropic drugs, the potential for drugs to inhibit or induce these enzyme systems has been poorly studied.

2. *Pharmacodynamic interactions* where the effects of one drug are altered by another drug via physiological mechanisms such as direct competition at receptor sites (e.g. dopamine agonists with dopamine blockers negate any therapeutic effect), augmentation of the same neurotransmitter pathway (e.g. fluoxetine with tramadol can lead to serotonin syndrome) or an effect on the physiological functioning of an organ/organ system in different ways (e.g. two different antiarrhythmic drugs). Most of these interactions can be easily predicted by a sound knowledge of pharmacology. A list can be found at the back of the *BNF*.

Pharmacodynamic interactions

Tricyclic antidepressants[8,9]:

- are H_1 blockers (sedative). This can be exacerbated by other sedative drugs or alcohol. Beware respiratory depression.

- are anticholinergic (dry mouth, blurred vision, constipation). This can be exacerbated by other anticholinergic drugs such as antihistamines or antipsychotics. Beware cognitive impairment and GI obstruction.

- are adrenergic α_1-blockers (postural hypotension). This can be exacerbated by other drugs that block α_1-receptors and by antihypertensive drugs in general. Adrenaline, in combination with α_1-blockers, can lead to hypertension.

- are arrhythmogenic. Caution is required with other drugs that can alter cardiac conduction directly (e.g. antiarrhythmics or phenothiazines) or indirectly through a potential to cause electrolyte disturbance (e.g. diuretics).

- lower the seizure threshold. Caution is required with other proconvulsive drugs (e.g. antipsychotics) and particularly if the patient is being treated for epilepsy (higher doses of anticonvulsants may be required).

- may be serotonergic (e.g. amitriptyline, clomipramine). There is the potential for these drugs to interact with other serotonergic drugs (e.g. tramadol, SSRIs, selegiline) to cause serotonin syndrome.

Table Pharmacokinetic interactions[3–7]

p4501A2	p4502C	p4502D6	p4503A
Genetic polymorphism	5–10% of Caucasians lack it	3–5% of Caucasians lack it	60% p450 content
Induced by: cigarette smoke charcoal cooking carbamazepine omeprazole phenobarbitone phenytoin	*Induced by:* phenytoin rifampicin	*Induced by:* carbamazepine phenytoin	*Induced by:* carbamazepine phenytoin prednisolone rifampicin
Inhibited by: cimetidine ciprofloxacin erythromycin fluvoxamine paroxetine	*Inhibited by:* cimetidine fluoxetine fluvoxamine sertraline	*Inhibited by:* chlorpromazine citalopram duloxetine fluoxetine fluphenazine haloperidol paroxetine sertraline tricyclics	*Inhibited by:* erythromycin fluoxetine fluvoxamine ketoconazole paroxetine sertraline tricyclics
Metabolises: clozapine haloperidol mirtazapine olanzapine theophylline tricyclics warfarin	*Metabolises:* diazepam omeprazole phenytoin tolbutamide tricyclics warfarin	*Metabolises:* clozapine codeine donepezil haloperidol methadone phenothiazines risperidone TCA secondary amines tramadol trazodone venlafaxine	*Metabolises:* benzodiazepines calcium blockers carbamazepine cimetidine clozapine codeine donepezil erythromycin galantamine mirtazapine risperidone steroids terfenadine tricyclics valproate venlafaxine Z-hypnotics

Depression & anxiety

SSRIs[10,11]:

- increase serotonergic neurotransmission. The main concern is serotonin syndrome (see page 171).

- inhibit platelet aggregation and increase the risk of bleeding, particularly of the upper GI tract. This effect is exacerbated by aspirin and NSAIDs.

MAOIs[12]:

- prevent the destruction of monoamine neurotransmitters. Sympathomimetic and dopaminergic drugs can lead to monoamine overload and hypertensive crisis. Pethidine and fermented foods can have the same effect.

- can interact with serotonergic drugs to cause serotonin syndrome.

Avoid/minimise problems by:

1. avoiding antidepressant polypharmacy

2. avoiding the co-prescription of other drugs with a similar pharmacology but not marketed as antidepressants (e.g. bupropion, sibutramine)

3. knowing your pharmacology (most interactions can be easily predicted).

References

1. Cashman JR. Human flavin containing mono-oxygenase: substrate specificity and role in drug metabolism. *Curr Drug Met* 2000; **1**: 181–191.
2. Anderson GD. A mechanistic approach to antiepileptic drug interactions. *Ann Pharmacother* 1998; **32**: 554–563.
3. Lin JH, Lu AYH. Inhibition and induction of cytochrome P450 and the clinical implications. *Clin Pharmacokinet* 1998; **35**: 361–390.
4. Mitchell PB. Drug interactions of clinical significance with selective serotonin reuptake inhibitors. *Drug Safety* 1997; **17**: 390–406.
5. Richelson E. Pharmacokinetic interactions of antidepressants. *J Clin Psychiatry* 1998; **59**(Suppl. 10): 22–26.
6. Greenblatt DJ, von Moltke LL, Harmatz JS *et al.* Drug interactions with newer antidepressants: role of human cytochromes P450. *J Clin Psychiatry* 1998; **59**(Suppl. 15): 19–27.
7. Taylor D. Pharmacokinetic interactions involving clozapine. *Br J Psychiatry* 1997; **171**: 109–112.
8. *British National Formulary*, 43rd edn. Appendix 1, pp. 618–658. London: British Medical Association and Royal Pharmaceutical Society of Great Britain, 2002.
9. Watsky EJ, Salzman C. Psychotropic drug interactions. *Hosp Community Psychiatry* 1991; **42**: 247–256.
10. Mitchell PB. Drug interactions of clinical significance with serotonin reuptake inhibitors. *Drug Safety* 1997; **17**: 390–406.
11. Edwards JG, Anderson I. Systematic review and guide to selection of serotonin reuptake inhibitors. *Drugs* 1999; **57**: 507–533.
12. Livingstone MG, Livingstone HM. Monoamine oxidase inhibitors: an update on drug interactions. *Drug Safety* **14**: 219–227.

Table	Antidepressants: relative adverse effects – a rough guide			
Drug	Sedation	Hypotension	Anticholinergic effects	Forms available
Tricyclics				
Amitriptyline	+++	+++	+++	tabs/caps, liq, inj
Clomipramlne	++	+++	++	tabs/caps, liq
Desipramine	+	++	+	tabs
Dothiepin	+++	+++	++	tabs, caps
Doxepin	+++	++	++	caps
Imipramine	++	+++	+++	tabs, liq
Lofepramine	+	+	+	tabs
Nortriptyline	+	++	+	tabs
Trimipramine	+++	+++	++	tabs, caps
Other antidepressants				
Duloxetlne	+/–	–	–	caps
Mianserin	++	–	–	tabs
Mirtazapine	+++	–	+	tabs
Reboxetine	+	–	+	tabs
Trazodone	+++	++	–	caps, liq
Venlafaxine	+/–	–	+	tabs
Selective serotonin reuptake inhibitors (SSRIs)				
Citalopram	+/–	–	–	tabs, liq
Escitalopram	+/–	–	–	tabs
Fluoxetine	–	–	–	caps, liq
Fluvoxamine	+	–	–	tabs
Paroxetine	+	–	+	tabs, liq
Sertraline	–	–	–	tabs
Monoamine oxidase inhibitors (MAOIs)				
Isocarboxazid	+	++	++	tabs
Phenelzine	+	+	+	tabs
Tranylcypromine	–	+	+	tabs
Reversible inhibitor of monoamine oxidase A (RIMA)				
Moclobemide	–	–	–	tabs

KEY: +++ High incidence/severity
++ Moderate
+ Low
– Very low/none

Depression & anxiety

185

Anxiety spectrum disorders

Anxiety is a normal emotion that is experienced by everyone at some time. Symptoms can be psychological, physical, or a mixture of both. Intervention is required when symptoms become disabling.

There are several disorders within the overall spectrum of anxiety disorders, each with its own characteristic symptoms. These are outlined briefly in the table below. Anxiety disorders can occur on their own, be part of other psychiatric disorders (particularly depression), be a consequence of physical illness such as thyrotoxicosis or be drug-induced (e.g. by caffeine)[1]. Co-morbidity with other psychiatric disorders is very common.

Anxiety spectrum disorders tend to be chronic and treatment is often only partially successful.

Benzodiazepines

Benzodiazepines provide rapid symptomatic relief from acute anxiety states. All guidelines and consensus statements recommend that this group of drugs should only be used to treat anxiety that is severe, disabling, or subjecting the individual to extreme distress. Due to their potential to cause physical dependence and withdrawal symptoms, these drugs should be used at the lowest effective dose for the shortest period of time (maximum 4 weeks), while medium/long-term treatment strategies are put in place. For the majority of patients these recommendations are sensible and should be adhered to. A very small number of patients with severely disabling anxiety may benefit from long-term treatment with a benzodiazepine and these patients should not be denied treatment[2]. NICE recommends that benzodiazepines should not be used to treat panic disorder[3]. They should be used with care in post-traumatic stress disorder (PTSD)[4].

SSRI dose and duration of treatment

When used to treat generalised anxiety disorder (**GAD**), SSRIs should initially be prescribed at half the normal starting dose for the treatment of depression and the dose titrated upwards into the normal antidepressant dosage range as tolerated (initial worsening of anxiety may be seen when treatment is started[5–7]). Response is usually seen within 6 weeks and continues to increase over time[8]. The optimal duration of treatment has not been determined but should be at least 6 months[9]. Effective treatment of GAD may prevent the development of major depression[10].

When used to treat **panic disorder**, the same starting dose and dosage titration as in GAD should be used. Doses of clomipramine[11], citalopram[12] and sertraline[13] towards the bottom of the antidepressant range give the best balance between efficacy and side-effects, whereas higher doses of paroxetine (40 mg and above) may be required[14]. Higher doses may be effective when standard doses have failed. Onset of action may take 6 weeks. There is some evidence that augmentation with clonazepam leads to a more rapid response (but not a greater magnitude of response overall)[14,15]. The optimal duration of treatment is unknown, but should be at least 8 months[16,17], with some authors recommending up to 18 months[18]. Less than 50% are likely to remain well after medication is withdrawn[18].

Lower starting doses are also required in post-traumatic stress disorder (**PTSD**), with high doses (e.g. fluoxetine 60 mg) often being required for full effect. Response is usually seen within 8 weeks[19], but can take up to 12 weeks[18]. Treatment should be continued for at least 6 months (relapse rate of 5% on active drug at this point versus 26% of those switched to placebo after acute treatment[20]) and probably longer[21,22].

Although the doses of SSRIs licensed for the treatment of obsessive compulsive disorder (**OCD**) are higher than those licensed for the treatment of depression (e.g. fluoxetine 60 mg, paroxetine 40–60 mg), lower (standard antidepressant) doses may be effective, particularly for maintenance treatment[23,24]. Initial response is usually slower to emerge than in depression (can take 10–12 weeks). The relapse rate in those who continue treatment for 2 years is half that of those who stop treatment after initial response (25–40% vs 80%)[25,26].

Standard antidepressant starting doses are well tolerated in **social phobia**[27-29], and upward dosage titration may benefit some patients but is not always required. Response is usually seen within 8 weeks and treatment should be continued for at least a year and probably longer[30].

SSRIs should not be stopped abruptly, as patients with anxiety spectrum disorders are particularly sensitive to discontinuation symptoms (see page 176). The dose should be titrated down as tolerated over several weeks to months.

Psychological approaches

There is good evidence to support the efficacy of some psychological interventions in anxiety spectrum disorders. Examples include exposure therapy in OCD and social phobia. Initial drug therapy may be required to help the patient become more receptive to psychological input, and some studies suggest that optimal outcome is achieved by combining psychological and drug therapies[1,3].

A discussion of the evidence base for psychological interventions is outside the scope of these guidelines. Further information can be found at www.doh.gov.uk[31]. There are often long waiting lists for psychological therapies and some specialist interventions may not be available at all in some areas. The table on the following pages does not list psychological interventions as first-line treatments for these reasons. It is recognised that for many patients their use as a first-line treatment would be appropriate, and indeed this is supported by NICE[3].

Summary of NICE guidelines for the treatment of generalised anxiety disorder and panic disorder[3]

1. Psychological therapy is more effective than pharmacological therapy and should be used as first line where possible. Details of the types of therapy recommended and their duration can be found in the NICE guidelines.

2. Pharmacological therapy is also effective. Most evidence supports the use of the SSRIs.

Panic disorder
- Benzodiazepines should not be used.
- A SSRI should be used as first line. If SSRIs are contraindicated or there is no response, imipramine or clomipramine can be used.
- Self-help (based on CBT principles) should be encouraged.

Generalised anxiety disorder
- Benzodiazepines should not be used beyond 2–4 weeks.
- A SSRI should be used as first line.
- Self-help (based on CBT principles) should be encouraged.

Table

Depression & anxiety

	Generalised anxiety disorder[3–9,32–40]	Obsessive compulsive disorder[24–27,41–53]
Clinical presentation	• Irrational worries • Motor tension • Hypervigilance • Somatic symptoms (e.g. hyperventilation, tachycardia and sweating)	• Obsessional thinking (e.g. constantly thinking that the door has been left unlocked) • Compulsive behaviour (e.g. constantly going back to check)
Emergency management	Benzodiazepines (normally for short-term use only: max. 2–4 weeks, but see ref. 2)	Not usually appropriate
First-line drug treatment Treatment of anxiety may prevent the subsequent development of depression[7]	• SSRIs (although may initially exacerbate symptoms. A lower starting is often required) • Venlafaxine (NICE recommend specialist referral) • Some TCAs (e.g. imipramine, clomipramine)	• SSRIs • Clomipramine
Other treatments (less well tolerated or weaker evidence base)	• Buspirone (has a delayed onset of action) • Hydroxyzine • β-Blockers (useful for somatic symptoms, particularly tachycardia) • Tiagabine	• Antipsychotics (evidence for quetiapine and risperidone as antidepressant augmentation, but not haloperidol) • Venlafaxine • Buspirone • Clomipramine (IV pulse loading) • Clonazepam (benzodiazepines in general are mainly useful in reducing associated anxiety) • Mirtazapine augmentation of SSRI
Non-drug treatments See www.doh.org.uk and NICE[3]	• Reassurance • Anxiety management, including relaxation training • CBT	• Exposure therapy • Behavioural therapy • CBT • Combined drug and psychological therapy may be the most effective option

Panic disorder[12–19,53–62]	Post-traumatic stress disorder[20–23,63–73]	Social phobia[28–30,74–78]
• Sudden unpredictable episodes of severe anxiety • Shortness of breath • Fear of suffocation/dying • Urgent desire to flee	• History of a traumatic life event (as perceived by the sufferer) • Emotional numbness or detachment • Intrusive flashbacks or vivid dreams • Disabling fear of re-exposure, causing avoidance of perceived similar situations	• Extreme fear of social situations (e.g. eating in public or public speaking) • Fear of humiliation or embarrassment • Avoidant behaviour (e.g. never eating in restaurants) • Anxious anticipation (e.g. feeling sick on entering a restaurant)
Benzodiazepines *(have a rapid effect, although panic symptoms return quickly if the drug is withdrawn)* NICE do *not* recommend	Not usually appropriate	Benzodiazepines (have a rapid effect and may be useful on a PRN basis)
• SSRIs (therapeutic effect can be delayed and patients can experience an initial exacerbation of panic symptoms) • Some TCAs (e.g. imipramine, clomipramine) • Reboxetine	• SSRIs • Serotonergic TCAs	• SSRIs • MAOIs
• MAOIs • Mirtazapine • Valproate • Inositol	• MAOIs • Valproate • Carbamazepine • Clonidine • Tiagabine • Olanzapine • Risperidone • Quetiapine • Mirtazapine • Phenytoin	• Moclobemide • Clonazepam • Propranolol (performance anxiety only) • Buspirone (adjunct to SSRIs only) • Venlafaxine • Valproate • Levetiracetam
• CBT • Anxiety management, including relaxation, training • Combined drug and psychological therapy may be the most effective option	• Debriefing should be available if desired • Counselling • Anxiety management • CBT, especially for avoidance behaviours or intrusive images	• CBT • Exposure therapy (combined drug and exposure therapy may be more effective)

References

1. Fineberg N, Drummond LM. Anxiety disorders: drug treatment or behavioural cognitive psychotherapy. *CNS Drugs* 1995; **3**: 448–466.
2. Royal College of Psychiatrists. Benzodiazepines: risks, benefits or dependence, a re-evaluation. Council Report CR 57. London: Royal College of Psychiatrists, 1997.
3. National Institute for Clinical Excellence. Anxiety: management of anxiety (panic disorder, with or without agoraphobia, and generalised anxiety disorder) in adults in primary, secondary and community care. 2004. www.nice.org.uk.
4. Davidson JRT. Use of benzodiazepines in social anxiety disorder, generalised anxiety disorder and posttraumatic stress disorder. *J Clin Psychiatry* 2004; **65**(Suppl. 5): 29–33.
5. Scott A, Davidson A, Palmer K. Antidepressant drugs in the treatment of anxiety disorders. *Adv Psychiatr Treat* 2001; **7**: 275–282.
6. Rocca P, Fonzo V, Scotta M *et al.* Paroxetine efficacy in the treatment of generalised anxiety disorder. *Acta Psychiatr Scand* 1997; **95**: 444–450.
7. Davidson JR. Pharmacotherapy of generalised anxiety disorder. *J Clin Psychiatry* 2001; **62**: 46–50.
8. Ballenger JC. Remission rates in patients with anxiety disorders treated with paroxetine. *J Clin Psychiatry* 2004; **65**: 1696–1707.
9. Stocchi F, Nordera G, Jokinen RH. Efficacy and tolerability of paroxetine for the long-term treatment of generalised anxiety disorder. *J Clin Psychiatry* 2003; **64**: 250–258.
10. Ballenger JC, Davidson JRT, Lecrubier Y *et al.* Consensus statement on generalised anxiety disorder from the international consensus group on depression and anxiety. *J Clin Psychiatry* 2001; **62**(Suppl. 11): 53–58.
11. Goodwin RD, Gorman JM. Psychopharmacologic treatment of generalised anxiety disorder and the risk of major depression. *Am J Psychiatry* 2002; **159**: 1935–1937.
12. Caillard V, Rouillon F, Viel JF *et al.* Comparative effects of low and high doses of clomipramine and placebo in panic disorder: a double-blind controlled study. *Acta Psychiatr Scand* 1999; **99**: 51–58.
13. Wade AG, Lepola U, Koponen HJ *et al.* The effect of citalopram in panic disorder. *Br J Psychiatry* 1997; **170**: 549–553.
14. Londborg PD, Wolkov R, Smith WT *et al.* Sertraline in the treatment of panic disorder: a multi-site, double-blind, placebo-controlled, fixed dose investigation. *Br J Psychiatry* 1998; **173**: 54–68.
15. Pollack MH, Simon NM, Worthington JJ *et al.* Combined paroxetine and clonazepam treatment strategies compared to paroxetine monotherapy for panic disorder. *J Psychopharmacol* 2003; **17**: 276–282.
16. Ballanger JC, Wheadon DE, Steiner M *et al.* Double blind, fixed dose, placebo controlled study of paroxetine in the treatment of panic disorder. *Am J Psychiatry* 1998; **155**: 36–42.
17. Ridels K, Schweizer E. Panic disorder: long term pharmacotherapy and discontinuation. *J Clin Psychopharmacol* 1998; **18**(Suppl. 2): 12–18.
18. Michelson D, Pollack M, Lydiard B *et al.* Continuing treatment of panic disorder after acute response: randomised, placebo-controlled trial with fluoxetine. *Br J Psychiatry* 1999; **174**: 213–218.
19. American Psychiatric Association. Practice Guideline for the Treatment of Panic Disorder. *Am J Psychiatry* 1998 (Suppl. 11).
20. Stein DJ, Zungu-Dinwayi N, van der Linden GHJ *et al.* Pharmacotherapy for posttraumatic stress disorder. Cochrane database of systematic reviews. Cochrane Library, Update Software, 2002.
21. Davidson J, Pearlstein T, Londborg P *et al.* Efficacy of sertraline in preventing relapse of posttraumatic stress disorder: results of a 28-week double-blind, placebo controlled study. *Am J Psychiatry* 2001; **158**: 1974–1981.
22. Ballenger JC, Davidson JRT, Lecrubier Y *et al.* Consensus statement update on posttraumatic stress disorder from the International Consensus Group on Depression and Anxiety. *J Clin Psychiatry* 2004; **65**(Suppl. 1): 55–62.
23. Martenyi F, Brown EB, Zhang H *et al.* Fluoxetine v placebo in prevention of relapse in post-traumatic stress disorder. *Br J Psychiatry* 2002; **181**: 315–320.
24. Ravizza L, Maina G, Bogetto F *et al.* Long term treatment of obsessive-compulsive disorder. *CNS Drugs* 1998; **10**: 247–255.
25. March JS. Treatment of obsessive compulsive disorder: the Expert Consensus Guideline Series. *J Clin Psychiatry* 1997; **58**(Suppl. 4).
26. Ravizza L, Barzega G, Bellino S *et al.* Drug treatment of obsessive compulsive disorder: long term trial with clomipramine and SSRIs. *Psychopharmacol Bull* 1996; **32**: 167–173.
27. Greist JH, Jefferson JW, Kobak KA *et al.* Efficacy and tolerability of serotonin transport inhibitors in OCD. *Arch Gen Psychiatry* 1995; **52**: 53–60.
28. Liebowitz MR, Stein MB, Tancer M *et al.* A randomized, double-blind, fixed-dose comparison of paroxetine and placebo in the treatment of generalised social anxiety disorder. *J Clin Psychiatry* 2002; **63**: 66–74.
29. Blomhoff S, Haug TT, Hellstrom K *et al.* Randomised controlled general practice trial of sertraline, exposure therapy and combined treatment in generalised social phobias. *Br J Psychiatry* 2001; **179**: 23–30.
30. Hood SD, Nutt DJ. Psychopharmacological treatments: an overview. In: Crozier R, Alden LE (eds). *International Handbook of Social Anxiety*. Oxford: John Wiley & Sons Ltd, 2001.
31. Treatment choice in psychological therapies and counselling. Evidence based clinical practice guideline. www.doh.org.uk.
32. Lader M. Treatment of anxiety. *BMJ* 1994; **309**: 321–324.
33. Allgulander C, Hackett D, Salinas E. Venlafaxine extended release (ER) in the treatment of generalised anxiety disorder. *Br J Psychiatry* 2001; **179**: 15–22.
34. Rickels K, Downing R, Schweizer E *et al.* Antidepressants for the treatment of generalised anxiety disorder: a placebo controlled comparison of imipramine, trazodone and diazepam. *Arch Gen Psychiatry* 1993; **50**: 884–895.

35. Lader M, Scotto JC. A multicentre double-blind comparison of hydroxyzine, buspirone and placebo in patients with generalised anxiety disorder. *Psychopharmacology* 1998; **139**: 402–406.
36. Kapczinski F, Lima MS, Souza JS *et al*. Antidepressants for generalized anxiety disorder (review). Cochrane Library 2005.
37. Rickels K, Zaninelli R, McCafferty J *et al*. Paroxetine treatment of generalized anxiety disorder: a double-blind, placebo controlled study. *Am J Psychiatry* 2003; **160**: 749–756.
38. Allgulander C, Dahl AA, Austin C *et al*. Efficacy of sertraline in a 12 week trial for generalized anxiety disorder. *Am J Psychiatry* 2004; **161**: 1642–1649.
39. Lenox-Smith AJ, Reynolds A. A double-blind, randomised, placebo controlled study of venlafaxine XL in patients with generalized anxiety disorder in primary care. *Br J Gen Pract* 2003; **53**: 772–777.
40. Rosenthal M. Tiagabine for the treatment of generalized anxiety disorder: a randomized, open-label, clinical trial with paroxetine as a positive control. *J Clin Psychiatry* 2003; **64**: 1245–1249.
41. Atmaca M, Kuloglu M, Tezcan E *et al*. Quetiapine augmentation in patients with treatment resistant obsessive-compulsive disorder: a single blind, placebo controlled study. *Int Clin Psychopharmacol* 2002; **17**: 115–119.
42. McDougle CJ, Epperson CN, Pelton GH *et al*. A double-blind placebo-controlled study of risperidone addition in serotonin reuptake inhibitor-refractory obsessive compulsive disorder. *Arch Gen Psychiatry* 2000; **57**: 794–801.
43. McDougle CJ, Goodman WK, Leckman JF. Haloperidol addition in fluvoxamine-refractory obsessive-compulsive disorder. *Arch Gen Psychiatry* 1994; **51**: 302–308.
44. Koran LM, Sallee FR, Pallanti S. Rapid benefit of intravenous pulse loading of clomipramine in obsessive-compulsive disorder. *Am J Psychiatry* 1997; **154**: 396–401.
45. Piccinelli M, Pini S, Bellantovonoc C *et al*. Efficacy of drug treatment in obsessive-compulsive disorder. A meta-analytic review. *Br J Psychiatry* 1995; **166**: 424–433.
46. Park LT, Jefferson JW, Greist JH. Obsessive-compulsive disorder: treatment options. *CNS Drugs* 1997; 7; 187–202.
47. Denys D, de Geus F, van Megen HJGM *et al*. A double-blind, randomised, placebo-controlled trial of quetiapine addition in patients with obsessive-compulsive disorder refractory to serotonin reuptake inhibitors. *J Clin Psychiatry* 2004; **8**: 1040–1048.
48. Shapira NA, Ward HE, Mandoki M *et al*. A double-blind, placebo-controlled trial of olanzapine addition in fluoxetine-refractory obsessive-compulsive disorder. *Biol Psychiatry* 2004; **550**: 553–555.
49. Maina G, Albert U, Ziero S *et al*. Antipsychotic augmentation for treatment resistant obsessive-compulsive disorder: what if antipsychotic is discontinued? *Int Clin Psychopharmacol* 2003; **18**: 23–28.
50. Hollander E, Rossi NB, Sood E *et al*. Risperidone augmentation in treatment-resistant obsessive-compulsive disorder: a double-blind, placebo controlled study. *Int J Neuropsychopharmacol* 2003; **6**: 397–401
51. Pallanti S, Quercioli L, Bruscoli M. Response acceleration with mirtazepine augmentation of citalopram in obsessive-compulsive disorder patients without comorbid depression: a pilot study. *J Clin Psychiatry* 2004; **65**: 1394–1399.
52. Hollander E, Friedberg J, Wasserman S *et al*. Venlafaxine in treatment-resistant obsessive-compulsive disorder. *J Clin Psychiatry* 2003; **64**: 546–550.
53. Johnson MR, Lydiard RB, Ballenger JC. Panic disorder: pathophysiology and drug treatment. *Drugs* 1995; **49**: 328–344.
54. Versiani M, Cassano G, Perugi G *et al*. Reboxetine, a selective norepinephrine reuptake inhibitor, is an effective and well-tolerated treatment for panic disorder. *J Clin Psychiatry* 2002; **63**: 31–37.
55. Bakker A, van Balkom AJLM, Spinhoven P *et al*. SSRIs V TCAs in the treatment of panic disorder: a meta-analysis. *Acta Psychiatr Scand* 2002; **106**: 163–167.
56. Wade A. Antidepressants in panic disorder. *Int Clin Psychopharmacol* 1999; 10(Suppl. 14): 13–17.
57. Benjamin J, Levine J, Fox M *et al*. Double-blind, placebo controlled, crossover trial of inositol treatment for panic disorder. *Am J Psychiatry* 1995; **152**: 1084–1086.
58. Baetz M, Bowen RC. Efficacy of divalproex sodium in patients with panic disorder and mood instability who have not responded to conventional therapy. *Can J Psychiatry* 1998; **43**: 73–77.
59. Otto MW, Tuby KS, Gould RA *et al*. An effect-size analysis of the relative efficacy and tolerability of serotonin selective reuptake inhibitors for panic disorder. *Am J Psychiatry* 2001; **158**: 1989–1992.
60. Bruce SE, Vasile RG, Goisman RM *et al*. Are benzodiazepines still the medication of choice for patients with panic disorder with or without agoraphobia. *Am J Psychiatry* 2003; **160**: 1432–1438.
61. Bandelow B, Behnke K, Lenoir S *et al*. Sertraline versus paroxetine in the treatment of panic disorder: an acute, double-blind noninferiority comparison. *J Clin Psychiatry* 2004; **65**: 405–413.
62. Sarchiapone M, Amore M, De Risio S *et al*. Mirtazepine in the treatment of panic disorder: an open label trial. *Int Clin Psychopharmacol* 2003; **18**: 35–38.
63. Connor KM, Sutherland SM, Tupler LA *et al*. Fluoxetine in post-traumatic stress disorder: randomised, double-blind study. *Br J Psychiatry* 1999; **175**: 17–22.
64. Davidson J. Drug therapy of post-traumatic stress disorder. *Br J Psychiatry* 1992; **160**: 309–314.
65. Taylor FB. Tiagabine for posttraumatic stress disorder; a case series of 7 women. *J Clin Psychiatry* 2003; **64**: 1421–1425.
66. Pivac N, Kovacic DK, Muck-Seler D. Olanzapine versus fluphenazine in an open trial in patients with psychotic combat-related post-traumatic stress disorder. *Psychopharmacology* (Berl). 2004 Oct; **175**: 451–456.
67. Fiteau MJ. Quetiapine reduces flashbacks in chronic posttraumatic stress disorder. *Can J Psychiatry* 2003; **48**: 282–283.
68. Sagud JM, Sagud M, Peles M. Olanzapine in the treatment-resistant, combat-related PTSD – a series of case reports. *Acta Psychiatr Scand* 2003; **107**: 394–396.
69. Otte C, Wiedemann K, Yassouridis A *et al*. Valproate monotherapy in the treatment of civilian patients with non-combat related posttraumatic stress disorder: an open label study. *J Clin Psychopharmacol* 2004; **24**: 106–108.
70. Davidson JRT, Weisler RH, Butterfield MI *et al*. Mirtazepine vs placebo in posttraumatic stress disorder: a pilot trial. *Biol Psychiatry* 2003; **53**: 188–191.

Depression & anxiety

71. Reich DD, Winternitz S, Hennen J *et al.* A preliminary study of risperidone in the treatment of posttraumatic stress disorder related to childhood abuse in women. *J Clin Psychiatry* 2004; **65**: 1601–1606.

72. Bremner JD, Mietzko T, Welter S *et al.* Treatment of posttraumatic stress disorder with phenytoin; an open-label pilot study. *J Clin Psychiatry* 2004; **65**: 1559–1564.

73. Schoenfeld FB, Marmar CR, Neylan TC. Current concepts in pharmacotherapy for posttraumatic stress disorder. *Psychiatr Serv* 2004; **55**: 519–531.

74. Blanco C, Schneirer FR, Schmidt A *et al.* Pharmacological treatment of social anxiety disorder: a meta-analysis. *Depress Anxiety* 2003; **18**: 29–40.

75. Stein MB, Pollack MH, Bystritsky A *et al.* Efficacy of low and higher dose extended-release venlafaxine in generalized social anxiety disorder: a 6-month randomized controlled trial. *Psychopharmacology* (Berl). 2005 Jan; **177**: 280–288.

76. Aarre TF. Phenelzine efficacy in refractory social anxiety disorder: a case series. *Nordic J Psychiat* 2003; **57**: 313–315.

77. Simon NM, Worthington JJ, Doyle AC *et al.* An open-label study of levetiracetam for the treatment of social anxiety disorder. *J Clin Psychiatry* 2004; **65**: 1219–1222.

78. Kinrys G, Pollack MH, Simon NM *et al.* Valproic acid for the treatment of social anxiety disorder. *Int Clin Psychopharmacol* 2003; **18**: 169–172.

Further reading

Hood SD, Argyroupoulos SV, Nutt DJ. Agents in development for anxiety disorders: current status and future potential. *CNS Drugs* 2000; **13**: 421–431.

Kaplan A, Hollander E. A review of pharmacological treatments for obsessive-compulsive disorder. *Psychiatr Serv* 2003; **54**: 1111–1118.

Depression & anxiety

Benzodiazepines

Benzodiazepines are normally divided into two groups depending on their half-life: hypnotics (short half-life) or anxiolytics (long half-life). Although benzodiazepines have a place in the treatment of some forms of epilepsy and severe muscle spasm, and as premedicants in some surgical procedures, the vast majority of prescriptions are written for their hypnotic and anxiolytic effects. A detailed account of the pharmacology of benzodiazepines, with respect to their anxiolytic and hypnotic properties, has been published by Nutt and Malizia[1]. Benzodiazepines are also used for rapid tranquillisation (see page 313) and, as adjuncts, in the treatment of depression and schizophrenia.

Anxiolytic effect

Benzodiazepines reduce pathological anxiety, agitation and tension. Although useful in the emergency management of anxiety, benzodiazepines are addictive, and in the majority of patients, use should be restricted to no more than 1 month[2]. In contrast with the commonly held belief that benzodiazepines should be avoided in bereavement as they inhibit psychological adjustment, an RCT by Warner et al.[3] found that benzodiazepines had no effect on the course of bereavement.

Repeat prescriptions should be avoided in those with major personality problems, whose difficulties are unlikely ever to resolve. Benzodiazepines should also be avoided, if possible, in those with a history of substance misuse.

Hypnotic effect

Benzodiazepines inhibit REM sleep and a rebound increase is seen when they are discontinued. There is a debate over the significance of this property[4].

Many people have unrealistic sleep expectations and hypnotics are effective drugs, at least in the short term. A high proportion of hospitalised patients are prescribed hypnotics[5]. Care should be taken to avoid using hypnotics regularly or for long periods of time[6]. Physical causes (pain, dyspnoea, etc.) or substance misuse (most commonly high caffeine consumption) should always be excluded before a hypnotic drug is prescribed. Be particularly careful to avoid prescribing hypnotics on discharge from hospital, as iatrogenic dependence may be the result.

Use in depression

Benzodiazepines are not a treatment for major depressive illness. The National Service Framework for Mental Health[7] highlights this point by including a requirement that GPs audit the ratio of benzodiazepines to antidepressants prescribed in their practice. NICE found no evidence to support the use of benzodiazepines alongside antidepressants in the initial treatment of depression[8].

Use in psychosis

Benzodiazepines have been shown to be effective in treating the prodromal symptoms of psychotic relapse[9]. The efficacy of benzodiazepines in RT, in conjunction with the fact that a significant minority of patients fail to respond adequately to antipsychotics alone, can result in benzodiazepines being prescribed on a chronic basis[10]. The literature in this area is confusing. There is evidence that

Depression & anxiety

some treatment-resistant patients may benefit from a combination of antipsychotics and benzodiazepines, either by showing a very marked antipsychotic response or by allowing the use of lower-dose antipsychotic regimens[11]. Alprazolam and clonazepam are possibly more effective than the other benzodiazepines in this regard[11].

Side-effects

Headaches, confusion, ataxia, dysarthria, blurred vision, gastrointestinal disturbances, jaundice and paradoxical excitement are all possible side-effects. A high incidence of reversible psychiatric side-effects, specifically loss of memory and depression, led to the withdrawal of triazolam[12]. The use of benzodiazepines has been associated with at least a 50% increase in the risk of hip fracture in the elderly[13,14]. The risk is greatest in the first few days and after 1 month of continuous use. High doses are particularly problematic. This would seem to be a class effect (the risk is not reduced by using short-half-life drugs). Benzodiazepines can cause anterograde amnesia[15] and can adversely affect driving performance[16].

Respiratory depression is rare with oral therapy but is possible when the IV route is used. A specific benzodiazepine antagonist, flumazenil, is available. Flumazenil has a much shorter half-life than diazepam, making close observation of the patient essential for several hours after administration.

IV injections can be painful and lead to thrombophlebitis, due to the low water solubility of benzodiazepines, and therefore it is necessary to use solvents in the preparation of injectable forms. Diazepam is available in emulsion form (Diazemuls) to overcome these problems.

Drug interactions

Benzodiazepines do not induce microsomal enzymes and so do not frequently precipitate pharmacokinetic interactions with any other drugs. Most benzodiazepines are metabolised by CYP3A4, which is inhibited by erythromycin, several SSRIs and ketoconazole. It is theoretically possible that co-administration of these drugs will result in higher serum levels of benzodiazepines. Pharmacodynamic interactions (usually increased sedation) can occur. Benzodiazepines are associated with an important interaction with methadone (see page 243).

References

1. Nutt DJ, Malizia AL. New insights into the role of the GABAa-benzodiazepine receptor in psychiatric disorder. *Br J Psychiatry* 2001; **179**: 390–396.
2. Committee on Safety of Medicines. Benzodiazepines, dependence and withdrawal symptoms. *Current Problems* 1988; **21**: 1–2.
3. Warner J, Metcalfe C, King M. Evaluating the use of benzodiazepines following recent bereavement. *Br J Psychiatry* 2001; **178**: 36–41.
4. Vogel GW, Buffenstein A, Minter K *et al*. Drug effects on REM sleep and on endogenous depression. *Neurosci Behav Rev* 1990; **14**: 49–63.
5. Mahomed R, Paton C, Lee E. Prescribing hypnotics in a mental health trust: what consultants say and what they do. *Pharm J* 2002; **268**: 657–659.
6. Royal College of Psychiatrists. *Benzodiazepines: Risks, Benefits or Dependence: a re-evaluation*. Council Report CR59. London: Royal College of Psychiatrists, 1997.
7. Department of Health. *The National Service Framework for Mental Health*. London: DoH, 1999.
8. National Institute for Clinical Excellence. Treatment guidelines for depression. 2004 www.nice.org.uk.
9. Carpenter WT, Buchanan RW, Kirkpatrick B *et al*. Diazepam treatment of early signs of exacerbation in schizophrenia. *Am J Psychiatry* 1999; **156**: 299–303.
10. Paton C, Banham S, Whitmore J. Benzodiazepines in schizophrenia: is there a trend towards long-term prescribing? *Psychiatr Bull* 2000; **24**: 113–115.
11. Wolkowitz OM, Pickar D. Benzodiazepines in the treatment of schizophrenia: a review and re-appraisal. *Am J Psychiatry* 1991; **148**: 714–726.

12. The sudden withdrawl of triazolam – reasons and consequences. *Drug Therap Bull* 1991; **29**: 89–90.
13. Wang PS, Bohn RL, Glynn RJ *et al.* Hazardous benzodiazepine regimens in the elderly: effects of half-life, dosage and duration on risk of hip fracture. *Am J Psychiatry* 2001; **158**: 892–898.
14. Cumming RG, Couteur DG. Benzodiazepines and risk of hip fracture in older people. A review of the evidence. *CNS Drugs* 2003; **17**: 825–837.
15. Verway B, Eling P, Wientjes H *et al.* Memory impairment in those who attempted suicide by benzodiazepine overdose. *J Clin Psychiatry* 2000; **61**: 456–459.
16. Barbone F, McMahon AD, Davey PG *et al.* Association of road-traffic accidents with benzodiazepine use. *Lancet* 1998; **352**: 1331–1336.

Further reading

Ashton H. Guidelines for the rational use of benzodiazepines. *Drugs* 1994; **48**: 25–40.
Chouinard G. Issues in the clinical use of benzodiazepines: potency, withdrawal and rebound. *J Clin Psychiatry* 2004; **65**(Suppl. 5): 7–12.
Summers J, Brown KW. Benzodiazepine prescribing in a psychiatric hospital. *Psychiatr Bull* 1998; **22**: 480–483.
Williams DDR, McBride A. Benzodiazepines: time for reassessment. *Br J Psychiatry* 1998; **173**: 361–362.

Depression & anxiety

Benzodiazepines and disinhibition

Unexpected increases in aggressive behaviour secondary to drug treatment are usually called disinhibitory or paradoxical reactions. These reactions may be characterised by acute excitement, hyperactivity, increased anxiety, vivid dreams, sexual disinhibition, hostility and rage. It is possible for a drug to have the potential both to decrease and increase aggressive behaviour. Examples include amphetamines, methylphenidate, benzodiazepines and alcohol (note that all are potential drugs of misuse).

How common are disinhibitory reactions with benzodiazepines?

The incidence of disinhibitory reactions varies widely depending on the population studied (see 'Who is at risk?' below). For example, a meta-analysis of benzodiazepine randomised, controlled trials (RCTs) that included many hundreds of patients with a wide range of diagnoses reported an incidence of less than 1% (similar to placebo)[1]; an RCT that recruited patients with panic disorder reported an incidence of 13%[2]; authors of case series (often reporting on use in high-risk patients) reported rates of 10–20%[1]; and an RCT that included patients with borderline personality disorder reported a rate of 58%[3].

Who is at risk?

Those who have learning disability, neurological disorder or CNS degenerative disease[4], are young (child or adolescent) or elderly[4,5], or have a history of aggression/poor impulse control[3,6] are at increased risk of experiencing a disinhibitory reaction. The risk is further increased if the benzodiazepine is a high-potency drug, has a short half-life, is given in a high dose or is administered intravenously (high and rapidly fluctuating plasma levels)[4,7]. Some people may be genetically predisposed[8].

What is the mechanism?[7,9,10]

Various theories of the mechanism have been proposed: the anxiolytic and amnesic properties of benzodiazepines may lead to a loss of the restraint that governs normal social behaviour, the sedative and amnesic properties of benzodiazepines may lead to a reduced ability to concentrate on the external social cues that guide appropriate behaviour and the benzodiazepine-mediated increases in GABA neurotransmission may lead to a decrease in the restraining influence of the cortex, resulting in untrammelled excitement, anxiety and hostility.

Subjective reports

People who take benzodiazepines rate themselves as being more tolerant and friendly, but respond more to provocation, than placebo-treated patients[11]. People with impulse control problems who take benzodiazepines may self-report feelings of power and overwhelming self-esteem[6]. Psychology rating scales demonstrate increased suggestibility, failure to recognise anger in others and reduced ability to recognise social cues.

Clinical implications

Benzodiazepines are frequently used in rapid tranquillisation and the short-term management of disturbed behaviour. It is important to be aware of their propensity to cause disinhibitory reactions.

Paradoxical/disinhibitory/aggressive outbursts in the context of benzodiazepine use:

- usually occur with high doses of high-potency drugs that are administered parenterally.
- are rare in the general population but more frequent in people with impulse control problems or CNS damage and in the very young or very old.
- usually occur in response to (very mild) provocation, the exact nature of which is not always obvious to others.
- are recognised by others but often not by the sufferer, who often believes that he is friendly and tolerant.

Suspected paradoxical reactions should be clearly documented in the clinical notes. In extreme cases, flumazenil can be used to reverse the reaction. If the benzodiazepine was prescribed to control acute behavioural disturbance, future episodes should be managed with parenteral antipsychotic drugs[12] or other non-benzodiazepine sedatives.

References

1. Dietch JT, Jennings RK. Aggressive dyscontrol in patients treated with benzodiazepines. *J Clin Psychiatry* 1998; **49**: 184–188.
2. O'Sullivan GH, Noshirvani H, Basoglu M *et al.* Safety and side effects of alprazolam: controlled study in agoraphobia with panic disorder. *Br J Psychiatry* 1994; **165**: 79–86.
3. Gardner DL, Cowdry RW. Alprazolam induced dyscontrol in borderline personality disorder. *Am J Psychiatry* 1985; **142**: 98–100.
4. Bond AJ. Drug-induced behavioural disinhibition. *CNS Drugs* 1998; **9**: 41–57.
5. Hawkridge SM, Stein DJ. A risk-benefit assessment of pharmacotherapy for anxiety disorders in children and adolescents. *Drug Safety* 1998; **19**: 283–297.
6. Daderman AM, Lidberg L. Flunitrazepam (Rohypnol) abuse in combination with alcohol causes premeditated, grievous violence in male juvenile offenders. *J Am Acad of Psychiat Law* 1999; **27**: 83–99.
7. van der Bijl P, Roelofse JA. Disinhibitory reactions to benzodiazepines: a review. *J Oral Maxillofac Surg* 1991; **49**: 519–523.
8. Short TG, Forrest P, Galletly DC. Paradoxical reactions to benzodiazepines – a genetically determined phenomenon? *Anaesth Intensive Care* 1987; **15**: 330.
9. Weisman AM, Berman ME, Taylor SP. Effects of chlorazepate, diazepam and oxazepam on a laboratory measurement of aggression in men. *Int Clin Psychopharmacol* 1998; **13**: 183–188.
10. Blair RJR, Curran HV. Selective impairment in the recognition of anger induced by diazepam *Psychopharmacology* 1999; **147**: 335–338.
11. Bond AJ, Curran HV, Bruce MS *et al.* Behavioural aggression in panic disorder after 8 weeks treatment with alprazolam. *J Affect Disorders* 1995; **35**: 117–123.
12. Paton C. Benzodiazepines and disinhibition: a review. *Psychiatr Bull* 2002; **26**: 460–462.

Depression & anxiety

Benzodiazepines: dependence and detoxification

Benzodiazepines are widely acknowledged as addictive and withdrawal symptoms can occur after 4–6 weeks of continuous use. At least a third of long-term users experience problems on dosage reduction or withdrawal[1]. Short-acting drugs such as lorazepam are associated with more problems on withdrawal than longer-acting drugs such as diazepam[1,2]. To avoid or lessen these problems, good practice dictates that benzodiazepines should not be prescribed as hypnotics or anxiolytics for longer than 4 weeks[3,4]. Intermittent use (i.e. not every day) may also help avoid problems of dependence and tolerance.

Problems on withdrawal[5]

Physical	Psychological
• Stiffness	• Anxiety/insomnia
• Weakness	• Nightmares
• GI disturbance	• Depersonalisation
• Paraesthesia	• Decreased memory and concentration
• Flu-like symptoms	• Delusions and hallucinations
• Visual disturbances	• Depression

In the majority, symptoms last no longer than a few weeks, although a minority experience disabling symptoms for much longer[1,3]. Continuing support can be required (e.g. psychological therapies or self-help groups).

If clinically indicated and assuming the patient is in agreement, benzodiazepines should be withdrawn as follows.

Confirming use

If benzodiazepines are not prescribed and patients are obtaining their own supply, use should be confirmed by urine screening (a negative urine screen in combination with no signs of benzodiazepine withdrawal, rules out physical dependence). Very short-acting benzodiazepines may not give a positive urine screen despite daily use.

Tolerance test

This will be required if the patient has been obtaining illicit supplies. No benzodiazepines/alcohol should be consumed for 12 hours before the test. A test dose of 10 mg diazepam should be administered (20 mg if consumption of >50 mg daily is claimed or suspected) and the patient observed for 2–3 hours. If there are no signs of sedation, it is generally safe to prescribe the test dose three times a day. Some patients may require much higher doses. Inpatient assessment may be desirable in these cases.

Switching to diazepam

Patients who take short- or intermediate-acting benzodiazepines should be offered an equivalent dose of diazepam (which has a long half-life and therefore provokes less severe withdrawal)[1]. Approximate 'diazepam equivalent'[1] doses are shown below.

Chlordiazepoxide	25 mg
Clonazepam	1–2 mg
Diazepam	**10 mg**
Lorazepam	1 mg
Lormetazepam	1 mg
Nitrazepam	10 mg
Oxazepam	30 mg
Temazepam	20 mg

The half-lives of benzodiazepines vary greatly. The degree of sedation that they induce also varies, making it difficult to determine exact equivalents. The above is an approximate guide only. Extra precautions apply in patients with hepatic dysfunction, as diazepam may accumulate to toxic levels. Diazepam substitution may not be appropriate in this group of patients.

Dosage reduction

- Reduce by 10 mg/day every 1–2 weeks, down to a daily dose of 50 mg.
- Reduce by 5 mg/day every 1–2 weeks, down to a daily dose of 30 mg.
- Reduce by 2 mg/day every 1–2 weeks, down to a daily dose of 20 mg.
- Reduce by 1 mg/day every 1–2 weeks until stopped.

Usually, no more than 1 week's supply (exact number of tablets) should be issued at any one time.

Anticipating problems[1,5,6]

Problematic withdrawal can be anticipated if previous attempts have been unsuccessful, the patient lacks social support, there is a history of alcohol/polydrug abuse or withdrawal seizures, the patient is elderly, or there is concomitant severe physical/psychiatric disorder or personality disorder. The acceptable rate of withdrawal may inevitably be slower in these patients. Some may never succeed. Risk–benefit analysis may conclude that maintenance treatment with benzodiazepines is appropriate[3]. Some patients may need interventions for underlying disorders masked by benzodiazepine dependence. If the patient is indifferent to withdrawal (i.e. is not motivated to stop), success is unlikely.

Adjunctive treatments

There is some evidence to support the use of antidepressant and mood-stabilising drugs as adjuncts during benzodiazepine withdrawal[1,7–10].

References

1. Schweizer E, Rickels K. Benzodiazepine dependence and withdrawal: a review of the syndrome and its clinical management. *Acta Psych Scand Suppl* 1998; **393**: 95–101.
2. Uhlenhuth EH, Balter MB, Ban TA *et al.* International study of expert judgement on therapeutic use of benzodiazepines and other psychotherapeutic medications. IV. Therapeutic dose dependence and abuse liability of benzodiazepines in the long-term management of anxiety disorders. *J Clin Psychopharmacol* 1999; **19**(Suppl. 2): 23–29.
3. Royal College of Psychiatrists. Benzodiazepines: risks, benefits or dependence: a re-evaluation. Council Report CR57. London: Royal College of Psychiatrists, 1997.
4. Committee on Safety of Medicines. Benzodiazepines, dependence and withdrawal symptoms. *Current Problems* 1988; **21**: 1–2.
5. Petursson H. The benzodiazepine withdrawal syndrome. *Addiction* 1994; **89**: 1455–1459.

Depression & anxiety

6. Tyrer P. Risks of dependence on benzodiazepine drugs: the importance of patient selection. *BMJ* 1989; **298**: 102–105.
7. Rickels K, DeMartinis N, Garcia-Espana F. Imipramine and buspirone in treatment of patients with generalised anxiety disorder who are discontinuing long-term benzodiazepine therapy. *Am J Psychiatry* 2000; **157**: 1973–1979.
8. Tyrer P, Ferguson B, Hallstrom C. A controlled trial of dothiepin and placebo in treating benzodiazepine withdrawal symptoms. *Br J Psychiatry* 1996; **168**: 457–461.
9. Schweizer E, Rickels K, Case WG *et al.* Carbamazepine treatment in patients discontinuing long term benzodiazepine therapy. *Arch Gen Psychiatry* 1991; **48**: 448–452.
10. Zitman FG, Couvee JE. Chronic benzodiazepine use in general practice patients with depression: an evaluation of controlled treatment and taper off. *Br J Psychiatry* 2001; **178**: 317–324.

Further reading

Department of Health. Drug misuse and dependence – guidelines on clinical management. London: Department of Health, 1999.
Gerada C, Ashworth M. ABC of mental health: addiction and dependence. Illicit drugs. *BMJ* 1997; **315**: 297–300.
Lader M. Withdrawal reactions after stopping hypnotics in patients with insomnia. *CNS Drugs* 1998; **10**: 425–440.
Mental Health Foundation. Guidelines for the prevention and treatment of benzodiazepine dependence. London: Mental Health Foundation, 1992.
Rickels K, DeMartinins N, Ryann M *et al.* Pharmacological strategies for discontinuing benzodiazepine treatment. *J Clin Psychopharmacol* 1999; **19**(Suppl. 2): 12–16.

Insomnia

A patient complaining of insomnia may describe one or more of the following symptoms:

- difficulty in falling asleep

- frequent waking during the night

- early morning wakening

- daytime sleepiness

- a general loss of well-being through the individual's perception of a bad night's sleep.

Insomnia is a common complaint affecting approximately one-third of the UK population in any one year[1]. It is more common in women, in the elderly (some reports suggest 50% of those over 65 years) and in those with medical or psychiatric disorders[2]. Population studies in the UK have found that the prevalence of symptoms of underlying psychiatric illness, particularly depression and anxiety, increases with the severity and chronicity of insomnia[3]. Insomnia that lasts for 1 year or more is an established risk factor for the development of depression[4]. Chronic insomnia rarely remits spontaneously[5].

Before treating insomnia with drugs, consider:

- Is the underlying cause being treated (depression, mania, breathing difficulties, urinary frequency, pain, etc.)?

- Is substance misuse or diet a problem?

- Are other drugs being given at appropriate times (i.e. stimulating drugs in the morning, sedating drugs at night)?

- Are the patient's expectations of sleep realistic (sleep requirements decrease with age)?

- Have all sleep hygiene approaches (see table below) been tried[1]?

Table Sleep hygiene approaches
- Increase daily exercise (not in the evening)
- Reduce daytime napping
- Reduce caffeine or alcohol intake, especially before bedtime
- Use the bed only for sleeping
- Use anxiety management or relaxation techniques
- Develop a regular routine of rising and retiring at the same time each day

Table	Guidelines for prescribing hypnotics[6]
1.	Use the lowest effective dose
2.	Use intermittent dosing (alternate nights or less) where possible
3.	Prescribe for short-term use (no more than 4 weeks) in the majority of cases
4.	Discontinue slowly
5.	Be alert for rebound insomnia/withdrawal symptoms
6.	Advise patients of the interaction with alcohol and other sedating drugs
7.	Avoid the use of hypnotics in patients with respiratory disease or severe hepatic impairment and in addiction-prone individuals

Short-acting hypnotics are better for patients who have difficulty dropping off to sleep, but tolerance and dependence may develop more quickly[4]. Long-acting hypnotics are more suitable for patients with frequent or early-morning wakening. These drugs may be less likely to cause rebound insomnia and can have next-day anxiolytic action, but next-day sedation and maybe loss of co-ordination are more likely to occur[6].

The most widely prescribed hypnotics are the benzodiazepines. Non-benzodiazepine hypnotics such as zopiclone and zolpidem are becoming more widely used but may be just as likely as the benzodiazepines to cause rebound, dependence and neuropsychiatric reactions[7–9]. Zopiclone may impair driving performance more than benzodiazepines[10]. NICE conclude that there is no difference in efficacy between zaleplon, zolpidem and zopiclone and that patients who fail to respond to one drug should not be offered another[11].

Table	Drugs used as hypnotics			
Drug	**Usual therapeutic dose (mg/day)**		**Time until onset (minutes)**	**Duration of action**
	Adult	*Elderly*		
Diazepam	5–10		30–60	Long
Lormetazepam	0.5–1.5		30–60	Short
Oxazepam	15–30		20–50	Medium
Nitrazepam	5–10		20–50	Long
Temazepam*	10–20	Quarter to half the adult dose	30–60	Short
Zaleplon	10		30	Very short
Zopiclone	3.75–7.5		15–30	Medium
Zolpidem	5–10		7–27	Short
Promethazine (not licensed)	25–50		Unclear, but may be 1–2 hours	Long

* Temazepam is a popular drug of misuse. Some of the Controlled Drug regulations apply to its prescription, supply and administration. Nursing paperwork can be simplified considerably by avoiding the use of this drug.

Although it is commonly believed that tolerance always develops rapidly to the hypnotic effect of benzodiazepines[11] and zopiclone, there are only limited objective data to support this, and the magnitude of the problem may have been overestimated[5]. Long-term treatment with hypnotics may be beneficial in a very small number of patients. Case reports, case series and consensus statements support this approach[4–6,12–14]. Long-term users may overestimate the benefits on continuing use: after a period of rebound symptoms immediately after withdrawal, may chronic users will return to the same sleep pattern (drug free) that they previously associated with hypnotic use[15]. As with all prescribing, the potential benefits and risks of hypnotic drugs have to be considered in the context of the clinical circumstances of each case.

References

1. Hajak G. A comparative assessment of the risks and benefits of zopiclone. *Drug Safety* 1999; **21**: 457–469.
2. Shapiro CM (ed.). *ABC of Sleep Disorders*. London: BMJ Publishing Group, 1993.
3. Nutt DJ, Wilson S. Evaluation of severe insomnia in the general population – implications for the management of insomnia: the UK perspective. *J Psychopharmacol* 1999; **13**(Suppl. 1): 33–34.
4. Moller HJ. Effectiveness and safety of benzodiazepines (benzodiazepine dependence and withdrawal: myths and management). *J Clin Psychopharmacol* 1999; **19**(Suppl. 2): 25–115.
5. Nowell PD, Mazumdar S, Buysse DJ *et al*. Benzodiazepines and zolpiderm for chronic insomnia. *J Am Med Assoc* 1997; **278**: 2170–2177.
6. Royal College of Psychiatrists. *Benzodiazepines: Risks, Benefits or Dependence: a re-evaluation.* Council Report CR59. London: Royal College of Psychiatrists, 1997.
7. Sikdar S, Ruben SM. Zopiclone abuse among polydrug users. *Addiction* 1996; **91**: 285–286.
8. Genick CA, Ludolph AC. Chronic abuse of zolpiderm. *J Am Med Assoc* 1994; **272**: 1721–1722.
9. Voshaar RCO, Balkom AJLM, Zitman FG. Zolpidem is not superior to temazepam with respect to rebound insomnia: a controlled study. *Eur Neuropsychopharmacol* 2004; **14**: 301–306.
10. Barbone F, McMahon AD, Davey PG *et al*. Association of road traffic accidents with benzodiazepine use. *Lancet* 1998; **352**: 1331–1336.
11. National Institute for Clinical Excellence. Zaleplon, zolpidem and zopiclone for the short-term management of insomnia. Technology Appraisal Guidance 77, 2004. www.nice.org.uk.
12. Lader M. Withdrawal reactions after stopping hypnotics in patients with insomnia. *CNS Drugs* 1998; **10**: 425–440.
13. Perlis ML, McCall V, Krystal AD *et al*. Long-term, non-nightly administration of zolpidem in the treatment of patients with primary insomnia. *J Clin Psychiatry* 2004; **68**: 1128–1137.
14. Mahomed R, Paton C, Lee E. Prescribing hypnotics in a mental health trust: what consultant psychiatrists say and what they do. *Pharm J* 2002; **268**: 657–659.
15. Poyares D, Guilleminault C, Ohayon MM *et al*. Chronic benzodiazepine usage and withdrawal in insomnia patients. *J Psychiatr Res* 2004; **38**: 327–334.

Further reading

Terzano MG, Rossi M, Palomba V *et al*. New drugs for insomnia: comparative tolerability of zopiclone, zolpidem and zaleplon. *Drug Safety* 2003; **26**: 261–282.

Depression & anxiety

chapter 5

Children and adolescents

Children and adolescents suffer from all the illnesses of adulthood. It is common for psychiatric illness to commence more diffusely, present 'atypically', respond less predictably and be associated with cumulative impairment more subtly. Childhood-onset illness is likely to be at least as severe and functionally disabling as adult-onset illness.

Very few psychotropic drugs are licensed for use in children. This should be carefully explained and informed consent sought from patients and their parents/carers.

Children

Principles of prescribing practice in childhood and adolescence[1]

1. **Target symptoms, not diagnoses.**
   Diagnosis can be difficult in children and co-morbidity is very common. Treatment should target key symptoms. While a working diagnosis is beneficial to frame expectations and facilitate communication with patients and parents, it should be kept in mind that it may take some time for the illness to evolve.

2. **Begin with less, go slow and be prepared to end with more.**
   In out-patient care, dosage will usually commence lower in mg/kg per day terms than adults and finish higher in mg/kg per day terms, if titrated to a point of maximal response.

3. **Multiple medications are often required in the severely ill.**
   Monotherapy is ideal. However, childhood-onset illness can be severe and may require treatment with psychosocial approaches in combination with more than one medication[2].

4. **Allow time for an adequate trial of treatment.**
   Children are generally more ill than their adult counterparts and will often require longer periods of treatment before responding. An adequate trial of treatment for those who have required in-patient care will therefore involve 8–12 weeks for most major conditions.

5. **Where possible, change one drug at a time.**

6. **Patient and family medication education is essential.**
   For some child and adolescent psychiatric patients the need for medication will be lifelong. The first experiences with medications are therefore crucial to long-term outcomes and adherence. It is important to adhere to the principles of CAAT (see page 362).

References

1. Nunn K, Dey C. *The Clinician's Guide to Psychotropic Prescribing in Children and Adolescents.* Sydney: Glade Publishing, 2004.
2. Luk E, Reed E. *Polypharmacy or pharmacologically rich? The Clinician's Guide to Psychotropic Prescribing in Children and Adolescents.* Sydney: Glade Publishing, 2004.

Children

Depression in children and adolescents

Psychological treatments should always be considered first-line. If these are inappropriate, have failed or are simply not available, **fluoxetine**[1,2] is the treatment of choice. Note that the placebo response rate is high in younger people[3] and that the benefits of active treatment are likely to be marginal: it is estimated that 1 in 6 may benefit[4]. The risk–benefit ratios for the other SSRIs are unfavourable (no proven efficacy, and increased risk of suicidal thoughts or acts). If there is no response to fluoxetine and drug treatment is still considered to be the most favourable option, **an alternative SSRI** may be used cautiously by specialists. Note that paroxetine and venlafaxine are considered to be unsuitable options[2]. It is important that the dose is increased slowly to minimise the risk of treatment-emergent agitation and that patients are monitored closely for the development of treatment-emergent suicidal thoughts and acts (number needed to harm (NNH) 60–80). Patients should be seen at least weekly in the early stages of treatment. See chapter 4 for more information.

Patients and their parents/carers should be well informed about the potential problems associated with SSRI treatment and know how to seek help in an emergency. They should be given a copy of the MHRA leaflet about the use of SSRIs in young people (available via the MHRA website)[2].

Tricyclic antidepressants are not effective in pre-pubertal children but may have marginal efficacy in adolescents[5]. Amitriptyline (up to 200 mg/day), imipramine (up to 300 mg/day) and nortriptyline have all been studied in RCTs. Note that due to more extensive metabolism, young people require higher mg/kg doses than adults. The side-effect burden associated with TCAs may be considerable. Vertigo, orthostatic hypotension, tremor and dry mouth limit tolerability. Tricyclics are also more cardiotoxic in young people than in adults. Baseline and on-treatment ECGs should be performed. Co-prescribing with other drugs known to prolong the QTc interval should be avoided. There is no evidence that adolescents who fail to respond to SSRIs respond to tricyclics.

Severe depression that is life-threatening or unresponsive to other treatments may respond to ECT[6]. ECT should not be used in children under 12[4]. The effects of ECT on the developing brain are unknown.

There is no good evidence to support the optimum duration of treatment. Adult guidelines are usually followed (see chapter 4). At the end of treatment, the antidepressant dose should be tapered down slowly to minimise discontinuation symptoms. Ideally this should be done over 6–12 weeks[4].

Note that up to a third of young people who present with an episode of depression will have a diagnosis of bipolar affective disorder within 5 years. When the presentation is of severe depression, associated with psychosis or rapid mood shifts and worsens on treatment with antidepressants, early bipolar illness should be suspected. Treatment with antidepressants alone is associated with new or worsening rapid cycling in as many as 23% of bipolar patients[7]. The younger the child, the greater the risk[8]. Early treatment with **mood-stabilisers** should be considered.

References

1. Whittington CJ, Kendall T, Cottrell D *et al.* Selective serotonin reuptake inhibitors in childhood depression: systematic review of published versus unpublished data. *Lancet* 2004; **363**: 1341–1345.
2. www.mhra.gov.uk
3. Jureidini JN, Doecke CJ, Mansfield PR *et al.* Efficacy and safety of antidepressants for children and adolescents. *BMJ* 2004; **328**: 879–883.
4. National Institute for Clinical Excellence, 2004. Depression in children (treatment guidelines). www.nice.org.uk
5. Hazell P, O'Connell D, Heathcote D *et al.* Tricyclic drugs for depression in children and adolescents. The Cochrane Database of Systematic Reviews, 2002.

Children

6. McKeough G. *Electroconvulsive therapy. The Clinician's Guide to Psychotropic Prescribing in Children and Adolescents.* Sydney: Glade Publishing, 2004.
7. Ghaemi SN, Boiman EE, Goodwin FK. Diagnosing bipolar disorder and the effect of antidepressants: a naturalistic study. *J Clin Psychiatry* 2000; **61**(10): 804–808.
8. Martin A, Young C, Leckman JF *et al.* Age effects on antidepressant-induced manic conversion. *Arch Pediatr Adolesc Med* 2004; **158**(8): 773–780.

Further Reading

Bloch Y, Levcovitch Y, Bloch AM. Electroconvulsive therapy in adolescents: similarities to and differences from adults. *J Am Acad Child Adolesc Psychiatry* 2001; **40**: 1332–1336.

Bipolar illness in children and adolescents

Bipolar illness with an onset in childhood or adolescence has a poorer prognosis than adult-onset illness[1]. The prevalence of comorbid psychiatric illness is high: anxiety disorders, conduct disorder, obsessive compulsive disorder (OCD) and substance abuse are common. Bipolar onset may precede substance abuse in many cases[2].

Medication	Comment
Valproate[5,9–14]	Effective in approximately 50% of acute manic or mixed episodes.
	More effective when combined with lithium or quetiapine.
	Marked weight gain can occur (association between weight gain, hyperandrogenism and polycystic ovarian syndrome. Adolescent girls may be more vulnerable than adults).
	Rare reports of serious hepatotoxicity in children.
	Very teratogenic (see page 268). Adequate contraception essential in sexually active adolescents.
Lithium [5,9,15–22]	Generally better at preventing manic episodes than depression.
	Often ineffective in rapid cycling.
	Younger children generally have more side-effects than older children (lower serum levels may be appropriate). Very toxic in overdose.
	Rapid withdrawal may precipitate a manic episode and this may be problematic in poor compliers. May be effective in reducing co-morbid substance abuse.
Carbamazepine[5]	High potential for drug interactions.
Lamotrigine[23–26]	Anecdotal reports of success in younger populations, with sometimes dramatic impact on reducing self-harm.
	Risk of Stevens–Johnson syndrome 1% (greatest in the first 8 weeks). Risk reduced with slow dose titration and special dosing guidelines for concomitant valproate – see manufacturer's guidelines. Safety data available from paediatric epilepsy populations.
	Evidence is lacking but, anecdotally, adolescent dosing similar to adults is appropriate (100–125 mg b.d.).
Olanzapine[27,28]	Open label study supports efficacy in acute mania.
	Dietician involvement recommended for weight management.
Quetiapine[12,27,29–31]	No published data. Expert opinion supports use in mania and agitation.
Antidepressants[32–36]	Should only be used when a combination of mood-stabilisers has failed.
	Can cause switching and increase rapidity of cycling even in the presence of mood-stabilisers.
	Avoid in rapid cycling.
	If commenced and patient is stabilised, use continuously as discontinuation may cause depressive relapse; i.e. acute treatment only in times of depression may be detrimental.

Children

Three or more untreated episodes may lead to cognitive impairment[3]. The more episodes, the more difficult they are to treat[4]. It is important to start treatment early and monitor carefully for the development of suicidal behaviour.

The evidence base supporting the use of mood-stabilizers in early-onset illness is poor. There are no adequately powered RCTs.

Valproate is usually the medication of first choice, followed by **lithium** and then **carbamazepine**. Response rates (total clinical global improvement and YMRS improvement) have been estimated to be: valproate 53%, lithium 38% and carbamazepine 38%[5]. **Lamotrigine** is used if treatment-resistant depressive episodes are present. Adolescents often respond poorly to monotherapy and more than one drug may be required to control symptoms[6,7]. **Antipsychotic** drugs may be required (see above).

Once symptomatic improvement occurs, treatment should be continued for at least 2 years to prevent relapse. Poor treatment response and recurrence are common[8].

Biochemical and physical monitoring should be carried out as for adults (see page 120).

References

1. Mick E, Biederman J, Faraone SV *et al.* Defining a developmental subtype of bipolar disorder in a sample of non-referred adults by age at onset *J Child Adolesc Psychopharmacol* 2003; **13**: 453–462.
2. Findling RL, Gracious BL, McNamara NK *et al.* Rapid, continuous cycling and psychiatric co-morbidity in paediatric bipolar I disorder. *Bipolar Disord* 2001; **3**: 202–210.
3. Vieta E, Benbarre A, Martinez-Aran A. Brain imaging correlates of cognitive dysfunction in bipolar disorder. *Bipolar Disord* 2004; **6**(Suppl. 1): 19.
4. Kessing LV, Anderson EW, Anderson PK. Predictors of recurrence of affective disorders in affective disorders – analysis accounting for individual heterogenicity. *J Affect Disorders* 2000; **57**(1–3): 139–145.
5. Kowatch RA, Suppes T, Carmody TJ *et al.* Effect size of lithium, divalproex sodium, and carbamazepine in children and adolescents with bipolar disorder. *J Am Acad Child Adolesc Psychiatry* 2000; **39**: 713–720.
6. Bhangoo RK, Myers FS *et al.* Medication use in children and adolescents treated in the community for bipolar disorder. *J Child Adolesc Psychopharmacol* 2003; **13**: 515–522.
7. Tillman R, Geller B. Definitions of rapid, ultrarapid, and ultradian cycling of episode duration in pediatric and adult bipolar disorders: a proposal to distinguish episodes from cycles. *J Child Adolesc Psychopharmacol* 2003; **13**: 267–271.
8. Weckerly J. Pediatric bipolar mood disorder. *J Dev Behav Pediatr* 2002; **23**: 42–56.
9. Findling RL, McNamara NK, Gracious BL *et al.* Combination lithium and divalproex sodium in paediatric bipolarity. *J Am Acad Child Psychiat* 2003; **42**: 895–901.
10. Isojarvi JIT, Laatikainen TJ, Pakarinen AJ *et al.* Polycystic ovaries and hyperandrogenism in women taking valproate for epilepsy. *New Engl J Med* 1993; **329**: 1383–1388.
11. Del Bello MP, Michael LS, Lee Rosenburg BS *et al.* A double-blind, randomised, placebo-controlled, study of quetiapine as adjuvant treatment for adolescent mania. *J Am Acad Child Psychiat* 2002; **41**: 1216–1223.
12. Bowden C. The effectiveness of divalproate in all forms of mania and the broader bipolar spectrum: many questions, few answers. *J Affect Disorders* 2004; **79**(Suppl.): S9–S14.
13. Freeman TW, Clothier JL, Pazzaglia P *et al.* A double-blind comparison of valproate and lithium in the treatment of acute mania. *Am J Psychiatry* 1992; **149**: 108–111.
14. Bowden CL. Valproate. *Bipolar Disord* 2003; **5**: 189–202.
15. Kafantaris V, Coletti DJ, Dicker R *et al.* Lithium treatment of acute mania in adolescents: a placebo-controlled discontinuation study. *J Am Acad Child Psychiat* 2004; **43**: 984–993.
16. Campbell M, Silva RR, Kafantaris V *et al.* Predictors of side effects associated with lithium administration in children. *Psychopharmacol Bull* 1991; **27**: 373–380.
17. Geller B, Cooper TB, Sun K *et al.* Double-blind and placebo-controlled study of lithium for adolescent bipolar disorders with secondary substance dependency. *J Am Acad Child Psychiat* 1998; **37**: 171–178.
18. Faedda GL, Tondo L, Baldessarini RJ *et al.* Outcome after rapid vs gradual discontinuation of lithium in bipolar disorders. *Arch Gen Psychiatry* 1993; **50**: 448–455.
19. Kafantaris V, Coletti DJ, Dicker R *et al.* Are childhood psychiatric histories of bipolar adolescents associated with family history, psychosis, and response to lithium treatment? *J Affect Disorders* 1998; **51**: 153–164.
20. Goodwin FK, Fireman B, Simon GE *et al.* Suicide risk in bipolar disorder during treatment with lithium and divalproex. *JAMA* 2003; **290**: 1467–1473.
21. Moore GM, Bebchuk JM, Wilds IB *et al.* Lithium-induced increase in human brain grey matter. *Lancet* 2000; **350**(9237): 1241–1242.

Children

22. Manji HK, Moore GJ, Chen G. Lithium at 50: have the neuroprotective effects of this unique cation been overlooked? *Biol Psychiatry* 1999; **46**: 929–940.
23. Carandang CG, Maxwell DJ, Robbins DR. Lamotrigine in adolescent mood disorders (Letter to the editor). *J Am Acad Child Psychiat* 2003; **42**: 750.
24. Calabrese JR, Vieta E, Shelton MD. Latest maintenance data on lamotrigine in bipolar disorder. *Eur Neuropsychopharm* 2003; **13**: S57–S66.
25. Calabrese JR, Supples T, Bowden CL *et al.* A double-blind, placebo-controlled prophylaxis study of lamotrigine in rapid-cycling bipolar disorder. Lamictal 614 Study Group. *J Clin Psychiatry* 2000; **61**: 841–850.
26. Rzany B, Correia O, Kelly JP *et al.* Risk of Stevens-Johnson syndrome and toxic epidermal necrolysis during first weeks of anti-epileptic therapy: a case-controlled study. *Lancet* 1999; **353**(9171): 2190–2194.
27. Kafantaris V, Coletti DJ, Dicker R *et al.* Adjunctive antipsychotic treatment of adolescents with bipolar psychosis. *J Am Acad Child Adolesc Psychiatry* 2001; **40**: 1448–1456.
28. Frazier JA, Biederman J, Tohen M *et al.* A prospective open label treatment trial of olanzapine monotherapy in children and adolescents with bipolar disorder. *J Child Adolesc Psychopharmacol* 2001; **11**: 239–250.
29. Vieta E, Parramon G, Padrell E *et al.* Quetiapine in the treatment of rapid cycling bipolar disorder. *Bipolar Disord* 2002; **4**: 335–340.
30. Sokolski KN, Denson TF. Adjunctive quetiapine in bipolar patients partially responsive to lithium or valproate. *Prog Neuro-Psychoph* 2003; **27**: 863–866.
31. Shaw J, Lewis JE, Shlomo P *et al.* A study of quetiapine: efficacy and tolerability in psychotic adolescents. *J Child Adolesc Psychopharmacol* 2001; **4**(11): 415–424.
32. Practice Guidelines for the Treatment of Patients with Bipolar Disorder (Revision). *Am J Psychiatry* 2002; **159**: 1–50.
33. Martin A, Young C, Leckman JF *et al.* Age effects on antidepressant-induced manic conversion. *Arch Pediatr Adolesc Med* 2004; **158**: 773–780.
34. Keck PE, Nelson EB, McElroy SL. Advances in pharmacologic treatment of bipolar depression. *Biol Psychiatry* 2003, **53**. 671–679.
35. Bottlender R, Rudolf D, Strauss A *et al.* Mood-stabilizers reduce the risk of developing antidepressant-induced maniform states in acute treatment of bipolar I depressed patients. *J Affect Disorders* 2001; **63**(1–3): 79–83.
36. Altshuler L, Supples T, Black D *et al.* Impact of antidepressant discontinuation after acute bipolar depression remission on rates of depressive relapse at 1-year follow-up. *Am J Psychiatry* 2003; **160**: 1252–1262.

Anxiety in children and adolescents

Where anxiety is the primary diagnosis, psychological interventions such as CBT are first-line treatment[1]. Where anxiety is secondary to another psychiatric disorder, treatment should target the primary illness.

Where anxiety is severe and disabling, and CBT is inappropriate or has failed, the use of medication is likely to be considered. The evidence base is poor. CBT should always be reconsidered if the young person makes a partial response to medication.

The treatment of anxiety in children and adolescents is generally the same as in adults (see page 186). The following additional considerations apply:

- Young people are more likely to develop disinhibition with benzodiazepines than are adults[2]. Extreme care is required.

- Young people treated with SSRIs are more likely to develop treatment-emergent suicidal thoughts and acts than are adults[3]. Venlafaxine is considered to be unsuitable for use in the treatment of depression in this age group[3]. Until further data are available, it would be wise to avoid using venlafaxine for the treatment of anxiety.

- Tricyclic antidepressants are generally poorly tolerated in young people[4]. They are more cardiotoxic than in adults.

- Buspirone can cause disinhibitory reactions and worsen aggression in children[5,6]. These risks are reduced in adolescents.

References

1. Compton SN, March JS, Brent D et al. Cognitive-behavioral psychotherapy for anxiety and depressive disorders in children and adolescents: an evidence-based medicine review. J Am Acad Child Psychiat 2004; 43: 930–959.
2. Paton C. Benzodiazepines and disinhibition: a review. Psychiatr Bull 2002; 26: 460–462.
3. National Institute for Clinical Excellence. Treatment of depression in children (treatment guideline). www.nice.org.uk
4. Hazell P, O'Connell D, Heathcote D et al. Tricyclic drugs for depression in children and adolescents. Cochrane Database of Systematic Reviews, 2002.
5. Kranzler HR. The use of buspirone in an adolescent with overanxious disorder. J Am Acad Child Psychiat 1988; 27: 789–790.
6. Pfeffer CR, Jiang H, Domeshek LJ. Buspirone treatment of psychiatrically hospitalized prepubertal children with symptoms of anxiety and moderately severe aggression. J Child Adolesc Psychopharmacol 1997; 7: 145–155.

Obsessive compulsive disorder (OCD) in children and adolescents

The treatment of OCD in children follows the same principles as in adults (see page 186). Note that **sertraline**[1-3] (from age 6 years) and **fluvoxamine** (from age 8 years) are the only SSRIs licensed in the UK for the treatment of OCD in young people. Care should be taken when prescribing SSRIs as this group of drugs has been linked with the development of suicidal thoughts and acts in children who are being treated for depression (see page 207).

Benzodiazepines should be avoided as the risk of disinhibitory reactions is high[4].

Note that Tourette's syndrome is known to be associated with OCD[5] (see page 221).

References

1. Cook EH, Wagner KD, March JS *et al.* Long-term sertraline treatment of children and adolescents with obsessive-compulsive disorder. *J Am Acad Child Psychiat* 2001; **40**: 1175–1181.
2. Pediatric OCD Treatment Study Team (POTS). Cognitive-behaviour therapy, sertraline, and their combination for children and adolescents with obsessive-compulsive disorder. *JAMA* 2004; **292**: 1969–1976.
3. Geller DA, Biederman J, Stewart SE. Which SSRI? A meta-analysis of pharmacotherapy trials in paediatric obsessive compulsive disorder. *Am J Psychiatry* 2003; **160**: 1919–1928.
4. Paton C. Benzodiazepines and disinhibition: a review. *Psychiatr Bull* 2002; **26**: 460–462.
5. Lenane MC, Swedo SE, Leonard HL. Psychiatric disorders in first-degree relatives of children and adolescents with obsessive compulsive disorder. *J Am Acad Child Psychiat* 1990; **29**: 17–23.

Further Reading

Lenane MC, Swedo SE, Leonard HL. Psychiatric disorders in first degree relatives of children and adolescents with obsessive compulsive disorders. *J Am Acad Child Adolesc Psychiatry* 1990; **29**: 407–412.

McDougle C, Epperson CN, Pelton GH *et al.* A double-blind, placebo-controlled study of risperidone addition in serotonin reuptake inhibitor-refractory obsessive-compulsive disorder. *Arch Gen Psychiatry* 2000; **57**: 794–801.

Nunn K, Dey C. *Medication Table. The Clinician's Guide to Psychotropic Prescribing in Children and Adolescents.* Sydney: Glade Publishing, 2004.

Children

Attention deficit hyperactivity disorder (ADHD)

Children

1. A diagnosis of ADHD should be made only after a comprehensive assessment by a child psychiatrist or paediatrician with expertise in ADHD[1]. Appropriate psychological, psychosocial and behavioural interventions should be put in place. Drug treatments should only be part of the overall treatment plan.

2. Stimulant drugs (**methylphenidate** and **dexamphetamine**) should be used first-line. Up to 90% of children will respond[2]. Stimulants are more effective in treating hyperactivity than inattention. Dosage regimes and monitoring are outlined below.

3. **Atomoxetine**[3,4] may be a suitable alternative for children who do not respond to stimulants or whose medication cannot be administered during the day. It may also be suitable where stimulant diversion is a problem. Monitoring of liver function is advisable.

4. Third-line drugs include **clonidine**[5] and **tricyclic antidepressants**[6]. Very few children should receive these drugs for ADHD alone. There is some evidence supporting the efficacy of **carbamazepine**[7]. There is no evidence to support the use of **atypical antipsychotics**[8].

5. Co-morbid psychiatric illness is common in ADHD children. Stimulants are often helpful overall[6] but are unlikely to be appropriate for children who have a psychotic illness or established problem with substance misuse[2].

6. Once stimulant treatment has been established, it is appropriate for repeat prescriptions to be supplied through general practitioners[1].

Adults

1. Although adult ADHD is recognised by both ICD-10 and DSM-IV, it remains a controversial diagnosis in the UK.

2. Up to 10% of ADHD children may still have symptoms at the age of 30. It is appropriate to **continue treatment started in childhood** in adults whose symptoms remain disabling.

3. A new diagnosis of ADHD in an adult should only follow a comprehensive assessment including interviews with adults who knew the patient as a child.

4. The prevalence of substance misuse and antisocial personality disorder are high in adults whose ADHD was not recognised in childhood[9]. Although methylphenidate is very effective in this population[10], most psychiatrists would feel uncomfortable about initiating stimulants in adults.

5. **Atomoxetine** is effective[11] but not licensed for initiation in adults. Monitoring of liver function is advisable.

References

1. National Institute of Clinical Excellence. Guidance on the use of methylphenidate (Ritalin/Equasym) for attention deficit hyperactivity disorder (ADHD) in childhood. NICE, 2000. www.nice.org.uk
2. Hutchins P, Nunn K, Hazell P. Attention deficit hyperactivity disorder. In: *The Clinician's Guide to Psychotropic Prescribing in Children and Adolescents.* Sydney: Glade Publishing, 2004.

3. Michelson D, Allen AJ, Busner J *et al.* Once daily atomoxetine treatment for children and adolescents with attention deficit hyperactivity disorder; a randomised, placebo-controlled trial. *Am J Psychiatry* 2002; **159**: 1896–1904.
4. Kratochvil CJ, Heiligenstein JH, Dittman R *et al.* Atomoxetine and methylphenidate treatment in children with ADHD: a prospective, randomised, open label trial. *J Am Acad Child Psychiat* 2002; **41**: 776–784.
5. Connor DF, Fletcher KE, Swanson JM. A meta-analysis of clonidine for symptoms of attention-deficit hyperactivity disorder. *J Am Acad Child Psychiat* 1999; **38**: 1551–1559.
6. Hazell P. Tricyclic antidepressants in children: is there a rationale for use? *CNS Drugs* 1996; **5**: 233–239.
7. Silva RR, Munoz DM, Alpert M. Carbamazepine use in children and adolescents with features of attention-deficit hyperactivity disorder – a meta-analysis. *J Am Acad Child Psychiat* 1996; **35**: 352–358.
8. Einarson TR, Iskedjian M. Novel antipsychotics for patients with attention-deficit hyperactivity disorder: a systematic review. Ottawa: Canadian Co-ordinating Office for Health Technology Assessments, 2001.
9. Cosgrove PVF. Attention deficit hyperactivity disorder: a review. *Prim Care Psychiatry* 1997; **3**: 101–113.
10. Spencer T, Wilens T, Biederman J *et al.* A double-blind, crossover comparison of methylphenidate and placebo in adults with childhood-onset attention-deficit hyperactivity disorder. *Arch Gen Psychiatry* 1995; **52**: 434–443.
11. Spencer T, Biederman J, Wilens T *et al.* Effectiveness and tolerability of atomoxetine in adults with attention deficit hyperactivity disorder. *Am J Psychiatry* 1998; **155**: 693–695.

Children

215

Table Prescribing in ADHD

Medication	Onset and duration of action	Dose	Comment	Recommended monitoring
Methylphenidate immediate release (Ritalin)[1,2]	Onset: 20–60 min Duration: 2–4 hours	Initially 5–10 mg daily titrated up to a maximum of 60 mg/day in divided doses using weekly increments of 5–10 mg.	Usually first-line treatment. Generally well tolerated[3]. "Controlled Drug".	BP Pulse Height and weight (risks probably overstated)[9–11]. Monitor for insomnia, mood and appetite change and the development of tics[12].
Methylphenidate sustained release (Concerta XL)[1,2]	Onset: 30 min–2 hours Duration: 12 hours	Initially 18 mg in the morning, titrated up to a maximum of 54 mg. 18 mg Concerta = 15 mg Ritalin	An afternoon dose of Ritalin may be required in some children to optimize treatment. "Controlled Drug".	Discontinue if no benefits seen in 1 month.
Dexamphetamine immediate release (Dexedrine)[3,4]	Onset: 20–60 min Duration: 3–6 hours	2.5–10 mg daily to start, titrated up to a maximum of 20 mg (occasionally 40 mg) in divided doses using weekly increments of 2.5 mg.	Considered to be less well tolerated than methylphenidate[3]. "Controlled Drug".	
Atomoxetine[5,6]	Approximately 4–6 weeks (atomoxetine is a NA reuptake inhibitor)	When switching from a stimulant, continue stimulant for first 4 weeks of therapy. For children <70 kg: Start with 0.5 mg/kg/day and increase after a minimum of 7 days to 1.2 mg/kg (single or divided doses) and increase up to 1.8 mg/kg/day if necessary. For children >70 kg: Start with 40 mg and increase after a minimum of 7 days to 80 mg.	Open, randomized study reports equal efficacy to methylphenidate[7]. May be useful where stimulant diversion is a problem[8]. Once-daily dosing convenient in schoolchildren. No longer licensed in adults. Not a CD.	Pulse BP Height Weight LFTs

References

1. Wolarich ML, Doffing MA. Pharmacokinetic considerations in the treatment of attention-deficit hyperactivity disorder with methylphenidate. *CNS Drugs* 2004; **18**: 243–250.
2. *British National Formulary*, September 2004, accessed via www.bnf.org/bnf
3. Efron D, Jarman F, Barker M. Side effects of methylphenidate and dexamphetamine in children with attention deficit hyperactivity disorder: a double-blind, crossover trial. *Pediatrics* 1997; **100**: 662–666.
4. Cyr M, Brown CS. Current drug therapy recommendations for the treatment of attention deficit hyperactivity disorder. *Drugs* 1998; **56**: 215–233.
5. Kelsey DK, Sumner CR, Casat CD *et al.* Once daily atomoxetine treatment for children with attention-deficit/hyperactivity disorder, including an assessment of evening and morning behaviour: a double-blind, placebo controlled trial. *Pediatrics* 2004; **114**: e1–e8.
6. Wernicke JF, Faries D, Girod D *et al.* Cardiovascular effects of atomoxetine in children, adolescents, and adults. *Drug Safety* 2003; **26**: 729–740.
7. Kratochvil CJ, Heiligenstein JH, Dittman R *et al.* Atomoxetine and methylphenidate treatment in children with ADHD: a prospective, randomised, open-label trial. *J Am Acad Child Psychiat* 2002; **41**: 776–784.
8. Heil SH, Holmes HW, Bickel WK *et al.* Comparison of the subjective, physiological and psychomotor effects of atomoxetine and methylphenidate in light drug users. *Drug Alcohol Depen* 2002; **67**: 149–156.
9. MTA Cooperative Group. A 14-month randomized clinical trial of treatment strategies for attention deficit/hyperactivity disorder. *Arch Gen Psychiatry* 1999; **56**: 1073–1086.
10. Kramer JR, Loney J, Ponto L *et al.* Predictors of adult height and weight in boys treated with methylphenidate for childhood behavior problems. *J Am Acad Child Psychiat* 2000; **39**: 517–524.
11. Poulton A, Cowell C. Slowing of growth in children starting treatment with stimulant medication. *J Paediatr Child Health* 2003; **39**: A7.
12. Gadow KD, Sverd J, Sprafkin J *et al.* Efficacy of methylphenidate for attention-deficit hyperactivity disorder in children with tic disorder. *Arch Gen Psychiatry* 1995; **52**: 444–455.

Children

Psychosis in children and adolescents

Schizophrenia is rare in children but the incidence increases rapidly in adolescence. Outcome in early-onset illness is generally poor[1]. While drug treatment is undoubtedly indicated, the evidence base underpinning the efficacy and tolerability of antipsychotic drugs in young people is poor.

Typical drugs, particularly haloperidol, have been subject to small RCTs. While haloperidol is effective, young people are more prone to EPSEs than adults[2]. Treatment-emergent dyskinesias can also be problematic[3].

Of the atypicals, only clozapine has been subject to a RCT[4]. While open studies and case series support a lower risk of treatment-emergent EPSEs with atypicals[1], this has to be balanced against the risk of significant weight gain[1,5,6] and all the physical (and psychological) health consequences thereof.

Clozapine seems to be effective in treatment-resistant psychosis in adolescents, although this population may be more prone to neutropenia and seizures than adults[4].

Overall, algorithms for treating psychosis in young people are the same as those for adult patients (see page 24).

References

1. Schulz SC, Findling RI, Friedman L *et al.* Treatment and outcomes in adolescents with schizophrenia. *J Clin Psychiatry* 1998; 59(Suppl.1): 50–54.
2. Findling RL, McNamara NK. Atypical antipsychotics in the treatment of chldren and adolescents: clinical applications. *J Clin Psychiatry* 2004; **65**: 30–44.
3. Connor DF, Fletcher KE, Wood JS. Neuroleptic related dyskinesias in children and adolescents. *J Clin Psychiatry* 2001; **62**: 967–974.
4. Kumra S, Frazier JA, Jacobsen LK *et al.* Childhood-onset schizophrenia: a double blind clozapine haloperidol comparison. *Arch Gen Psychiatry* 1996; **53**: 1090–1097.
5. Theisen FM, Linden A, Geller F *et al.* Prevalence of obesity in adolescent and young adult patients with and without schizophrenia and in relationship to antipsychotic medication. *J Psychiatric Res* 2001; **35**: 339–345.
6. Toren P, Ratner S, Nathaniel L *et al.* Benefit-risk assessment of atypical antipsychotics in the treatment of schizophrenia and comorbid disorders in children and adolescents. *Drug Safety* 2004; **27**: 1135–1156.

Children

Autism

Autism is a chronic and debilitating, pervasive developmental disorder involving deficits in language, social interaction and behaviour. Onset is before 3 years of age and the aetiology is unclear. Prevalence is estimated at 6 cases per 1000 children[1], with boys being affected at least three times as frequently as girls[2]. As few as 10% of children with autism may be able to live independently as adults[3].

Deficits in communication make it difficult directly to elicit psychopathology in people with autism. Co-morbid conditions such as mood disorders and ADHD often have to be diagnosed solely from observing behaviour. It therefore follows that case reports and case series should be interpreted with caution. Besides the obvious bias associated with the reporting of open data, the patients included may not be representative of people with autism as a whole.

SSRIs

Case reports and open-case series suggest that SSRIs may be effective in ameliorating repetitive and aggressive behaviours[4]. A double-blind study of fluvoxamine in adults confirmed these findings and also reported improvements in language and social interaction for active drug over placebo[5]. The efficacy and tolerability of SSRIs in the treatment of autistic symptoms are at the time of writing being investigated in a Cochrane Review. No results are yet available[6].

Antipsychotics

Small, placebo-controlled studies have found haloperidol to be effective in reducing social withdrawal, stereotypies, overactivity mood dysregulation and irritability, and pimozide effective in reducing aggression[4]. There are 13 publications reporting on the efficacy of risperidone in autism, only one of which is a randomised, double-blind, placebo-controlled study[7]. Risperidone is probably effective in the treatment of hyperactivity, aggression and repetitive behaviour and possibly effective in the treatment of depression and irritability[7]. Evidence supporting the efficacy of other atypicals is scant. Note that haloperidol is associated with a high prevalence of EPSEs in young people and all atypicals can cause significant weight gain.

Anticonvulsants/mood-stabilisers

Approximately 30% of people with autism have comorbid epilepsy[8] and affective illness is also thought to be common[9]. In a review of the literature on the use of anticonvulsant drugs in people with autism and epilepsy, Di Martino and Tuchman[9] report that irritability, aggressiveness and communication improve irrespective of whether or not seizures improve. It is possible that the effect of these drugs in regulating mood is relevant. Caution, however, is required. A case series reported improvements in behaviour with lamotrigine but this finding was not replicated in a double-blind, placebo-controlled trial[10]. There are no randomised, placebo-controlled studies of other anticonvulsant drugs.

Other drugs

Small, controlled studies have reported beneficial effects with clomipramine (for aggression, repetitiveness and irritability), methylphenidate (for overactivity), clonidine (for overactivity, irritability and aggression) and naltrexone (for overactivity)[4]. Large doses of vitamin B_6 (200 mg/day per 70-kg adult) in combination with magnesium (100 mg/day per 70-kg adult) have been reported to lead to improvements in communication and interpersonal skills. A Cochrane Review concludes that there is insufficient evidence to make any recommendation regarding the use of high doses of B_6[11]. Note that there are unresolved concerns regarding the safety of high doses of B_6. Further information can be found in the *BNF*.

The future

There is some evidence that glutamate antagonists (e.g. phencyclidine) and $5HT_{2a}$ agonists (e.g. LSD) can mimic the symptoms of autism[12]. These observations may lead to the development of novel treatments. It may be of note that lamotrigine (a glutamate antagonist) is probably ineffective and risperidone (a $5HT_{2a}$ antagonist) probably effective in ameliorating symptoms of autism.

References

1. Bertrand J, Mars A, Boyle C *et al.* Prevalence of autism in a United States population: the Brick Township, New Jersey, investigation. *Pediatrics* 2001; **108**: 1155–1161.
2. Lotter V. Epidemiology of autistic conditions in young children. I. Prevalence. *Social Psychiatry* 1974; **1**: 124–137.
3. Wing L. *Diagnosis and Treatment of Autism.* New York: Plenum, 1989.
4. Palermo MT, Curatolo P. Pharmacologic treatment of autism. *J Child Neurol* 2004; **19**: 155–164.
5. McDougle CJ, Naylor ST, Cohen DJ *et al.* A double blind, placebo controlled study of fluvoxamine in adults with autistic disorder. *Arch Gen Psychiatry* 1996; **53**: 1001–1008.
6. Wheeler DM, Hazell P, Silove N *et al.* Selective serotonin reuptake inhibitors for the treatment of autism spectrum disorders (protocol for a Cochrane Review). In The Cochrane Library, Issue 3, 2004.
7. Barnard L, Young AH, Pearson J *et al.* A systematic review of the use of atypical antipsychotics in autism. *J Psychopharmacol* 2002; **16**: 93–101.
8. Olsson I, Steffenburg S, Gillberg C. Epilepsy in autism and autistic like conditions. A population based study. *Arch Neurol – Chicago* 1988; **45**: 666–668.
9. Di Martino A, Tuchman RF. Antiepileptic drugs: affective use in autism spectrum disorders. *Pediatr Neurol* 2001; **25**: 199–207.
10. Belsito M, Kirk K, Landa R *et al.* Lamotrigine therapy for childhood autism. A randomised, double blind, placebo controlled trial. *J Autism Dev Disord* 2001; **31**: 175–181.
11. Nye C, Brice A. Combined vitamin B_6-magnesium treatment in autistic spectrum disorders. In The Cochrane Library, Issue 3, 2004.
12. Carlsson ML. Hypothesis: is infantile autism a hypoglutamatergic disorder? Relevance of glutamate–serotonin interactions for pharmacotherapy. *J Neural Transm* 1998; **105**: 525–535.

Children

Tourette's syndrome

Tourette's syndrome is defined by persistent motor and vocal tics. These tics wax and wane over time and are known to be exacerbated by external factors such as stress, anxiety and fatigue. The pathophysiology of Tourette's syndrome is not completely understood. Dopamine, acetylcholine, noradrenaline, sex hormones, GABA, serotonin and opiate pathways have all been implicated.

The prevalence of Tourette's syndrome in children and adolescents is estimated to be 1:1000 boys and 1:10,000 girls[1]. Co-morbid depression, anxiety, attention deficit disorder, OCD and behavioural problems are more prevalent than would be expected by chance association alone[2]. These co-morbid conditions are usually treated first before assessing the level of disability caused by the tics. Treatment aimed primarily at reducing tics is warranted if they cause distress to the patient or are functionally disabling.

Studies of pharmacological interventions in Tourette's syndrome are difficult to interpret for several reasons[3]:

1. There is a large interindividual variation in tic frequency and severity. Small, randomised studies may include patients that are very different at baseline.
2. The severity of tics in a given individual varies markedly over time, making it difficult to separate drug effect from natural variation.
3. The placebo effect is large.
4. The bulk of the literature consists of case reports, case series, open studies and hugely underpowered, randomised studies. Publication bias is also likely to be an issue.
5. A high proportion of patients have co-morbid psychiatric illness. It is difficult to disentangle any direct effect on Tourette's syndrome from an effect on the co-morbid illness. For example, patients with co-morbid OCD would be expected to fare better on a SSRI than placebo or an antipsychotic. This makes it difficult to interpret studies that report improvements in global functioning rather than specific reductions in tics.

The bulk of the published literature concerns children and adolescents. It is commonly believed that younger people are more responsive to treatment than adults but this observation is poorly supported by objective evidence.

Antipsychotics

A 24-week, double-blind, placebo-controlled double crossover study of 22 children and adolescents found pimozide (mean dose 3.4 mg/day) to be statistically superior to placebo in controlling tics[4]. Outcome in the haloperidol arm of this study (mean dose 3.5 mg) was numerically superior to placebo but did not reach statistical significance. Although this study is widely quoted as being positive for pimozide and negative for haloperidol, the absolute difference in response between the two active treatment arms was small. Two children developed severe anxiety and depression during the haloperidol phase that resulted in early termination of treatment. Haloperidol tends to be poorly tolerated by children and adolescents[5]. The high burden of side-effects leads to less than a third being willing to continue treatment in the longer term[6].

Risperidone has been shown to be more effective than placebo in a small (N=34), randomised study[7]. Fatigue and increased appetite were problematic in the risperidone arm and a mean weight gain of 2.8 kg over 8 weeks was reported. Although there is a suggestion that risperidone[8] and olanzapine[9] may be more effective than pimozide, weight gain may be more pronounced in children and adolescents than in adults and this may limit the use of atypicals in young people[8].

Sulpiride has been shown to be effective and relatively well tolerated[10], as has ziprasidone[11]. Open studies support the efficacy of quetiapine[12] and olanzapine[13]. One very small crossover study (N=7) found no effect for clozapine[14].

Other drugs

Clonidine has been shown in open studies to reduce the severity and frequency of tics but this effect does not seem to be convincingly larger that placebo[15]. There may be an age-specific effect, with clonidine being more effective than placebo in adults[16]. Motor tics may be more responsive than vocal tics[16]. Guanfacine (also an adrenergic alpha 2 agonist) has been shown to lead to a 30% reduction in tic-rating-scale scores[17]. Problems with underpowering and the subsequent interpretation of the literature in this area are illustrated by a randomised, controlled trial that found risperidone and clonidine to be equally effective[18].

A small (N=10), double-blind, placebo-controlled, crossover trial of baclofen was suggestive of beneficial effects in overall impairment rather than a specific effect on tics[19]. The numerical benefits shown in this study did not reach statistical significance. Similarly, a double-blind, placebo-controlled trial of nicotine augmentation of haloperidol found beneficial effects in overall impairment rather than a specific effect on tics[20]. These benefits persisted for several weeks after nicotine (in the form of patches) was withdrawn. Nicotine patches were associated with a high prevalence of nausea and vomiting (71% and 40% respectively). The authors suggest that PRN use may be appropriate. Pergolide (a D1-D2-D3 agonist) given in low dose significantly reduced tics in a double-blind, placebo-controlled, crossover study in children and adolescents[21]. Side-effects included sedation, dizziness, nausea and irritability. Flutamide, an antiandrogen, has been the subject of a small RCT in adults with TS. Modest, short-lived effects were seen in motor but not phonic tics[3].

Case reports or case series describing positive effects for ondansetron[22], clomiphene[23], tramadol[24], ketanserin[25], topiramate[26], cyproterone[27] and cannabis[28] have been published. Many other drugs have been reported to be effective in single case reports. Patients in these reports all had co-morbid psychiatric illness, making it difficult to determine the effect of these drugs on Tourette's syndrome alone.

References

1. Awaad Y. Tics in Tourette syndrome: new treatment options. *J Child Neurol* 1999; **14**: 316–319.
2. Riddle MA, Carlson J. Clinical psychopharmacology for Tourette syndrome and associated disorders. In: *Tourette Syndrome*, pp 343–354 Cohen DJ, Goetz G, Jankovic J *et al.* (eds). Philadelphia: Lippincott Williams & Wilkins, 2001.
3. Peterson B, Zhang H, Anderson G *et al.* A double blind, placebo controlled, crossover trial of an antiandrogen in the treatment of Tourette's syndrome. *J Clin Psychopharm* 1988; **18**: 324–331.
4. Sallee FR, Nesbitt L, Jackson C *et al.* Relative efficacy of haloperidol and pimozide in children and adolescents with Tourette's disorder. *Am J Psychiatry* 1997; **154**: 1057–1062.
5. Richardson MA, Haugland G, Craig TJ. Neuroleptic use, parkinsonian symptoms, tardive dyskinesia and associated factors in child and adolescent psychiatric patients. *Am J Psychiatry* 1991; **148**: 1322–1328.
6. Chappell PB, Leckman JF, Riddle MA. The pharmacological treatment of tic disorders. *Chil Adolesc Psychiat Clin N Am* 1995; **4**: 197–216.
7. Scahill L, Leckman JF, Schultz RT *et al.* A placebo controlled trial of risperidone in Tourette syndrome. *Neurology* 2003; **60**: 1130–1135.
8. Bruggeman R, van der Linden C, Buitelaar JK. Risperidone versus pimozide in Tourette's disorder: a comparative double blind parallel group study. *J Clin Psychiatry* 2001; **62**: 50–56.
9. Onofrj M, Paci C, D'Andreamatteo G *et al.* Olanzapine in severe Gilles de la Tourette syndrome: a 52 week double-blind cross-over study vs low-dose pimozide. *J Neurol* 2000; **247**: 443–446.

10. Robertson MM, Schnieden V, Lees AJ. Management of Gilles de la Tourette syndrome using sulpiride. *Clin Neuropharmacol* 1990; **3**: 229–235.
11. Sallee FR, Kurlan R, Goetz G *et al.* Ziprasidone treatment of children and adolescents with Tourette's syndrome: a pilot study. *J Am Acad Child Adolesc Psychiatry* 2000; **39**: 292–299.
12. Mukaddes NM, Abali O. Quetiapine treatment of children and adolescents with Tourette's disorder. *J Child Adolesc Psychopharmacol* 2003; **13**: 295–299.
13. Budman CL, Gayer A, Lesser M. An open label study of the treatment efficacy of olanzapine for Tourette's disorder. *J Clin Psychiatry* 2001; **62**: 290–294.
14. Caine ED, Polinsky RJ, Kartzinel R *et al.* The trial use of clozapine for abnormal involuntary movement disorders. *Am J Psychiatry* 1979; **136**: 317–320.
15. Goetz CG, Tanner CM, Wilson RS *et al.* Clonidine and Giles de la Tourette syndrome: double blind study using objective rating methods. *Ann Neurol* 1987; **21**: 307–310.
16. Leckman JF, Hardin MT, Riddle MA *et al.* Clonidine treatment of Gilles de la Tourette's syndrome. *Arch Gen Psychiatry* 1991; **48**: 324–328.
17. Scahill L, Chappell PB, Kim YS *et al.* Guanfacine in the treatment of children with tic disorders and ADHD: a placebo-controlled study. Presented at American Academy of Child and Adolescent Psychiatry, October 1999.
18. Gaffney GR, Perry PJ, Lund BC. Risperidone versus clonidine in the treatment of children and adolescents with Tourette's syndrome. *J Child Adolesc Psychopharmacol* 2002; **41**: 330–336.
19. Singer HS, Wendlandt J, Krieger M *et al.* Baclofen treatment in Tourette syndrome: a double blind, placebo controlled, crossover trial. *Neurology* 2001; **56**: 599–604.
20. Silver AA, Shytle D, Philipp MK *et al.* Transdermal nicotine and haloperidol in Tourette's disorder: a double blind placebo controlled study. *J Clin Psychiatry* 2001; **62**: 707–714.
21. Gilbert DL, Sethuraman G, Sine L *et al.* Tourette's syndrome improvement with pergolide in a randomised, double blind, crossover trial. *Neurology* 2000; **54**: 1310–1315.
22. Toren P, Laor N, Cohen DJ. Ondansetron treatment in patients with Tourette's syndrome. *Int Clin Psychopharmacol* 1999; **14**: 373–376.
23. Sandyk R. Clomiphene citrate in Tourette's syndrome. *Int J Neurosci* 1988; **43**: 103–106.
24. Shapira NA, McConville BJ, Pagnucco ML *et al.* Novel use of tramadol hydrochloride in the treatment of Tourette's syndrome. *J Clin Psychiatry* 1998; **58**: 174–175.
25. Singer HS, Walkup JT. Ketanserin treatment of Tourette's syndrome in children. *Am J Psychiatry* 1999; **156**: 1122–1123.
26. Abbuzahab FS, Brown VL. Topiramate for clozapine induced seizures. *Am J Psychiatry* 2001; **158**: 968–969.
27. Izmir M, Dursun SM. Cyproterone acetate treatment of Tourette's syndrome. *Can J Psychiatry* 1999; **44**: 710–711.
28. Sandyk R, Awerbuch G. Marijuana and Tourette's syndrome. *J Clin Psychopharm* 1988; **8**: 444–445.

Children

Melatonin in the treatment of insomnia in children and adolescents

Insomnia is a common problem in children with sensory deficits and some learning disability syndromes. It is also a symptom of childhood psychiatric disorders such as depression and ADHD. Approximately 10% of otherwise normal children[1] and up to 80% of children with developmental disorders[2] suffer from delayed sleep phase syndrome.

Melatonin is a hormone that is produced by the pineal gland in a circadian manner. The evening rise in melatonin, enabled by darkness, precedes the onset of natural sleep by about 90 minutes[3]. There is no direct evidence that melatonin is involved in sleep consolidation. Given its association with circadian rhythms and the fact that it is a 'natural' product, melatonin is commonly prescribed to treat insomnia in children and adolescents. Melatonin is not a licensed medicine in the UK.

Efficacy

Five placebo-controlled studies have been published to date. Four studies demonstrated improvements in the time taken to fall asleep[1-6]. The fifth study recruited children with fragmented sleep and melatonin had no effect[7]. In the four positive RCTs there was no consistent effect on total sleep duration or number of awakenings.

Side-effects

Many of the children who have received melatonin in RCTs and published case series had developmental problems and/or sensory deficits. The scope for detecting subtle adverse effects in this population is limited. Screening for side-effects was not routine in all studies. Melatonin has been reported to worsen seizures[1,8] and may also exacerbate asthma[9,10] in the short term. Other reported side-effects include headache, depression, restlessness, confusion, nausea, tachycardia and pruritis[11,12]. Long-term side-effects have not been evaluated.

Dose

The cut-off point between physiological and pharmacological doses in children is less than 500 µg. Physiological doses of melatonin result in very high receptor occupancy. The doses used in RCTs and published case series vary hugely, between 500 µg and 5 mg being the most common although much lower and higher doses have been used. The optimal dose is unknown and there is no evidence to support a direct relationship between dose and response. Pharmacological doses may mediate their effect via GABA receptors[13].

References

1. Smits MG, Nagtegaal EE, van der Heijden J *et al.* Melatonin for chronic sleep onset disorder in children: a randomised placebo controlled trial. *J Child Neurol* 2001; **16**: 86–92.
2. Jan JE, O'Donnell ME. Use of melatonin in the treatment of paediatric sleep disorders. *J Pineal Res* 1996; **21**: 193–199.
3. Tzischinsky O, Lavie P. Melatonin possesses time-dependent hypnotic effects. *Sleep* 1994; **17**: 638–645.
4. McArthur AJ, Budden SS. Sleep dysfunction in Rett syndrome: a trial of exogenous melatonin treatment. *Dev Med Child Neurol* 1998; **49**: 186–192.
5. Dodge NN, Wilson GA. Melatonin for treatment of sleep disorders in children with developmental disabilities. *J Child Neurol* 2001; **16**: 581–584.

6. Smits MG, van Stel HF, van der Heijden K *et al.* Melatonin improves health status and sleep in children with idiopathic chronic sleep-onset insomnia: a randomised placebo-controlled trial. *J Am Acad Child Psychiat* 2003; **42**: 1286–1293.
7. Camfield P, Gordon K, Dooley J. Melatonin appears ineffective in children with intellectual deficits and fragmented sleep. Six 'N of 1' trials. *J Clin Neurol* 1996; **11**: 341–343.
8. Sheldon SH. Pro-convulsant effects of oral melatonin in neurologically disabled children. *Lancet* 1998; **351**: 1254.
9. Maestroni GJM. The immunoendocrine role of melatonin. *J Pineal Res* 1993; **14**: 1–10.
10. Sutherland ER, Ellison MC, Kraft M *et al.* Elevated serum melatonin is associated with the nocturnal worsening of asthma. *J Allergy Clin Immun* 2003; **112**: 513–517.
11. Chase JE, Gidal BE. Melatonin: therapeutic uses in sleep disorders. *Ann Pharmacother* 1997; **31**: 1218–1226.
12. Jan JE, Freeman RD, Fast DK. Melatonin treatment of sleep-wake cycle disorders in children and adolescents. *Dev Med Child Neurol* 1999; **41**: 491–500.
13. Sack RL, Hughes RJ, Edgar DM *et al.* Sleep-promoting effects of melatonin: at what dose, in whom, under what conditions and by what mechanisms? *Sleep* 1997; **20**: 908–911.

Children

Rapid tranquillisation (RT) in children and adolescents

As in adults, a comprehensive mental state assessment and appropriately implemented treatment plan along with staff skilled in the use of de-escalation techniques and appropriate placement of the patient are key to minimising the need for enforced parenteral medication.

Oral medication should always be offered before resorting to IM. Monitoring after RT is the same as in adults (see page 316).

Table Recommended drugs for RT

Medication	Dose	Onset of action	Comment
Olanzapine IM[1,2]	2.5–10 mg	15–30 min IM	Possibly increased risk of respiratory depression when administered with benzodiazepines.
Haloperidol[3]	0.025–0.075 mg/kg/dose (max 2.5 mg) IM Adolescents > 12 years can receive the adult dose	20–30 min IM	Must have parenteral anticholinergics present in case of laryngeal spasm (young people more vulnerable to severe EPSEs).
Lorazepam[3,4]	0.05–0.1 mg/kg/dose IM	20–40 min	Slower onset of action than midazolam. Flumazenil is the reversing agent. Risk of disinhibitory reactions.
Midazolam[4,5]	0.1–0.15 mg/kg	10–20 min IM (1–3 min IV)	Quicker onset and shorter duration of action than lorazepam or diazepam. Shorter onset and duration of action than haloperidol. Flumazenil is the reversing agent.
Diazepam–IV only (Not for IM administration)[6]	0.1 mg/kg/dose by slow IV injection. Max 40 mg total daily dose <12 years and 60 mg >12 years	5–10 min	Long half-life that does not correlate with length of sedation. Possibility of accumulation. Flumazenil is the reversing agent. **Never give as IM injection**

References

1. Breier A, Meehan K, Birkett M *et al*. A double-blind, placebo-controlled dose-response comparison of intramuscular olanzapine and haloperidol in the treatment of acute agitation in schizophrenia. *Arch Gen Psychiatry* 2004; 59: 441–448.
2. Lindborg SR, Beasley CM, Alaka K *et al*. Effects of intramuscular olanzapine vs haloperidol and placebo on QTc intervals in

acutely agitated patients. *Psychiatry Res* 2003; **119**: 113–123.

3. Sorrentino A. Chemical restraints for the agitated, violent, or psychotic paediatric patient in the emergency department: controversies and recommendations. *Curr Opin Pediatr* 2004; **16**: 201–205.
4. Nobay F, Simon BC, Levitt A *et al*. A prospective, double-blind, randomized trial of midazolam versus haloperidol versus lorazepam in the chemical restraint of violent and severely ill patients. *Acad Emerg Med* 2004; **11**: 744–749.
5. Kennedy RM, Luhmann JD. The 'ouchless' emergency department. Getting closer: advances in decreasing distress during painful procedures in the emergency department. *Pediatr Clin N Am* 1999; **46**: 1215–1247.
6. Nunn K, Dey C. *Medication Table. The Clinician's Guide to Psychotropic Prescribing in Children and Adolescents*. Sydney: Glade Publishing, 2004.

Persistent aggression in children and adolescents

As in adults, persistent aggression may be secondary to a number of underlying psychiatric illnesses. The most common primary diagnoses in children include conduct disorder, bipolar illness, autism and psychotic illness. It is important to understand what drives the aggressive behaviour and to intervene appropriately.

There is most evidence supporting the use of risperidone in aggressive behaviour[1,2]. There are fewer data for olanzapine, quetiapine and clozapine. Risperidone can cause significant EPSEs in young people[1] and all atypicals can cause considerable weight gain.

Lithium may also be effective[3–5].

References

1. Schur S, Sikich L, Findling R *et al*. Treatment recommendations for the use of antipsychotics for aggressive youth (TRAAY). I. A review. *J Am Acad Child Psychiat* 2003; **42**: 132–144.
2. Pappadopulos E, Macintyre J, Crismon ML *et al*. Treatment recommendations for the use of antipsychotics for aggressive youth (TRAAY). II. *J Am Acad Child Psychiat* 2003; **42**: 147–161.
3. Campbell M, Adams P, Small A *et al*. Lithium in hospitalized children with conduct disorder: a double-blind and placebo controlled study. *J Am Acad Child Psychiat* 1995; **34**: 445–453.
4. Malone RP, Delaney MA, Luebbert JF *et al*. A double-blind placebo-controlled study of lithium in hospitalized aggressive children and adolescents with conduct disorder. *Arch Gen Psychiatry* 2000; **57**: 649–654.
5. Campbell M, Silva RR, Kafantaris V *et al*. Predictors of side effects associated with lithium administration in children. *Psychopharmacol Bull* 1991; **27**: 373–380.

Further reading

Kranzler H, Roofeh D, Gerbino-Rosen G *et al*. Clozapine: its impact on aggressive behaviour among children and adolescents with schizophrenia. *J Am Acad Child Adolesc Psychiatry* 2005; **44**: 55–63.

Children

chapter 6

Substance misuse

Alcohol

Pharmacotherapy for alcohol withdrawal

- Alcohol withdrawal is associated with significant morbidity and mortality when improperly managed.
- All patients need general support; a proportion will need pharmacotherapy to manage withdrawal symptoms.
- Benzodiazepines are recognised as the treatment of choice for alcohol withdrawal. They are cross-tolerant with alcohol and have anticonvulsant properties.
- Parenteral vitamin replacement is an important adjunctive treatment for the prophylaxis and/or treatment of Wernicke Korsakoff syndrome and other vitamin-related neuropsychiatric conditions.

Alcohol detoxification

Before alcohol detoxification there should be consideration of the following;

- Does the client want to undergo detoxification? Detoxification from alcohol should not be done without assessing the goals of treatment.
- Are the intended goals of detoxification symptom suppression, prevention of complications or a prelude to abstinence? Detoxification should be considered within the wider context of the ongoing care/treatment package.
- Are plans in place for the post-detoxification period?

In addition a risk assessment should be carried out to determine the appropriate setting of the detoxification (see guidelines for in-patient detoxification below). Care is required with older patients – it may be preferable to arrange in-patient withdrawal.

The majority of patients can be detoxified in the community. However, in-patient detoxification is indicated where there is:

- severe dependence
- history of DTs and alcohol withdrawal seizures
- history of failed community detoxification
- poor social support
- cognitive impairment
- psychiatric co-morbidity
- poor physical health, e.g. diabetes, liver disease, hypertension.

The alcohol withdrawal syndrome

In alcohol-dependent drinkers, the central nervous system has adjusted to the constant inhibitory presence of alcohol in the body. When the blood alcohol concentration (BAC) is suddenly lowered, the brain is left in a hyperactive and hyperexcited state, causing the withdrawal syndrome.

The alcohol withdrawal syndrome is not a uniform entity. It varies significantly in clinical manifestations and severity. Symptoms can range from mild insomnia to delirium tremens (DTs) and convulsions.

The first symptoms and signs occur within hours of the last drink and peak within 24–48 hours. They include restlessness, tremor, sweating, anxiety, nausea, vomiting, loss of appetite and insomnia. Tachycardia and systolic hypertension are also evident. Generalised seizures occur rarely, usually within 24 hours of cessation. In DTs there is confusion, disorientation, agitation, tachycardia and hypertension. Fever is common. Visual and auditory hallucinations and paranoid ideation are also seen.

DTs often present insidiously with night-time confusion. The mortality is approximately 1–2%. Treatment of DTs requires early diagnosis and prompt transfer to the general medical setting. Intravenous diazepam, fluid and electrolyte replacement and parenteral thiamine can be administered safely there. A full medical assessment is required.

In most patients, symptoms of alcohol withdrawal are mild-to-moderate and disappear within 5–7 days after the last drink. In more severe cases (about 5% of cases), DTs may develop.

Risk factors for DTs and seizures

- severe alcohol dependence
- past experience of DTs
- long-standing history of alcohol dependence with previous episodes of in-patient treatment
- older age
- concomitant acute illness
- severe withdrawal symptoms when presenting for treatment.

Alcohol withdrawal assessment

1. history (including history of previous episodes of alcohol withdrawal)
2. physical examination
3. time of most recent drink

4. concomitant drug intake
5. severity of withdrawal symptoms
6. co-existing medical/psychiatric disorders
7. laboratory investigations: BAC, FBC, U&E, LFTs, INR, urinary drug screen.

Withdrawal scales can be helpful. They can be used as a baseline against which withdrawal severity can be measured over time. Use of these scales can minimise over- and under-dosing with benzodiazepines.

The Clinical Institute Withdrawal Assessment for Alcohol–Revised Version (CIWA-Ar) is a 10-item scale that can be used to monitor the clinical course of alcohol withdrawal. (Items 1–9 are scored from 0–7 and item 10 from 0–4; maximum possible score of 67.)

1. nausea and vomiting
2. tremor
3. paroxysmal sweats
4. anxiety
5. agitation
6. tactile disturbances
7. auditory disturbances
8. visual disturbances
9. headache and fullness in head
10. orientation and clouding of sensorium

Severity of alcohol withdrawal	CIWA-Ar score
mild	<10
moderate	10–20
severe	20+

Community detoxification

1. Discuss the treatment plan with the patient and the person who will be supporting him or her. This should include contingency plans. Put a copy in the notes, give a copy to the patient and send a copy to the GP.
3. Arrange for medication to be picked up on a daily basis.
4. If a patient resumes drinking, stop the medication used for detoxification.
5. Give patients and their carers contact details so they can contact you if there are any problems.

Use of benzodiazepines

Longer-acting benzodiazepines may be more effective in preventing seizures and delirium, but there is a risk of accumulation in elderly patients, and those with liver failure[1]. Additional titration using PRN or as-required medication may be used to achieve complete symptom suppression in the first 2 days[2].

Dose of benzodiazepines

The dose needed will depend on an assessment of:

1. severity of alcohol dependence (clinical history, number of units per drinking day and the score on Severity of Alcohol Dependence Questionnaire (SADQ)).
2. severity of alcohol withdrawal symptoms. CIWA-Ar (above) or Short Alcohol Withdrawal Scale (SAWS)[3].

Table Short Alcohol Withdrawal Scale (SAWS)

	None (0)	Mild (1)	Moderate (2)	Severe (3)
Anxious				
Sleep disturbance				
Problems with memory				
Nausea				
Restless				
Tremor (shakes)				
Feeling confused				
Sweating				
Miserable				
Heart pounding				

The SAWS is a self-completion questionnaire. Symptoms cover the previous 24-hour period. Scores above 12 require pharmacotherapy.

Use of chlordiazepoxide

Mild dependence usually requires very small doses of chlordiazepoxide, or it may be managed without medication.

Moderate dependence requires a larger dose of chlordiazepoxide. A typical regime might be 10–20 mg q.d.s., reducing gradually over 5–7 days. Note that this is usually adequate *and longer treatment is rarely helpful or necessary.*

Example – moderate dependence

Day 1 .... 20 mg q.d.s.
Day 2 .... 15 mg q.d.s.
Day 3 .... 10 mg q.d.s.
Day 4 .... 5 mg q.d.s.
Day 5 .... 5 mg b.d.

Severe dependence requires even larger doses of chlordiazepoxide and will often require specialist/in-patient treatment. Daily monitoring is advised for the first 2–3 days, especially for severe dependence (see below). This may require special arrangements over a weekend. Prescribing should not start if the patient is heavily intoxicated, and in such circumstances the patient should be advised to return in a sober state at an early opportunity.

In-patient protocol for alcohol detoxification

The approach should be flexible with regard to the number of days prescribed, depending on the individual. Severely dependent patients should get 7 days treatment with the flexibility of as-required medication in the first 2 days. If symptoms are controlled within the first 2 days, it will be easier to implement the reducing regime. Patients who have a history of DTs, head injury or cognitive impairment may need lengthier withdrawal regimes, e.g. lasting 10 days.

Chlordiazepoxide should be prescribed according to a flexible regimen over the first 24 (up to 48) hours, with dosage titrated against the rated severity of withdrawal symptoms. This is followed by a fixed, 5-day reducing regimen, based upon the dosage requirement estimated during the first 24 (–48) hours.

Occasionally (e.g. in DTs) the flexible regime may need to be prolonged beyond the first 24 hours. However, rarely (if ever) is it necessary to resort to the use of other drugs, such as antipsychotics (associated with reduced seizure threshold) or intravenous diazepam (associated with risk of overdose).

The intention of the flexible protocol for the first 24 hours is to titrate dosage of chlordiazepoxide against severity of alcohol withdrawal symptoms. It is necessary to avoid either under-treatment (associated with patient discomfort and a higher incidence of complications such as seizures or DTs), or over-treatment (associated with excessive sedation and risk of toxicity/interaction with alcohol consumed before admission).

In the in-patient setting it is possible to be more responsive, with constant monitoring of the severity of withdrawal symptoms, linked to the administered dose of chlordiazepoxide.

Prescribing in alcohol withdrawal – in-patient protocol

First 24 hours (day 1)

On admission, the patient should be assessed by a doctor and prescribed chlordiazepoxide. (Diazepam is used in some centres and may be used for those with a history of sensitivity to chlordiazepoxide although some metabolites are shared.) Three doses of chlordiazepoxide must be specified:

FIRST DOSE (STAT)

This is the first dose of chlordiazepoxide which will be administered by ward staff immediately following admission, as a fixed 'stat' dose. It should be estimated upon:

- clinical signs and symptoms of withdrawal (see below)
- breath alcohol concentration on admission and 1 hour later.

The dose prescribed should usually be within the range of 5–50 mg. However, if withdrawal symptoms on admission are mild, or if the breath alcohol is very high, or rising, the initial dose may be 0 mg (i.e. nothing). It is the relative fall in blood alcohol concentration that determines the need for medication, not the absolute figure (hence the need to take two Alcometer readings at an interval soon after admission). Caution is needed if a patient shows a high Alcometer level.

INCREMENTAL DOSE (RANGE)

This is the range within which subsequent doses of chlordiazepoxide should be administered during the first 24 hours (see below). A dose of 5–40 mg will cover almost all circumstances.

MAXIMUM DOSE IN 24 HOURS

This is the maximum cumulative dose that may be given during the first 24 hours. It may be estimated according to clinical judgement, but **250 mg should be adequate for most cases.** Doses above 250 mg should not be prescribed without prior discussion with a consultant or specialist registrar.

The cumulative chlordiazepoxide dose administered during the initial 24-hour period assessment is called the *baseline dose*, and this is used to calculate the subsequent reducing regime.

Days 2–5

After the initial 24-hour assessment period a standardised reducing regime is used. Chlordiazepoxide is given in divided doses, four times daily. The afternoon and evening doses can be proportionately higher in order to provide night sedation (but note that the effect of chlordiazepoxide and its metabolites is long-lived). The dose should be reduced each day by approximately 20% of the baseline dose, such that no chlordiazepoxide is given on day 6. **However, a longer regime may be required in the case of patients who have DTs or a history of DTs. This should be discussed with a specialist registrar or consultant, and the dose tailored according to clinical need.**

> ### Note
> Chlordiazepoxide should not routinely be prescribed on a PRN basis after the initial assessment is complete. Patients exhibiting significant further symptoms may have psychiatric (or other) complications and should be seen by the ward or duty doctor.

Observations and administration

After chlordiazepoxide has been prescribed as above, the first 'stat' dose is given immediately. Subsequent doses during the first 24 hours are administered with a frequency and dosage that depend upon the observations of alcohol withdrawal status rated by the ward staff.

OBSERVATIONS

Each set of observations consists of:
- applying an alcohol withdrawal scale (e.g. CIWA-Ar) and/or clinical observations
- BP
- pulse
- Alcometer reading (first and second observations only).

Observations should be recorded:
- during the admission procedure, immediately after the patient has arrived on the ward
- throughout the first 24 hours, at a frequency depending upon:
  - severity of withdrawal
  - whether or not chlordiazepoxide has been administered
- twice daily from days 2–6.

If patients are asleep (and this is not due to intoxication), they should not be woken up for observations. However, it should be recorded that they were asleep.

During the first 24 hours chlordiazepoxide should be administered when withdrawal symptoms are considered significant (usually a CIWA-Ar score of >15). If a patient suffers hallucinations or agitation, an increased dose should be administered, according to clinical judgement.

Table Alcohol withdrawal treatment interventions

Severity	Supportive care	Medical care	Pharmacotherapy to assist detoxification	Setting
Mild CIWA-Ar <10	Moderate-to-high level required	Little required	Little to none required – maybe symptomatic treatment only (e.g. paracetamol)	Home
Moderate CIWA-Ar 10–20	Moderate-to-high level required	Little required	Little to none required – maybe symptomatic treatment only	Home or community
Severe CIWA-Ar >20	High level required	Medical monitoring	Usually required – probably symptomatic and substitution treatment (e.g. chlordiazepoxide)	Community or hospital
Complicated CIWA-Ar >10 plus medical problems	High level required	Specialist medical care required	Substitution and symptomatic treatments probably required	Hospital

Substance misuse

Example of a chlordiazepoxide regimen – severe dependence

		Total (mg)
Day 1 (first 24 hours)	40 mg q.d.s. + 40 mg PRN	200
Day 2	40 mg q.d.s.	160
Day 3	30 mg t.d.s. and 40 mg nocte (or 30 mg q.d.s.)	120–130
Day 4	30 mg b.d. and 20 mg b.d. (or 25 mg q.d.s.)	100
Day 5	20 mg q.d.s.	80
Day 6	20 mg b.d. and 10 mg b.d.	60
Day 7	10 mg q.d.s.	40
Day 8	10 mg t.d.s. or 10 mg b.d. and 5 mg b.d.	30
Day 9	10 mg b.d. (or 5 mg q.d.s.)	20
Day 10	10 mg nocte	10

Vitamin supplementation

All patients undergoing in-patient detoxification should be given parenteral thiamine as prophylaxis for Wernicke's encephalopathy. This is probably best given for 5 days. Clients undergoing community detoxification should also be considered for parenteral prophylaxis with Pabrinex because oral thiamine is not adequately absorbed. There is considerable doubt about the usefulness of oral replacement.

IM thiamine preparations have a lower incidence of anaphylactoid reactions than IV preparations. This is approximately 1 per 5 million pairs of ampoules of Pabrinex, which is far lower than many frequently used drugs which carry no special warning in the *BNF*. This risk has resulted in fears about using parenteral preparations, and the inappropriate use of oral thiamine preparations. Given the nature of Wernicke's encephalopathy, the benefit-to-risk ratio strongly favours parenteral thiamine[2,4].

However according to the *BNF* parenteral vitamin supplements should only be administered where suitable resuscitation facilities are available. The IM route is usually used. Intravenous administration should be by dilution in 50–100 ml normal saline and infused over 15–30 minutes. This allows immediate discontinuation should anaphylaxis occur. Anaphylaxis is extremely rare after IM administration and this is the preferred route in most centres.

The classical triad of ophthalmoplegia, ataxia and confusion is rarely present in Wernicke's encephalopathy, and the syndrome is much more common than is widely believed. A presumptive diagnosis of Wernicke's encephalopathy should therefore be made in any patient undergoing detoxification who experiences any of the following signs:

- ataxia
- hypothermia and hypotension
- confusion

- ophthalmoplegia/nystagmus
- memory disturbance
- coma/unconsciousness.

Parenteral B-complex must be administered before glucose is administered in all patients presenting with altered mental status.

Prophylactic treatment for Wernicke's encephalopathy should be:

> **One pair IM/IV ampoules high-potency B-complex vitamins (Pabrinex) daily for 3–5 days**
> (*Or:* **thiamine 200–300 mg IM daily, if Pabrinex unavailable).**

Note: All patients should receive this regime as an absolute minimum.

Therapeutic treatment: Wernicke's encephalopathy (undertaken within the general medical hospital) consists of:

At least two pairs of IM/IV ampoules high-potency B-complex vitamins daily for 2 days.
- If no response, discontinue treatment.
- If signs/symptoms respond, continue one pair ampoules daily for 5 days or for as long as improvement continues.

For out-patient detoxification, the options available are:
- Oral vitamin supplementation with vitamin B Compound Strong, one tablet three times daily (but this is unlikely to be absorbed effectively and is therefore of little or no benefit to alcohol-dependent patients).
- Parenteral supplementation, as above, in a clinical setting where appropriate resuscitation facilities are available.

Seizure prophylaxis

Meta-analyses of trials assessing the efficacy of drugs preventing alcohol withdrawal seizures demonstrated that benzodiazepines, particularly long-acting preparations such as diazepam and chlordiazepoxide, significantly reduced seizures[5]. Most clinicians prefer to use diazepam for medically assisted withdrawal in those with a previous history of seizures. Some units advocate carbamazepine loading in patients with untreated epilepsy; that is, those with a history of more than two seizures during previous withdrawal episodes, or previous seizures despite adequate diazepam loading. Phenytoin does not prevent alcohol-withdrawal seizures and is therefore not indicated. Note that there is no need to continue an anticonvulsant if it has been used to treat or prevent an alcohol-withdrawal seizure.

Those who have a seizure for the first time should be investigated to rule out an organic disease or structural lesion.

Liver disease

For individuals with impaired liver function, oxazepam (a short-acting benzodiazepine) may be preferred to chlordiazepoxide, in order to avoid excessive build-up of metabolites and over-sedation.

Hallucinations

Mild perceptual disturbances usually respond to chlordiazepoxide. However, frank hallucinations should be treated with oral haloperidol. Haloperidol may also be given intramuscularly or (very rarely) intravenously if necessary. Caution is needed because haloperidol can reduce seizure threshold. Have parenteral procyclidine available in case of dystonic reactions. Note also haloperidol's effect on the QT interval (see page 87). Given this known effect, IV treatment should probably be avoided.

Symptomatic pharmacotherapy

Dehydration:	Ensure adequate fluid intake in order to maintain hydration and electrolyte balance. Dehydration can lead to cardiac arrythmia and death.
Pain:	Paracetamol.
Nausea and vomiting:	Metoclopramide (Maxolon) 10 mg or prochlorperazine (Stemetil) 5 mg 4–6 hourly.
Diarrhoea:	Diphenoxylate and atropine (Lomotil). Loperamide (Imodium).
Hepatic encephalopathy:	Lactulose (within the general medical hospital).
Skin itching	(occurs commonly and not only in individuals with alcoholic liver disease): Antihistamines.

Relapse prevention

Acamprosate and supervised disulfiram should be considered as adjuncts to psychosocial treatment. These should be initiated by a specialist service. After 12 weeks, transfer of the prescribing to the GP may be appropriate, though specialist care may continue (shared care). Naltrexone does not have a marketing authorisation for the treatment of alcohol dependence in the UK.

References

1. Mayo-Smith MF. Pharmacological management of alcohol withdrawal. *JAMA* 1997; **278**: 144–151.
2. Lingford-Hughes A, Welch S, Nutt DJ. Evidence-based guidelines for the pharmacological management of substance misuse, addiction and co-morbidity: recommendations from the British Association for Psychopharmacology. *J Psychopharmacol* 2004; **18**: 293–339.
3. Gossop M, Keaney F, Stewart D *et al.* A Short Alcohol Withdrawal Scale (SAWS): development and psychometric properties. *Addict Biol* 2002; 7: 37–43.
4. Thomson A, Cook C, Touquet R *et al.* The Royal College of Physicians report on alcohol; guidelines for managing Wernicke's encephalopathy in the accident and emergency department. *Alcohol Alcohol* 2002; **37**: 513–521.
5. Hillbom M, Pieninkeroinen I, Leone M. Seizures in alcohol-dependent patients: epidemiology, pathophysiology and management. *CNS Drugs* 2003; **17**: 1013–1030.

Further reading

Claassen CA, Adinoff B. Alcohol withdrawal syndrome: guidelines for management. *CNS Drugs* 1999; **12**: 279–291.
Duncan D, Taylor D. Chlormethiazole or chlordiazepoxide in alcohol detoxification. *Psychiatr Bull* 1996; **20**: 599–601.
Edwards G, Marshall EJ, Cook CCH. *The Treatment of Drinking Problems,* 4th edition. Cambridge: Cambridge University Press, 2003.

Substance misuse

Opioid dependence

Note: treatment of opioid dependence usually requires specialist intervention – generalists should always contact substance misuse services (where available) before attempting to treat opioid dependence.

Treatment aims
- to reduce or prevent withdrawal symptoms
- to reduce or eliminate non-prescribed drug use
- to stabilise drug intake and lifestyle
- to reduce drug-related harm (particularly injecting behaviour)
- to help maintain contact and provide an opportunity to work with the patient.

Treatment
This will depend upon:
- what is available
- patient's previous history of drug use and treatment
- patient's current drug use and circumstances.

Evidence of opioid dependence
Patient's self-reporting of opioid dependence must be confirmed by positive urine results for opioids, and objective signs of withdrawal or general restlessness should be present before considering prescribing any substitute pharmacotherapy. Recent sites of injection may also be present.

Table Objective opioid withdrawal scales

Symptoms	Absent/normal	Mild-moderate	Severe
Lactorrhoea	Absent	Eyes watery	Eyes streaming/wiping eyes
Rhinorrhoea	Absent	Sniffing	Profuse secretion (wiping nose)
Agitation	Absent	Fidgeting	Can't remain seated
Perspiration	Absent	Clammy skin	Beads of sweat
Piloerection	Absent	Barely palpable hairs standing up	Readily palpable, visible
Pulse rate (BPM)	<80	>80 but <100	>100
Vomiting	Absent	Absent	Present
Shivering	Absent	Absent	Present
Yawning/10 min	<3	3–5	6 or more
Dilated pupils	Normal <4 mm	Dilated 4–6 mm	Widely dilated >6 mm

Subjective opioid withdrawal symptoms can include nausea, stomach cramps, muscular tension, muscle spasms/twitching, aches and pains, and insomnia.

Substance misuse

> *Note:* Untreated heroin withdrawal symptoms typically reach their peak 32–36 hours after the last dose and symptoms will have subsided substantially after 5 days. Untreated methadone withdrawal typically reaches its peak at 4–6 days and symptoms do not substantially subside for 10–12 days.[1]

Induction and stabilisation of substitute prescribing

It is usually preferable to use a longer-acting opioid agonist or partial agonist (e.g. methadone or buprenorphine respectively) in opioid dependence, as it is generally easier to maintain stability[1]. However, patients with a less severe opioid dependency (e.g. history of using codeine or dihydrocodeine-containing preparations only) may in some cases be better managed by maintaining/detoxifying them using that preparation or an equivalent.

Choosing between buprenorphine and methadone for substitute treatment

Current evidence has not identified particular groups of patients who routinely do better on buprenorphine or methadone. So, the decision should be made after discussion with the patient and taking the following into consideration:

- Buprenorphine appears to have a milder withdrawal syndrome than methadone and therefore may be preferred for detoxification programmes[2,3].

- Side-effects: differences in side-effect profiles (e.g. buprenorphine is often described as less sedating) may affect patient preference.

- Buprenorphine appears to provide greater 'blockade' effects than doses of methadone less than 60 mg[4-7]. This may be considered an advantage or a disadvantage by patients. In particular, patients with chronic pain conditions that frequently require additional opioid analgesia may have difficulties in being treated with buprenorphine.

- Buprenorphine is more effective than placebo for reducing opioid use and retaining patients. Buprenorphine is comparable to methadone at lower doses (30–60 mg). Higher-dose methadone maintenance treatment (>60 mg) appears more effective than buprenorphine. However, there are no adequate trials of high-dose buprenorphine (16–32 mg) compared with high-dose methadone maintenance treatment[8].

- Methadone levels may be altered by drugs that inhibit/induce CYP3A4 such as erthromycin, several SSRIs, ribovarin and some anticonvulsants. This may make dose assessment difficult if patients are not consistent in their use of these CYP3A4-inhibiting drugs. Buprenorphine is less affected by such medications and may be preferable for such patients.

- Women who are pregnant or planning a pregnancy should consider methadone treatment, as the safety of buprenorphine in pregnancy has not been demonstrated.

- Methadone clients unable to reduce to doses of methadone less than 60 mg without becoming 'unstable' cannot easily be transferred to buprenorphine.

- Patients with a history of diversion of medication may be better served with methadone treatment which has the capacity for daily supervised administration. Sublingual buprenorphine tablets can be more easily diverted with the risk of injecting tablets.

Methadone

Methadone is a Controlled Drug with a high dependency potential and a low lethal dose. The initial 2 weeks of treatment with methadone are associated with a substantially increased risk of overdose mortality[1,9–12]. It is vitally important that appropriate assessment, titration of doses and monitoring are performed during this period.

Prescribing should commence only if:

- opioid drugs are being taken on a regular basis (typically daily)
- there is convincing evidence of dependence (see above)
- consumption of methadone can be supervised, especially for the initial doses.

Supervised daily consumption is recommended for new prescriptions, for a minimum of 3 months, if possible[1]. Alternatively, instalment prescriptions for daily dispensing and collection should be used. Certainly no more than 1 week's supply should be dispensed at one time, except in very exceptional circumstances[1].

Methadone should be prescribed in the oral liquid formulation (mixture or linctus). Tablets are likely to be crushed and inappropriately injected and therefore should not be prescribed[1,13].

> **Important:** All patients starting a methadone treatment programme must be informed of the risks of toxicity and overdose, and the necessity for safe storage[1,11–13].

Methadone and risk of torsade de pointes/QT prolongation

Recent evidence has pointed to methadone being a risk factor for developing torsade de pointes, which can lead to sudden death. Several case reports and retrospective studies have documented methadone-related torsades/QT prolongation[14–21]. In addition prospective studies have documented significant increases in QT prolongation following methadone induction for maintenance treatment[22]. This suggests that methadone may be a risk factor for QT prolongation and torsades. A limitation to the evidence may be confounding variables that predispose to increasing the QT interval. Other illicit (cocaine) and prescribed drugs (lofexidine) have also been linked to QT interval prolongation. Methadone combined with other QT-prolonging agents may increase the likelihood of QT prolongation and torsades (see page 87).

Risk factors for QT prolongation

In combination with other QT risk factors (see page 89)

high-dose methadone >100 mg
injectable methadone
illicit drugs with QT effect such as cocaine.

Indications for ECG monitoring

- new clients with other risks for QT prolongation (see page 90)
- methadone maintenance: existing clients with:
  - risk factors as above
  - current cardiac symptoms or history.

Induction of methadone:

- baseline ECG
- ECG after methadone stabilisation (4 weeks after stabilisation).

Maintenance treatment:
ECG 6–12-monthly depending on risk factors above.

DOSE

For patients who are *currently prescribed* methadone and if *all* the criteria listed below are met, then it is safe to prescribe the same dose:

- Dose confirmed by prescriber.

- Last consumption confirmed (e.g. pharmacy contacted) and is within last 3 days.

- Prescriber has stopped prescribing and current prescription is completed or cancelled to date.

- Patient is comfortable on dose (no signs of intoxication/withdrawal).

- No other contraindications or cautions are present.

Otherwise the following recommendations should be followed.

STARTING DOSE

Consideration must be given to the potential for opioid toxicity, taking into account:

- Tolerance to opioids can be affected by a number of factors and it obviously significantly influences an individual's risk of toxicity[23]. Tolerance should be assessed on the history of quantity, frequency and route of administration (be aware of the likelihood of over-reporting). As patients' tolerance to methadone can be significantly reduced within 3–4 days of not using, caution must be exercised when re-instating their dose.

- Use of other drugs, particularly depressants (e.g. alcohol and benzodiazepines).

- Long half-life of methadone, as cumulative toxicity may develop[24,25].

- Inappropriate dosing can result in potentially fatal overdose, particularly in the first few days[10–13]. Deaths have occurred following the commencement of a daily dose of 40 mg methadone[1]. It is safer to keep to a low dose that can subsequently be increased at intervals if this dose proves to be insufficient.

> *Note:* Opioid withdrawal is *not* a life-threatening condition. Opioid toxicity is.

Direct conversion tables for opioids and methadone should be viewed cautiously, as there are a number of factors influencing the values at any given time. It is much safer to titrate the dose against presenting withdrawal symptoms.

The **initial total** daily dose in most cases will be in the range of 10–40 mg methadone, depending on the level of tolerance (low: 10–20 mg; moderate: 25–40 mg). Starting doses of >30 mg should be prescribed with caution because of the risk of overdose. It is safer to use a starting dose of 10–20 mg and reassess the patient after a period of 2–4 hours. Further incremental doses of 5–10 mg can be given, depending on the severity of the withdrawal symptoms. *Note:* onset of action should be evident within half an hour, with peak plasma levels being achieved after approximately 4 hours of dosing.

Heavily dependent users with high tolerance may require larger doses. A starting dose, not exceeding 30 mg can be given, followed by a second dose after a minimum interval of 2–4 hours. The second dose can be up to 30 mg, depending on the persisting severity of withdrawal symptoms. High doses should be prescribed only by specialists in substance misuse.

Table Methadone dose after initial dose	
Severity of withdrawal after initial dose	*Additional dosage*
Mild	Nil
Moderate (muscle aches and pains, pupil dilation, nausea, yawning, clammy skin)	5–10 mg
Severe (vomiting, profuse sweating, piloerection, tachycardia, elevated BP)	20–30 mg

STABILISATION DOSE

- First week
  Out-patients should attend daily for the first few days to enable assessment by the prescriber and any dose titration against withdrawal symptoms. Dose increases should not exceed 5–10 mg/day and 30 mg/week above the initial starting dose. Note that steady-state plasma levels are achieved only approximately 5 days after the last dose increase. Once the patient has been stabilised on an adequate dose, methadone should be prescribed as a single daily dose. It should not be prescribed on a PRN basis.

- Subsequent period
  Subsequent increases should not exceed 10 mg per week beyond the induction period[1] up to a total daily dose of 60–120 mg. Stabilisation is usually achieved within 6 weeks but may take longer. However, it is important to consider that some patients may require a quicker stabilisation. This would need to be balanced by a high level of supervision, thereby allowing the ability to increase doses more rapidly.

CAUTIONS

- **Intoxication.** Methadone should not be given to any patient showing signs of intoxication, especially when due to alcohol or other depressant drugs (e.g. benzodiazepines)[23]. Risk of fatal overdose is greatly enhanced when methadone is taken concomitantly with alcohol and other respiratory depressant drugs. Concurrent alcohol and illicit drug consumption must be borne in mind when considering subsequent prescribing of methadone because of the increased risk of overdose associated with polysubstance misuse[9,12,26,27].

- **Severe hepatic/renal dysfunction**. Metabolism and elimination of methadone may be affected, in which case the dose or dosing interval should be adjusted accordingly against clinical presentation. Because of extended plasma half-life, the interval between assessments during initial dosing may need to be extended.

OVERDOSE

In the event of methadone overdose, naloxone should be administered, following *BNF* guidelines.

Dose: by intravenous injection, 0.8–2 mg repeated at intervals of 2–3 minutes to a maximum of 10 mg if respiratory function does not improve.

By subcutaneous or intramuscular injection: as intravenous injection but only if intravenous route not feasible (onset of action slower).

By continuous intravenous infusion, 2 mg diluted in 500 ml intravenous infusion solution at a rate adjusted according to response.

Always Call Emergency Services

Pregnancy and breast-feeding

There is no evidence of an increase in the incidence of congenital defects with methadone; however, the newborn may suffer withdrawal syndrome[28]. It is important to prevent the patient from going into a withdrawal state, since this is dangerous for both mother and foetus. Specialist advice should be obtained before prescribing or detoxifying, particularly with regard to management and treatment plan during pregnancy.

Methadone is considered compatible with breast-feeding, with no adverse effects to the nursing infant when the mother is consuming 20 mg/24 hours or less[28].

Analgesia for methadone-prescribed patients

Non-opioid analgesics should be used in preference (e.g. paracetamol, NSAIDs). If opioid analgesia is indicated (e.g. codeine, dihydrocodeine, MST), this should be titrated accordingly against pain relief, with the methadone dose remaining constant to alleviate withdrawal symptoms. Avoid titrating the methadone dose to provide analgesia.

Injectable opioid maintenance treatment

At present there is insufficient evidence supporting the use of injectable opioid drugs for maintenance treatment[19]. However, it may be considered as a 'second-line' treatment option in some patients for whom an adequate trial (e.g. at least 6 months) of optimised methadone maintenance treatment is failing (e.g. doses > 80 mg, regular supervised dosing, regular attendance at key worker and medical reviews, and appropriate management of medical or psychiatric co-morbidity). Injectable methadone or diamorphine treatment should only be initiated by a substance misuse specialist. National Treatment Agency (NTA) guidelines[29] advocate that all clients currently on injectable opioids should be physically assessed (supervised) while taking their prescribed drug on a regular basis, enabling assessment of a patient's tolerance and injecting techniques.

There appears to be considerable individual variation in appropriate dose conversions between oral and injectable methadone. Oral methadone has a bioavailability of approximately 80% (ranging from 40% to 99%). It is estimated that the injectable methadone dose = 80% × oral methadone dose. Clients should be regularly monitored in the early stages and the dose titrated (up or down) as clinically indicated.

Dose conversions between oral methadone and injectable diamorphine vary between 3:1 and 6:1 according to the dose[29].

Buprenorphine (Subutex)[30–32]

Buprenorphine is a synthetic opioid. It is a partial opioid agonist with low intrinsic activity and high affinity at μ-opioid receptors. It is effective in treating opioid dependence because:

- It alleviates/prevents opioid withdrawal and craving.
- It reduces the effects of additional opioid use because of its high receptor affinity[4–6].
- It is long-acting, allowing daily (or less) dosing. The duration of action is related to the buprenorphine dose administered: low doses (e.g. 2 mg) exert effects for up to 12 hours; higher doses (e.g. 16–32 mg) exert effects for as long as 48–72 hours.

STARTING DOSE

The same principles as for methadone apply when starting treatment with buprenorphine. However, of particular interest with buprenorphine is the phenomenon of precipitated withdrawal. Patient education is an important factor in reducing the problems during induction.

INDUCTING HEROIN USERS

The first dose of buprenorphine should be administered when the patient is experiencing opioid withdrawal symptoms to reduce the risk of precipitated withdrawal. The initial dose recommendations are as follows:

patient in withdrawal and no risk factors	8 mg buprenorphine
patient not experiencing withdrawal and no risk factors	4 mg buprenorphine
patient has concomitant risk factors (e.g. medical condition, polydrug misuse, low or uncertain severity of dependence)	2–4 mg buprenorphine

Transferring from methadone

Patients transferring from methadone are at risk of experiencing precipitated withdrawal symptoms that may continue at a milder level for 1–2 weeks. Factors affecting precipitated withdrawal are listed in the table below.

Table Factors affecting risk of precipitated withdrawal with buprenorphine

Factor	Discussion	Recommended strategy
Dose of methadone	More likely with doses of methadone above 30 mg Generally, the higher the dose, the more severe the precipitate withdrawal[33]	Attempt transfer only from doses of methadone <40 mg Transfer from >60 mg should not be attempted
Time between last methadone dose and first buprenorphine dose	Interval should be at least 24 hours. Increasing the interval reduces the incidence and severity of withdrawal[34,35]	Cease methadone and delay first dose until patient experiencing withdrawal from methadone
Dose of buprenorphine	Very low doses of buprenorphine (e.g. 2 mg) are generally inadequate to substitute for methadone. High first doses of buprenorphine (e.g. 8 mg) are more likely to precipitate withdrawal	First dose should generally be 4 mg; review patient 2–3 hours later
Patient expectancy	Patients not prepared for precipitated withdrawal are more likely to become distressed and confused by the effect	Inform patients in advance Have contingency plan for severe symptoms
Use of other medications	Symptomatic medication (e.g. lofexidine) can be useful to relieve symptoms	Prescribe in accordance to management plan

Substance misuse

Transferring from methadone dose of <40 mg

Methadone should be ceased abruptly, and the first dose of buprenorphine given at least 24 hours after the last methadone dose. The following conversion rates are recommended:

Last methadone dose	Initial buprenorphine dose	Day 2 buprenorphine dose
20–40 mg	4 mg	6–8 mg
10–20 mg	4 mg	4–8 mg
1–10 mg	4 mg	4 mg

Transferring from methadone dose of 40–60 mg

- The methadone dose should be reduced as far as possible without the patient becoming unstable or chaotic, and then abruptly stopped.

- The first buprenorphine dose should be delayed until the patient displays clear signs of withdrawal, generally 48–96 hours after the last dose of methadone. Symptomatic medication (lofexidine) may be useful to provide transitory relief.

- An initial dose of 4 mg should be given. The patient should then be reviewed 2–3 hours later.

- If withdrawal has been precipitated, further symptomatic medication can be prescribed.

- If there has been no precipitation or worsening of withdrawal, an additional 2–4 mg of buprenorphine can be dispensed and given on the same day.

- The patient should be reviewed the following day, at which point the dose should be increased to 8–12 mg.

Transferring from methadone doses of >60 mg

Such transfers should not be attempted in an out-patient setting. Consider referral to in-patient unit if required.

Transferring from other prescribed opioids

There is little experience in transferring patients from other prescribed opioids (e.g. codeine, dihydrocodeine, morphine). Basic principles suggest that transferring from opioids with short half-lives should be similar to inducting heroin users, whereas transferring from opioids with longer half-lives will be similar to transferring from methadone.

Stabilisation dose of buprenorphine

Out-patients should attend regularly for the first few days to enable assessment by the prescriber and any dose titration. Dose increases should be made in increments of 2–4 mg at a time, daily if necessary, up to a maximum daily dose of 32 mg. Effective maintenance doses are usually in the range of 12–24 mg daily[30], and patients should generally be able to achieve maintenance levels within 1–2 weeks of starting buprenorphine.

Less than daily dosing

Buprenorphine is registered in the UK as a medication to be taken daily. International evidence and experience indicate that many clients can be comfortably maintained on one dose every 2–3 days[32,36–38]. This may be pertinent to patients in buprenorphine treatment who are considered unsuitable for take-away medication because of the risk of diversion. The following conversion rate is recommended:

2-day buprenorphine dose = 2 × daily dose of buprenorphine (maximum 32 mg)
3-day buprenorphine dose = 3 × daily dose of buprenorphine (to a maximum 32 mg)

Note: In the event of patients being unable to stabilise comfortably on buprenorphine (often those transferring from methadone), the option of transferring to methadone should be available. Methadone can be commenced 24 hours after the last buprenorphine dose. Doses should be titrated according to clinical response, being mindful of the residual 'blockade' effect of buprenorphine, which may last for several days.

Cautions with buprenorphine

- **Liver function:** There is some evidence that high-dose buprenorphine can cause changes in liver function in individuals with a history of liver disease[39]. Such patients should have LFTs measured before commencing with follow-up investigations conducted 6–12 weeks after commencing buprenorphine. More frequent testing should be considered in patients of particular concern, e.g. severe liver disease or those at risk of injecting the tablets.
- **Intoxication:** Buprenorphine should not be given to any patient showing signs of intoxication, especially due to alcohol or other depressant drugs (e.g. benzodiazepines). Buprenorphine in combination with other sedative drugs can result in respiratory depression, sedation, coma and death. Concurrent alcohol and illicit drug consumption must be borne in mind when considering subsequent prescribing of buprenorphine due to the increased risk of overdose associated with polysubstance misuse.

Overdose with buprenorphine
Buprenorphine as a single drug in overdose is generally regarded as safer than methadone and heroin because it causes less respiratory depression. However, in combination with other respiratory depressant drugs, the effects may be harder to manage. Very high doses of naloxone (e.g. 10–15 mg) may be needed to reverse buprenorphine effects (although lower doses such as 0.8–2 mg may be sufficient); hence, ventilator support is often required in cases where buprenorphine is contributing to respiratory depression (e.g. in polydrug overdose).

Always Call Emergency Services

Pregnancy and breast-feeding
Currently, there is insufficient evidence regarding the use of buprenorphine as an opioid substitute treatment during pregnancy or breast-feeding to define its safety profile[28]. More evidence is available on the safety of methadone, which for that reason makes it the preferred choice. Further evaluation and consideration would have to be made for individual cases.

Analgesia for buprenorphine-prescribed patients
Non-opioid analgesics should be used in preference (e.g. paracetamol, NSAIDs). Buprenorphine reduces or blocks the effect of full agonist opioids, therefore complicating their use as analgesics in patients on buprenorphine. If adequate pain control cannot be achieved, it may be necessary to transfer the patient to a stable methadone dose so that an opioid analgesic can be effectively used for pain control (see note on analgesia for methadone-prescribed patients).

Substance misuse

Opioid detoxification and reduction regimes

COMMUNITY SETTING
- **Methadone**
  Following a period of stabilisation with methadone, a contract should be negotiated between the patient and prescriber to reduce the daily methadone dose by 5–10 mg weekly or fortnightly. However, this should be reviewed regularly and remain flexible to adjustments and changes in the patient's readiness for total abstinence. Factors such as an increase in heroin or other drug use, or worsening of the patient's physical, psychological or social well-being, may warrant a temporary increase, stabilisation or slowing-down of the reduction rate.
- **Buprenorphine**
  The same principles for methadone apply when planning a buprenorphine detoxification regime. Dose reduction should be gradual to minimise withdrawal discomfort. A suggested reduction regime follows.

Daily buprenorphine dose	*Reduction rate*
Above 16 mg	4 mg every 1–2 weeks
8–16 mg	2–4 mg every 1–2 weeks
2–8 mg	2 mg per week or fortnight
Below 2 mg	Reduce by 0.4–0.8 mg per week

- **Lofexidine**
  Lofexidine is licensed for the management of symptoms of opioid withdrawal. It is non-opioid and therefore less liable to misuse and diversion. Its use in community detoxification is more likely to be successful for patients with an average daily heroin use of up to 0.5 g (or 30 mg methadone equivalent), for non-polydrug users and for those with shorter drug and treatment histories, or for those at an end stage of methadone detoxification (patients taking not more than 20 mg daily).
  - *Precautions:* severe coronary insufficiency, recent MI, bradycardia, cerebrovascular disease, chronic renal failure, pregnancy and breast-feeding.
    QT prolongation has been reported[40]. Consider ECG monitoring during treatment based on other cardiac risk factors.
  - *Interactions:* alcohol and other CNS depressants – lofexidine may enhance the effects. Tricyclic antidepressants – concomitant use may reduce the efficacy of lofexidine.
  - *Side-effects:* drowsiness, dryness of mouth, throat and nose, hypotension, bradycardia and rebound hypertension on withdrawal.
    Before commencing treatment with lofexidine, baseline blood pressure should be measured and monitored over the first few days. If there is a significant drop in BP (systolic less than 90 mmHg or 30 mmHg below baseline), or pulse is below 55, lofexidine should be withheld. Treatment should be reviewed with the option either to continue at a reduced dose or discontinue.
  - *Dose:* Initially, 0.4–0.6 mg twice daily, increased as necessary, to control withdrawal symptoms, in steps of 0.2–0.4 mg daily, to a maximum total daily dose of 2.4 mg. The total daily dose should be given in 2–4 divided doses, with one dose at bedtime to offset insomnia associated with opioid withdrawal. Treatment course should be 7–10 days, followed by a gradual withdrawal over 2–4 days.

Low, reducing doses of methadone (e.g. 15 mg/10 mg/5 mg daily) may be given over the initial days of treatment with lofexidine as a cross-over period, to minimise withdrawal symptoms. This is appropriate only for patients currently taking methadone before detoxification.

Additional short-term medication may be required for nausea, stomach cramps, diarrhoea and insomnia.

IN-PATIENT SETTING

- **Methadone**
  Patients should have a starting dose assessment of methadone over 48 hours following the same guidelines listed above. The dose may then be reduced following a linear regime over 10 days.
- **Buprenorphine**
  Buprenorphine can be used effectively for short-term in-patient detoxifications following the same principles as for methadone.
- **Lofexidine** *(see community detoxification regimes above for more information)*
  Higher doses of lofexidine (up to the maximum daily dose of 2.4 mg) may be given initially, particularly for patients with an average daily heroin use over 0.5 g (or 30 mg methadone equivalent). This is provided there is adequate monitoring of BP, pulse and adverse effects, and appropriate action can be taken in any such event. If there is a significant drop in BP or pulse (systolic less than 90 mmHg or 30 mmHg below baseline, or pulse is below 55), lofexidine should be withheld until normal measurements are obtained and then reintroduced cautiously at a lower dose. In certain cases lofexidine may need to be discontinued and alternative detoxification treatment regimes considered.

  The total daily dose should be given in four divided doses over the first 2–3 days with the full treatment course continuing for 7–10 days. This should then be followed by a gradual withdrawal over 2–4 days.

  Additional short-term medication may be required for nausea, stomach cramps, diarrhoea and insomnia.

Relapse prevention – naltrexone

Evidence for the effectiveness of naltrexone as a treatment for relapse prevention in opioid misusers is inconclusive[41]. Combined use of naltrexone and psychosocial therapy has proved to be more effective than either therapy alone in improving post-treatment outcomes[42]. The available trials do not yet provide a final evaluation of naltrexone maintenance treatment. A trend in favour of treatment with naltrexone has been observed with highly motivated client groups only[41]. There is a risk of adverse events such as fatal overdose in those who relapse to opioid use. Therefore this should be used with extreme caution.

INITIATING TREATMENT

Naltrexone has the propensity to cause a severe withdrawal reaction in patients who are either currently taking opioid drugs or who were previously taking opioid drugs and have not allowed a sufficient wash-out period prior to administering naltrexone.

The minimum recommended interval between stopping the opioid and starting naltrexone depends on the opioid used, duration of use and the amount taken as a last dose. Opioid agonists with long half-lives such as methadone will require a wash-out period of up to 10 days, whereas shorter-acting opioids such as heroin may only require up to 7 days.

Experience with buprenorphine indicates that a wash-out period of up to 7 days is sufficient (final buprenorphine dose of >2 mg; duration of use of >2 weeks) and in some cases naltrexone may be started within 2–3 days of a patient's stopping (final buprenorphine dose of <2 mg; duration of use of <2 weeks).

A test dose of naloxone (0.2–0.8 mg), which has a much shorter half-life than naltrexone, may be given to the patient prior to starting naltrexone treatment. Any withdrawal symptoms precipitated will be of shorter duration than if precipitated by naltrexone.

Substance misuse

Patients *must* be advised of the risk of withdrawal prior to giving the dose. It is worth thoroughly questioning patients as to whether they have taken any opioid-containing preparation unknowingly (e.g. an over-the-counter analgesic).

Patients must also be warned of the risk of acute opioid toxicity occurring in any attempt to overcome the blockade effect of naltrexone. Changes in the individual's opioid tolerance level are likely to be very significant particularly following a detoxification programme and any period of abstinence.

Dose of naltrexone

An initial dose of 25 mg naltrexone should be administered after a suitable opioid-free interval (and naloxone challenge if appropriate). The patient should be monitored for 4 hours after the first dose for symptoms of opioid withdrawal. Symptomatic medication for withdrawal (lofexidine) should be available for use on the first day of naltrexone dosing (withdrawal symptoms may last up to 4–8 hours). Once the patient has tolerated this low naltrexone dose, subsequent doses can be increased to 50 mg daily as a maintenance dose.

References

1. Department of Health, Scottish Office Department of Health, Welsh Office, Department of Health and Social Services, Northern Ireland. Drug Misuse and Dependence – Guidelines on Clinical Management, 1999.
2. Seifert J, Metzner C, Paetzold W *et al.* Detoxification of opiate addicts with multiple drug abuse: a comparison of buprenorphine vs. methadone. *Pharmacopsychiatry* 2002; **35**: 159–164.
3. Jasinski DR, Pevnick JS, Griffiths JD. Human pharmacology and abuse potential of the analgesic buprenorphine: a potential agent for treating narcotic addiction. *Arch Gen Psychiatry* 1978; **35**: 501–516.
4. Bickel WK, Stitze ML, Bigelow GE *et al.* Buprenorphine: dose-related blockade of opioid challenge effects in opioid dependent humans. *J Pharmacol Exp Ther* 1988; **247**: 47–53.
5. Walsh SL, Preston KL, Bigelow GE *et al.* Acute administration of buprenorphine in humans: partial agonist and blockade effects. *J Pharmacol Exp Ther* 1995; **274**: 361–372.
6. Comer SD, Collins ED, Fischman MW. Buprenorphine sublingual tablets: effects on IV heroin self-administration by humans. *Psychopharmacology* 2001; **154**: 28–37.
7. Donny EC, Walsh SL, Bigelow GE *et al.* High-dose methadone produces superior opioid blockade and comparable withdrawal suppression to lower doses in opioid-dependent humans. *Psychopharmacology* 2002; **161**: 202–212.
8. Mattick RP, Kimber J, Breen C *et al.* Buprenorphine maintenance versus placebo or methadone maintenance for opioid dependence. *Cochrane Database of Systematic Reviews,* 2003, Issue 3.
9. Harding-Pink D. Methadone: one person's maintenance dose is another's poison. *Lancet* 1993; **341**: 665–666.
10. Drummer OH, Opeskin K, Syrjanen M *et al.* Methadone toxicity causing death in ten subjects starting on methadone maintenance program. *Am J Forensic Med Pathol* 1992; **13**: 346–350.
11. Caplehorn J. Deaths in the first two weeks of maintenance treatment in NSW in 1994: identifying cases of iatrogenic methadone toxicity. *Drug Alcohol Rev* 1998; **17**: 9–17.
12. Zador D, Sunjic S. Deaths in methadone maintenance treatment in NSW, Australia 1990–1995. *Addiction* 2000; **95**: 77–84.
13. Task Force to Review Services for Drug Misusers. *Report of an Independent Review of Drug Treatment Services in England.* London: DoH Publication, 1996.
14. Vodoz JF, Jaquier F, Lamy O. Torsade de pointes: a severe and unknown adverse effect in a patient taking methadone. *Schweizerische Rundschau für Medizin Praxis* 2003; **92**: 1748–1750.
15. Sala M, Anguera I, Cervantes M. Torsade de pointes due to methadone. *Ann Intern Med* 2003; **139**: 307.
16. Mokwe EO, Ositadinma O. Torsade de pointes due to methadone. *Ann Intern Med* 2003; **139**: W64.
17. De Bels D, Staroukine M, Devriendt J. Torsade de pointes due to methadone. *Ann Intern Med* 2003; **139**: E156.
18. Krantz MJ, Lewkowiez L, Hays H *et al.* Torsade de pointes associated with very-high-dose methadone. *Ann Intern Med* 2002; **137**: 501–504. Summary for patients. *Ann Intern Med* 2002; **137**: 142.
19. Lingford-Hughes AR, Welch S, Nutt AJ. Evidence-based guidelines for the pharmacological management of substance misuse, addiction and comorbidity: recommendations from the British Association for Psychopharmacology. *J Psychopharmacol* 2004; **18**: 293–335.
20. Hall W. Reducing the toll of opioid overdose deaths in Australia. *Drug Alcohol Rev* 1999; **18**: 213–220.
21. Kornick CA, Kilborn MJ, Santiago-Palma J *et al.* QTc interval prolongation associated with intravenous methadone. *Pain* 2003; **105**: 499–506.

Substance misuse

22. Martell BA, Arnsten JH, Ray B *et al.* The impact of methadone induction on cardiac conduction in opiate users. *Ann Intern Med* 2003; **139**: 154–155.
23. White J, Irvine R. Mechanisms of fatal opioid overdose. *Addiction* 1999; **94**: 961–972.
24. Wolff K, Rostami-Hodjegan A, Shires S *et al.* The pharmacokinetics of methadone in healthy subjects and opiate users. *Br J Clin Pharmacol* 1997; **44**: 325–334.
25. Rostami-Hodjegan A, Wolff K, Hay A *et al.* Population pharmacokinetics in opiate users: characterisation of time dependent changes. *Br J Clin Pharmacol* 1999; **47**: 974–986.
26. Farrell M, Neeleman J, Griffiths P *et al.* Suicide and overdose among opiate addicts. Editorial. *Addiction* 1996; **91**: 321–323.
27. Neal J. Methadone, methadone treatment and non-fatal overdose. *Drug Alcohol Depen* 2000; **58**: 117–124.
28. Briggs GG, Freeman RK, Yaffe SJ (eds). *Drugs in Pregnancy and Lactation*, 6th edition. Philadelphia: Lippincott, Williams and Wilkins, 2002.
29. NTA guidelines http://www.nta.nhs.uk/ http://www.nta.nhs.uk/programme/national/IOT_trial_guidance.pdf
30. Ling W, Charuvastra C, Collins JF *et al.* Buprenorphine maintenance treatment of opiate dependence: a multicenter, randomized clinical trial. *Addiction* 1998; **93**: 475–486.
31. Mattick RP, Kimber J, Breen C *et al.* Buprenorphine maintenance versus placebo or methadone maintenance for opioid dependence. Cochrane Database of Systematic Reviews, 4, Oxford, 2002.
32. Amass L, Bickel WK, Higgins ST *et al.* Alternate day dosing during buprenorphine treatment of opioid dependence. *Life Sci* 1994; **54**: 1215–1228.
33. Walsh SL, June HL, Schuh KJ *et al.* Effects of buprenorphine and methadone in methadone-maintained subjects. *Psychopharmacology* 1995; **119**: 268–276.
34. Strain EC, Preston KL, Liebson IA *et al.* Acute effects of buprenorphine, and hydromorphone and naloxone in methadone maintained volunteers. *J Pharmacol Exp Ther* 1992; **261**: 985–993.
35. Strain EC, Preston KL, Liebson IA *et al.* Buprenorphine effects in methadone maintained volunteers: effects at 2 hours after methadone. *J Pharmacol Exp Ther* 1995; **272**: 628–638.
36. Amass L, Bickel WK, Crean JP *et al.* Alternate day buprenorphine dosing is preferred to daily dosing by opioid dependent humans. *Psychopharmacology* 1998; **136**: 217–225.
37. Johnson RE, Eissenberg T, Stitzer ML *et al.* Buprenorphine treatment of opioid dependence: clinical trial of daily versus alternate day dosing. *Drug Alcohol Depen* 1995; **40**: 27–35.
38. Eissenberg TR, Johnson RE, Bigelow GE *et al.* Controlled opioid withdrawal evaluation during 72-hr dose omission in buprenorphine maintained patients. *Drug Alcohol Depen* 1997; **45**: 81–91.
39. Berson A, Gervais A, Cazals D *et al.* Hepatitis after intravenous buprenorphine misuse in heroin addicts. *J Hepatol* 2001; **34**: 346–350.
40. Schmittner J, Schroeder JR, Epstein DH *et al.* QT interval increased after single dose of lofexidine. *BMJ* 2004; **329**: 1075.
41. Kirchmayer U, Davoli M, Verster A. Naltrexone maintenance treatment for opioid dependence. Cochrane Database of Systematic Reviews, Issue 2, Oxford, 2003.
42. Tucker T, Ritter A. Naltrexone in the treatment of heroin dependence: a comprehensive review. *Drug Alcohol Rev* 2000; **19**: 73–82.

Substance misuse

Drugs of misuse – a summary

One in ten adults use illicit drugs in any one year[1], and at least a third of those with mental illness can be classified as having a 'dual diagnosis'[2,3]. It is therefore important to be aware of the main mental state changes associated with drugs of abuse. Urine-testing for illicit drugs is routine on many psychiatric wards. It is important to be aware of the duration of detection of drugs in urine and of other commonly used substances and drugs that can give a false-positive result.

References

1. Ramsey M, Spiller J. *Drug Misuse Declared in 1996: Latest Results from the British Crime Survey*. London: Home Office, 1996.
2. Menenzes PR, Johnson S, Thornicroft G *et al.* Drug and alcohol problems among individuals with severe mental illness in south London. *Br J Psychiatry* 1996; **168**; 612–619.

Drug	Physical signs/ symptoms of intoxication	Most common mental state changes[8]	Withdrawal symptoms
Amphetamine[4]	Tachycardia Increased BP Anorexia	Visual/tactile/ olfactory auditory hallucinations Paranoia Decreased concentration Elation	Extreme fatigue Hunger Depression
Benzodiazepines	Sedation Dizziness Respiratory depression	Relaxation Visual hallucinations Disorientation Sleep disturbance	Seizures Psychosis Paraesthesia
Barbiturates	Headache Hypotension Respiratory depression	Restlessness/ataxia Confusion/ excitement Drowsiness	Similar to alcohol: tremor, vomiting, seizures, delirium tremens
Cannabis[5,6]	Tachycardia Lack of co-ordination Red eyes Postural hypotension	Elation, psychosis Perceptual distortions Disturbance of memory/ judgement, twofold increase in risk of developing schizophrenia[11]	Restlessness Irritability Insomnia Anxiety[7]
Cocaine	Tachycardia/tachypnoea Increased BP/headache Respiratory depression	Euphoria Paranoid psychosis Panic attacks/anxiety Insomnia/excitement	Profound lethargy Decreased consciousness
Heroin	Pinpoint pupils Clammy skin Respiratory depression	Drowsiness Euphoria Hallucinations	Nausea General aches and pains/gooseflesh Runny nose/eyes Diarrhoea
Methadone	Respiratory depression Pulmonary oedema	As above	As above but milder and longer lasting

3. Phillips P, Johnson S. Drug and alcohol misuse among inpatients with psychotic illnesses in 3 inner London psychiatric units. *Psychiatr Bull* 2003; **27**: 217–220.
4. Srisuraponont M, Kittiratanapaiboon P, Jarusuraisin N. Treatment for amphetamine dependence and abuse. Cochrane Database of Systematic Reviews, Oxford, Update Software, 2001.
5. Hall W, Solowij N. Long-term cannabis use and mental health. *Br J Psychiatry* 1997; **171**: 107–108.
6. Johns A. Psychiatric effects of cannabis. *Br J Psychiatry* 2001; **178**: 116–122.
7. Budney AJ, Hughes JR, Moore BA *et al.* Review of the validity and significance of cannabis withdrawal syndrome. *Am J Psychiatry* 2004; **161**: 1967–1977.
8. *Micromedex Healthcare*, Vol. 17. Thomson Ltd, USA, 2004.
9. Euromed Ltd. info@euromed.ltd.uk.
10. HM Prison Service. *Non-instrumental Drug Screen Test Cross-reactivity Manual.* Drug Strategy Unit, Prison Service Headquarters, 2001
11. Arseneault L, Cannon M, Witton J *et al.* Causal association between cannabis and psychosis: examination of the evidence. *Br J Psychiatry* 2004; **184**: 110–117.

Duration of withdrawal	Duration of detection in the urine[6, 7]	Other substances which give a positive result[9,10]
Peaks 7–34 hours Lasts maximum of 5 days	Up to 72 hours	Cough and decongestant preparations, selegiline, large quantities of tryamine, tranylcypromine, chloroquine, ranitidine
Usually short-lived but may last weeks to months	2–21 days: depending on half-life of drug taken	Zopiclone (possible)
Depends on half-life – likely to be at least several days	24 hours–14 days, depending on half-life	None known
Uncertain Probably less than 1 month[6] (longer in heavy users[7])	Single use: 3 days Chronic heavy use: up to 4 weeks	Passive 'smoking' of cannabis
12–18 hours	2–3 days	Food/tea containing coco leaves
Peaks after 36–72 hours	Up to 48 hours	Food/tea containing poppy seed Procaine Any opiate analgesic Diphenoxylate, naltrexone
Peaks after 4–6 days Can last 3 weeks	Up to 7 days with chronic use	Imipramine Meperidine

Substance misuse

Interactions between 'street drugs' and prescribed psychotropic drugs

There are some significant interactions between 'street drugs' and drugs that are prescribed for the treatment of mental illness. Information comes from case reports or theoretical assumptions, rarely from systematic investigation. A summary can be found in the table opposite, but remember that the knowledge base is poor. Always be cautious.

In all patients who misuse street drugs:

- Infection with hepatitis B and C is common. This may lead to a reduced ability to metabolise other drugs and increased sensitivity to side-effects.
- Prescribed drugs may be used in the same way as illicit drugs (i.e. erratically and not as intended). Large quantities of prescribed drugs should not be given to out-patients.

Acute behavioural disturbance

Acute intoxication with street drugs may result in behavioural disturbance. Non-drug management is preferable. If at all possible, a urine drug screen should be done to determine the drugs that have been taken, before prescribing any psychotropic. A physical examination should be done if possible (BP, TPR and ECG).

If intervention with a psychotropic is unavoidable, haloperidol 5 mg *or* olanzapine 10 mg po/IM is probably the safest option. Temperature, pulse, respiration and blood pressure *must* be monitored afterwards. Benzodiazepines are commonly misused with other street drugs and so standard doses may be ineffective in tolerant users. Interactions are also possible (see table opposite). Try to avoid.

References for table overleaf

1. Johns A. Psychiatric effects of cannabis. *Br J Psychiatry* 2001; **178**: 116–122.
2. Ashton S. Pharmacology and effects of cannabis: a brief review. *Br J Psychiatry* 2001; **178**: 101–106.
3. Zullino DF, Delessert D, Eap CB *et al.* Tobacco and cannabis smoking cessation can lead to intoxication with clozapine or olanzapine. *Int Clin Psychopharm* 2002; **17**: 141–143.
4. Benowitz NL, Jones RT. Effects of delta-9-tetrahydrocannabinol on drug distribution and metabolism. *Clin Pharmacol Ther* 1977; **22**: 259–268.
5. Annex 14, Drug interactions. In: *Drug Misuse and Dependence – Guidelines on Clinical Management.* Department of Health. Norwich: HMSO.
6. Wines JD, Weiss RD. Opioid withdrawal during risperidone treatment. *J Clin Psychopharm* 1999; **11**: 198–203.
7. Eap CB, Bertschy G, Powell K. Fluvoxamine and fluoxetine do not interact in the same way with the metabolism of the enantiomers of methadone. *J Clin Psychopharm* 1997; **17**: 113–117.
8. Ketter TA, Post RM, Worthington K. Principles of clinically important drug interactions with carbamazepine. I. *J Clin Psychopharm* 1991; **11**: 198–203.
9. Miller BL, Mena I, Giombetti R *et al.* Neuropsychiatric effects of cocaine: SPECT measurements. In: Miller EB (ed). *Cocaine: Physiological and Physiopathological Effects.* New York: Haworth Press, 1992.
10. Gowing LR, Henry-Edwards SM, Irvine RJ *et al.* The health effects of ecstasy: a literature review. *Drug Alcohol Revs* 2002; **21**: 53–63.
11. Newton TF, Ling W, Kalechstein AD *et al.* Risperidone pre-treatment reduces the euphoric effects of experimentally administered cocaine. *Psychiatry Res* 2001; **102**: 227–233.
12. Grabowski J, Rhoades H, Silverman P *et al.* Risperidone for the treatment of cocaine dependence: randomised double-blind trial. *J Clin Psychopharm* 2000; **20**: 305–310.
13. Vuori E, Henry JA, Ojanpera L *et al.* Death following ingestion of MDMA (ecstasy) and moclobemide. *Addiction* 2003; **98**: 365–368.
14. O'Dell LE, George FR, Ritz MC. Antidepressant drugs appear to enhance cocaine-induced toxicity. *Exp Clin Psychopharmacol* 2000; **8**: 133–141.
15. Macedo DS, Santos RS, Belchior LD *et al.* Effect of anxiolytic, antidepressant, and antipsychotic drugs on cocaine-induced seizures and mortality. *Epilepsy and Behavior* 2004; **5**: 852–856.

Substance misuse

16. Liechti ME, Baumann C, Gamma A *et al.* Acute psychological effects of 3,4-methylendioxymethamphetamine (MDMA, "Ecstasy") are attenuated by the serotonin uptake inhibitor citalopram. *Neuropsychopharmacology* 2000; **22**: 513–521.
17. Balki SL. Antidepressants in the treatment of cocaine dependence. Cochrane Database of Systematic Reviews. Oxford: Update Software, 2001.
18. Rowbotham MC, Jones RT, Benowitz NL *et al.* Trazodone–oral cocaine interactions. *Arch Gen Psychiatry* 1984; **41**: 895–899.
19. Roldan CJ, Habal R, Hnatiuk OW *et al.* Toxicity of cocaine. 2004; www.emedicine.com/med/topic400.htm

Further reading

Howard LA, Sellers EM, Tyndale RF. The role of pharmacogenetically variable cytochrome P450 enzyme in drug abuse and dependence. *Pharmacogenomics* 2002; **3**: 185–199.
Ley A, Jeffery DP, McLaren S *et al.* Treatment programmes for people with both severe mental illness and substance misuse. Cochrane Database of Systematic Reviews. Update Software, Oxford, 2002.
Williams R, Cohen J. Substance use and misuse in psychiatric wards. *Psychiatr Bull* 2000; **24**: 43–46.

Substance misuse

Substance misuse

Table Interactions between 'street drugs' and psychotropics (for references, see page 254)

	Cannabis	Heroin/methadone[5]	Cocaine Amphetamines Ecstasy	Alcohol
General considerations	• Usually smoked in cigarettes (induces CYP1A2) • Can be sedative[1] • Dose-related tachycardia[2]	• Can produce sedation/ respiratory depression • QTc prolongation also reported with methadone (see page 241)	• Stimulants (cocaine can be sedative in higher doses) • Arrhythmia possible • Cerebral/cardiac ischaemia with cocaine[9] • Hyperthermia/ dehydration with ecstasy[10]	• Sedative • Liver damage possible
Older antipsychotics	• Antipsychotics reduce the psychotropic effects of almost all drugs of abuse by blocking dopamine receptors (dopamine is the neurotransmitter responsible for 'reward') • Patients prescribed antipsychotics may increase their consumption of illicit substances to compensate • Patients who have taken ecstasy may be more prone to EPSEs • Cardiotoxic or very sedative antipsychotics are best avoided, at least initially. Sulpiride is a reasonably safe first choice			
Atypicals	• Risk of additive sedation • Cannabis can reduce serum levels of olanzapine and clozapine via induction of CYP1A2[3]	• Risk of additive sedation • Case report of methadone withdrawal being precipitated by risperidone[6]	• Risperidone may reduce the euphoric effects of cocaine[11], but does not reduce cocaine use[12]	• Increased risk of hypotension with olanzapine (and possibly other β-blockers)
Antidepressants	• Tachycardia has been reported (monitor pulse and take care with TCAs[4])	• Avoid very sedative antidepressants • Some SSRIs can increase methadone plasma levels[7] (citalopram is SSRI of choice)	• Avoid TCAs (arrhythmia) • MAOIs contraindicated (hypertension) • Moclobemide and SSRIs may increase stimulant toxicity[13-15] and SSRIs may attenuate psychological effects[16] • Various antidepressants have been used in 'crack' withdrawal and may lower the 'high' experienced with stimulants. They are ineffective for cocaine dependence[17]. One small study suggests no interaction between cocaine and trazodone[18]	• Avoid very sedative antidepressants • Avoid antidepressants that are toxic in OD • Impaired psychomotor skills (not SSRIs)
Anticholinergics	• Misuse is likely. Try to avoid if at all possible (by using an atypical if an antipsychotic is required) • Can cause hallucinations, elation and cognitive impairment			

256

Lithium	• Very toxic if taken erratically • Always consider the effects of dehydration (particularly problematic with alcohol or ecstasy)			
Carbamazepine/valproate		• Carbamazepine (CBZ) decreases methadone levels[8] (danger if CBZ stopped suddenly) • Valproate seems less likely to interact	• Carbamazepine induces CYP3A4, which leads to increased formation of norcocaine (hepatotoxic and more carciotoxic than cocaine)[19]	• Monitor LFTs
Benzodiazepines (Always remember that benzodiazapines are liable to misuse)	• Monitor level of sedation	• Oversedation (and respiratory depression possible) • Concomitant use can lead to accidental overdose • Possible pharmacokinetic interaction (increased methadone levels)	• Oversedation (if high doses of cocaine have been taken) • Widely used after cocaine intoxication	• Oversedation (and respiratory depression) possible • Future misuse possible • Widely used in alcohol detoxification

chapter 7

Use of psychotropics in special patient groups

Depression and psychosis in epilepsy

The prevalence of clinical depression in people with epilepsy varies from 9% to 22%[1,2], and depressive symptoms may occur in up to 60% of people with intractable epilepsy[3]. Suicide rates have been estimated to be 4–5 times that of the general population[1,2]. The prevalence of psychotic illness in people with epilepsy is at least 4%[4]. Peri-ictal depression or psychosis (that is, symptoms temporally related to seizure activity) should initially be treated by optimising anticonvulsant therapy[4]. Interictal depression or psychosis (symptoms occurring independently of seizures) is likely to require treatment with antidepressants or antipsychotics[2,4].

Use of antidepressants and antipsychotics in epilepsy

The majority of antipsychotics and antidepressants can reduce the seizure threshold[1,2,5,6] and the risk is dose-related. Treatment with an antidepressant or antipsychotic drug increases the risk of *de novo* seizures in non-epileptic subjects 10-fold[5]. There are few systematic studies of antipsychotics or antidepressants in people with epilepsy. Data are mainly derived from animal studies, clinical trials, case reports and CSM reports. The table below gives some general guidance. Treatment should be commenced at the lowest dose and this should be gradually increased until a therapeutic dose is achieved[2,6,7]. As a general rule, the more sedating a drug is, the more likely it is to induce seizures[6].

Electroconvulsive therapy (ECT) has anticonvulsive properties and is worth considering in the treatment of depression in patients with unstable epilepsy[1,2].

Depression and psychosis associated with anticonvulsant drugs

Anticonvulsant drugs have been associated with new-onset depression and psychosis[1]. If anticonvulsants have recently been changed, this should always be considered as a potential cause of a new/worsening depressive or psychotic illness. Lowering of folate levels by some anticonvulsants may also influence the expression of depression[1]. Folate levels should be checked.

Special groups

Psychosis[8]

Product data sheets and case reports associate the following anticonvulsants with the onset of psychotic symptoms: carbamazepine, ethosuximide, tiagabine, topiramate, valproate and vigabatrin. There are case reports in the literature describing psychosis related to topiramate[9], zonisamide[10] and

Table Psychotropics in epilepsy		
Antidepressant	**Safety in epilepsy**	**Special considerations**
Moclobemide[14]	Good choice	Not known to be proconvulsive
SSRIs[15] Trazodone[15]	Good choice	Low proconvulsive effect[2,16], but SSRIs have many potential interactions with anticonvulsant drugs (see above). Seizure risk is dose-related Citalopram may be the safest SSRI[17] but seizures have been reported in overdose[18]
Mirtazapine/reboxetine/ venlafaxine[19,20]	Care required	Very limited data and clinical experience Use with care. Mirtazapine may affect EEG
Amitriptyline Dothiepin[21] Clomipramine[22]	Avoid	Most are epileptogenic Ideally, should be avoided completely
Lithium[2]	Care required	Low proconvulsive effect at therapeutic doses Marked proconvulsive activity in overdose
Antipsychotic		
Trifluoperazine/ haloperidol[2,6,23,24]	Good choice	Low proconvulsive effect. Carbamazepine increases the metabolism of some antipsychotics and larger doses of an antipsychotic may be required
Sulpiride	Good choice	Low proconvulsive effect (less clinical experience) No known interactions with anticonvulsants
Risperidone[20] Olanzapine[25,26] Quetiapine[27,28] Amisulpride	Care required	Limited clinical experience Use with care. Olanzapine may affect EEG[29] Seizures rarely reported with quetiapine
Chlorpromazine[4,30,31] Loxapine[32]	Avoid	Most epileptogenic of the older drugs Ideally best avoided completely
Clozapine[4,5,33]	Avoid	Very epileptogenic. Approximately 4–5% who receive more than 600 mg/day develop seizures Sodium valproate is the anticonvulsant of choice as it has a lower incidence of leukopenia than carbamazepine
Zotepine[34]	Avoid	Has established dose-related proconvulsive effect Best avoided completely
Depot antipsychotics	Avoid	None of the depot preparations currently available are thought to be epileptogenic, however: • the kinetics of depots are complex (seizures may be delayed) • if seizures do occur, the offending drug may not be easily withdrawn Depots should be used with extreme care

levetiracetam[11]. Some of these reports may relate to the process of 'forced normalisation' in which a diminished frequency of seizures allows psychotic symptoms to emerge.

Depression[8,12]
Product data sheets and case reports associate the following anticonvulsants with the onset of depressive symptoms: acetazolamide, barbiturates, carbamazepine, ethosuximide, gabapentin, phenytoin, piracetam, tiagabine, topiramate and vigabatrin.

Interactions
Pharmacokinetic interactions between anticonvulsants and antidepressants/antipsychotics are common. These interactions are primarily mediated through cytochrome P450 enzymes[1,2]. Fluoxetine and paroxetine are potent inhibitors of several hepatic CYP enzyme systems (CYP2D6, CYP3A4). Sertraline is a less potent inhibitor, but this effect is dose-related and higher doses of sertraline are commonly used. Citalopram is a weak inhibitor. Carbamazepine and phenytoin have a narrow therapeutic index and plasma levels can be increased by enzyme inhibitors. This is particularly dangerous with phenytoin. Plasma levels should be monitored and dosage adjustment may be required.

Carbamazepine is an enzyme inducer (mainly CYP3A4) and can lower serum levels of some antipsychotic drugs[13]. Many other medicines can cause problems in people with epilepsy by raising or reducing the seizure threshold or interacting with anticonvulsant drugs. Check Appendix 1 of the *BNF* or contact pharmacy for advice (see also page 263 for a summary).

Epilepsy and driving

People with epilepsy may not drive a car if they have had a seizure while awake in the previous year or, if seizures occur only during sleep, this has been an established nocturnal pattern for at least 3 years. The consequences of inducing seizure with antidepressants or antipsychotics can therefore be significant. For further information see www.dvla.gov.uk.

References

1. Harden CL, Goldstein MA. Mood disorders in patients with epilepsy; epidemiology and management. *CNS Drugs* 2002; **16**(Suppl. 5): 291–302.
2. Curran S, de Pauw K. Selecting an antidepressant for use in a patient with epilepsy; safety considerations. *Drug Saf* 1998; **18**(Suppl. 2): 125–133.
3. Lambert MV, Robertson MM. Depression in epilepsy: etiology, phenomenology and treatment. *Epilepsia* 1999; **40**(Suppl.10): 21–47.
4. Blumer D, Wakhu S, Montouris G *et al*. Treatment of the interictal psychosis. *J Clin Psychiatry* 2000; **61**(Suppl. 2): 110–122.
5. Pisani F, Oteri G, Costa C *et al*. Effects of psychotropic drugs on seizure threshold. *Drug Saf* 2002; **25**: 91–110.
6. Marks RC, Luchins DJ. Antipsychotic medications and seizures. *Psychiatr Med* 1991; **9**: 37–52.
7. Donald L, Rosentein MD, Craig J *et al*. Seizures associated with antidepressants: a review. *J Clin Psychiatry* 1993; **54**(Suppl. 8): 289–299.
8. http://emc.vhn.net.
9. Hofer A, Fleischhacker WW, Hummer M. Worsening of psychosis after replacement of adjunctive valproate with topiramate in schizophrenia patient. *J Clin Psychiatry* 2003; **64**: 1267–1268.
10. Miyamoto T, Kohsaka M, Koyama T. Psychotic episodes during zonisamide treatment. *Seizure* 2000; **9**: 65–70.
11. Youroukos S, Lazopoulou D, Michelakou D *et al*. Acute psychosis associated with levetiracetam. *Epileptic Disord* 2003; **5**: 117–119.
12. Besag FM. Behavioural effects of the newer antiepileptic drugs: an update. *Expert Opin Drug Saf* 2004; **3**: 1–8.
13. Tihonen J, Vartiainen H, Hakola P. Carbamazepine induced changes in plasma levels of neuroleptics. *Pharmacopsychiatry* 1995; **28**: 26–28.
14. Schiwy W, Heath WR, Delini-Stula A. Therapeutic and side effect profile of a selective and reversible MAOI inhibitor: results of dose finding trials in depressed patients. *J Neural Transm* 1989; **28**: 33–44.

Special groups

15. Weden OP, Oderda GM, Klein-Schwartz W *et al.* Relative toxicity of cyclic antidepressants. *Ann Emerg Med* 1986; **15**: 797–804.
16. Duncan D, Taylor D. Which is the safest antidepressant to use in epilepsy? *Psychiatr Bull* 1995; **19**: 355–357.
17. Specchio LM, Iudice A, Specchio N *et al.* Citalopram as treatment of depression in patients with epilepsy. *Clin Neuropharmacol* 2004; **27**: 133–136.
18. Cuenca PJ, Holt KR, Hoefle JD. Seizure secondary to citalopram overdose. *J Emerg Med* 2004; **26**: 177–181.
19. Juckel G, Schule C, Pogarell O *et al.* Epileptiform EEG patterns induced by mirtazapine in both psychiatric patients and healthy volunteers. *J Clin Psychopharmacol* 2003; **23**: 421–422.
20. Alldredge BK. Seizure risk associated with psychotropic drugs: clinical and pharmacokinetic considerations. *Neurology* 1999; **53**(Suppl. 2): 68–75.
21. Buckley NA, Dawson AH, Whyte IM *et al.* Greater toxicity in overdose of dothiepin than other tricyclic antidepressants. *Lancet* 1994; **343**: 159–162.
22. Stimmel GL, Dopheide JA. Psychotropic drug-induced reductions in seizure threshold: incidence and consequences. *CNS Drugs* 1996; **5**: 37–50.
23. Markowitz JC, Brown RP. Seizures with neuroleptics and antidepressants. *Gen Hosp Psychiatry* 1987; **9**: 135–141.
24. Darbk JK, Pasta DJ, Dabin L. Haloperidol dose and blood level variability: toxicity and interindividual and intraindividual variability in the nonresponder patient in the clinical practice setting. *J Clin Psychopharmacol* 1995; **15**: 334–340.
25. Beasley CM, Tollefson GD, Tran PV. Safety of olanzapine. *J Clin Psychiatry* 1997; **58**(Suppl. 10): 13–17.
26. Lee JW, Crismon ML, Dorson PG. Seizure associated with olanzapine. *Ann Pharmacother* 1999; **33**: 554–556.
27. Dogu O, Sevim S, Kaleagasi HS. Seizures associated with quetiapine treatment. *Ann Pharmacother* 2003; **37**:1224–1227.
28. Hedges DW, Jeppson KG. New-onset seizure associated with quetiapine and olanzapine. *Ann Pharmacother* 2002; **36**: 437–439.
29. Amann BL, Pogarell O, Mergl R *et al.* EEG abnormalities associated with antipsychotics: a comparison of quetiapine, olanzapine, haloperidol and healthy subjects. *Hum Psychopharmacol* 2003; **18**: 641–646.
30. Itil TM, Soldatos C. Epileptogenic side effects of psychotropic drugs. *JAMA* 1980; **244**: 1460–1463.
31. Logothetis J. Spontaneous epileptic seizures and EEG changes in the course of phenothiazine therapy. *Neurology* 1967; **17**: 869–877.
32. Peterson CD. Seizures induced by acute loxapine overdose. *Am J Psychiatry* 1981; **138**: 1089–1091.
33. Toth P, Frankenberg FR. Clozapine and seizures: a review. *Can J Psychiatry* 1994; **39**: 236–238.
34. Tscuchiya H, Kawahara R, Tanaka Y *et al.* Generalised seizure during treatment of schizophrenia with zotepine. *Yonago Acta Med* 1986; **29**: 103–171.

Further reading

Centorrino F, Price BH, Tuttle MMS *et al.* EEG abnormalities during treatment with typical and atypical antipsychotics. *Am J Psychiatry* 2002; **159**: 109–115.

Schmitz B. Antidepressant drugs: indications and guidelines for use in epilepsy. *Epilepsia* 2002; **43**(Suppl. 2): 14–18.

Van der Feltz-Cornelis CM. Treatment of interictal psychiatric disorder in epilepsy. I. Affective and anxiety disorders. *Acta Neuropsychiatr* 2002; **14**: 39–43.

Van der Feltz-Cornelis CM. Treatment of interictal psychiatric disorder in epilepsy. II. Chronic psychosis. *Acta Neuropsychiatr* 2002; **14**: 44–48.

Van der Feltz-Cornelis CM. Treatment of interictal psychiatric disorder in epilepsy. III. Personality disorder, aggression and mental retardation. *Acta Neuropsychiatr* 2002; **14**: 49–54.

Special groups

Drug interactions between antiepileptic drugs and other psychotropic drugs

Antiepileptic drug	Increases level of	Decreases level of	Level increased by	Level decreased by
Carbamazepine	Phenytoin	Clonazepam Clobazam Ethosuximide Primidone Valproic acid Lamotrigine Tiagabine Topiramate Phenytoin Haloperidol Clozapine Olanzapine Risperidone Quetiapine Zotepine TCAs ?Sertraline ?Citalopram Bupropion Donepezil Methylphenidate Thyroxine Methadone Benzodiazepines	Valproic acid and primidone increase levels of 10,11-epoxide, metabolite of carbamazepine Fluoxetine Fluvoxamine	Phenobarbitone Phenytoin
Phenytoin	Carbamazepine Phenobarbitone Valproate	Carbamazepine Valproate Phenobarbitone Lamotrigine Tiagabine Topiramate Benzodiazepines Haloperidol Clozapine Quetiapine TCAs Paroxetine Methadone Donepezil Bupropion	Carbamazepine Phenobarbitone Valproate Topiramate Phenothiazines ?Zotepine Fluoxetine Fluvoxamine Trazodone TCAs Sertraline Diazepam Benzodiazepines Disulfiram Methylphenidate Alcohol (acute)	Vigabatrin Carbamazepine Phenobarbitone Valproate Alcohol (chronic)

cont.

Antiepileptic drug	Increases level of	Decreases level of	Level increased by	Level decreased by
Lamotrigine	None known	None known	Valproate Sertraline	Phenytoin Carbamazepine Oxcarbazepine Phenobarbitone Primidone
Valproate	Phenobarbitone Primidone Free phenytoin TCAs Benzodiazepines	Total phenytoin Topiramate 10-monohydroxy metabolite of oxcarbazepine	Lamotrigine Oxcarbazepine Topiramate ?Fluoxetine	Phenytoin Phenobarbitone Carbamazepine ?Fluoxetine
Gabapentin	None known	None known	None known	None known
Levetiracetam	?Phenytoin	None known	None known	None known
Vigabatrin	Carbamazepine	Phenytoin ?Phenobarbitone	None known	None known
Oxcarbazepine	10,11-epoxide, metabolite of carbamazepine Phenobarbitone Phenytoin	Carbamazepine Lamotrigine		Phenobarbitone Carbamazepine Phenytoin Valproate
Phenobarbitone	Phenytoin	Carbamazepine Clonazepam Lamotrigine Tiagabine Valproate Ethosuximide Phenytoin Haloperidol ?Chlorpromazine Clozapine Quetiapine Zotepine Mianserin TCAs Paroxetine ?Donepezil Bupropion Benzodiazepines Methadone	Valproate Oxcarbazepine Phenytoin Alcohol (acute)	Vigabatrin Alcohol (chronic)
Tiagabine	None known	Valproate	?Fluoxetine ?Valproate	Phenytoin Phenobarbitone Carbamazepine Primidone
Topiramate	Phenytoin	?Valproate	?Valproate	Phenytoin Carbamazepine Phenobarbitone

cont.

Antiepileptic drug	Increases level of	Decreases level of	Level increased by	Level decreased by
Ethosuximide	?Phenytoin ?Valproate	None known	Valproate	Carbamazepine Phenobarbitone Phenytoin
Tiagabine	?Valproate	Valproate	?Fluoxetine	Phenytoin Phenobarbitone Carbamazepine Primidone

Further reading

British Medical Association and Royal Pharmaceutical Society. *British National Formulary*, Issue 49, Appendix 1, 2004.

Patsalos PN, Fröscher W, Pisani F *et al.* The importance of drug interactions in epilepsy therapy. *Epilepsia* 2002; **43**: 365–385.

Schmitz B. Antidepressant drugs. indications and guidelines for use in epilepsy. *Epilepsia* 2002; **43**(Suppl. 2): 14–18.

Special groups

Withdrawing anticonvulsant drugs

Patients with epilepsy

Optimal treatment with anticonvulsant drugs will render two-thirds of people with epilepsy seizure-free[1,2]. Many patients ask about drug withdrawal. It should be noted that this is a specialist area of practice, and it is strongly recommended that patients are referred for a neurological opinion.

The withdrawal of anticonvulsants in people with epilepsy has been associated with relapse rates of 12–63%[2]. This wide variation probably reflects the heterogeneous nature of the patients studied. It should be noted that patients who remain on anticonvulsant drugs also relapse[3].

The following factors are associated with unsuccessful withdrawal[2,4,5].

Onset of epilepsy during or after adolescence.
Family history of epilepsy.
Epilepsy of proven or suspected organic origin.
Mental retardation.
Abnormal neurological examination.
Poor initial response to treatment.
Ongoing seizures during treatment.
Prescription of two or more anticonvulsant drugs.
Ongoing abnormal EEG.
Abnormal EEG developing during withdrawal period.

The dose of anticonvulsant drugs should be gradually tapered down over a period of 6 months. If the patient is taking more than one anticonvulsant (note that such a patient is at increased risk of relapse), they should be withdrawn sequentially. The risk of seizure recurrence is greatest during the period of anticonvulsant withdrawal and steadily decreases over the first year; 70–80% of relapses occur within a year[3].

Recommendation

Patients with epilepsy should be referred to a neurologist for advice about withdrawing anticonvulsant drugs.

Patients with affective disorders

There is no systematic research that addresses the risk of relapse in patients who take anticonvulsant drugs for their mood-stabilising properties. There are three possibilities:

1. The natural course of the illness is improved by a period of treatment with mood-stabilising drugs. There is no evidence to suggest that this is true. Patients with bipolar illness tend to have more episodes and shorter periods of stability as they get older.

2. The illness resumes its natural course. It then follows that the more effective the mood-stabilising medication has been, the greater the chance of relapse when it is stopped.

3. Prognosis may be worsened in some way that is poorly understood. This has been demonstrated for lithium (see page 110). Treatment with lithium for at least 3 years followed by gradual taper over at least 1 month minimises this risk. It is unknown if these observations hold true for anticonvulsant drugs. There is some evidence to suggest that the risk of completed suicide is high in the month after (presumably abrupt) discontinuation of either lithium or valproate[6].

Recommendation

When used as mood-stabilisers, it would be prudent to withdraw anticonvulsant drugs slowly. The optimum duration of taper is unknown. A period of at least 1 month is suggested.

References

1. Cockerell OC, Johnson AL, Saunder JW *et al*. Remission of epilepsy: results from the National General Practice Study of Epilepsy. *Lancet* 1995; **346**: 140–4.
2. Cockerell OC, Johnson AL, Saunder JW *et al*. Prognosis of epilepsy: a review and further analysis of the first nine years of the British National General Practice Study of Epilepsy, a prospective population-based study. *Epilepsia* 1997; **38**: 31–46.
3. Britton JW. Antiepileptic drug withdrawal: literature review. *Mayo Clin Proc* 2002; 77: 1378–1388.
4. Medical Research Council. Antiepileptic Drug Withdrawal Study Group. Randomised study of antiepileptic drug withdrawal in patients in remission. *Lancet* 1991; **337**: 1175–1180.
5. Schmidt D, Gram L. A practical guide to when (and how) to withdraw antiepileptic drugs in seizure-free patients. *Drugs* 1996; 52: 870–874.
6. Goodwin FK, Fireman B, Simon GE et al. Suicide risk in bipolar disorder during treatment with lithium and divalproex. *JAMA* 2003; **290**: 1467–1473.

Special groups

Drug choice in pregnancy

A 'normal' outcome to pregnancy can never be guaranteed. The spontaneous abortion rate in confirmed early pregnancy is 10–20% and the risk of spontaneous major malformation is 2–3% (approx. 1 in 40 pregnancies)[1]. Drugs account for a very small proportion of abnormalities (approximately 5% of the total). Potential risks of drugs include major malformation (first-trimester exposure), neonatal toxicity (third-trimester exposure) and long-term neurobehavioural effects.

The safety of psychotropics in pregnancy cannot be clearly established because robust, prospective trials are obviously unethical. Individual decisions on psychotropic use in pregnancy are therefore dependent upon an imperfect retrospective database and a 'best guess' assessment of the risks and benefits associated with withdrawal or continuation of drug treatment. The patient's view of risks and benefits will have paramount importance. This section provides a brief summary of knowledge to date.

General principles of prescribing in pregnancy

- Treat only when absolutely necessary (potential benefit outweighs potential harm), but remember: mentally ill women who are pregnant are very likely to require treatment.
- Ensure that the prospective parents are fully involved in all discussions.
- Always take into account the risk of relapse when considering discontinuing psychotropics – relapse may ultimately be more harmful to the mother and child than continued, effective drug therapy.
- Try to avoid all drugs in the first trimester (when major organs are being formed).
- Use an established drug at the lowest effective dose.
- Avoid polypharmacy whenever possible.
- Be prepared to adjust doses as pregnancy progresses and drug handling is altered. Dose increases are frequently required in the 3rd trimester when blood volume expands by around 30%. Plasma level monitoring is helpful, where available.
- Ensure adequate foetal screening during pregnancy.
- Be aware of potential problems with individual drugs around the time of delivery.
- Inform obstetric team of psychotropic use and possible complications.
- Monitor the neonate for withdrawal effects after birth.
- Document all decisions.

Risk of psychosis during pregnancy and postpartum[2–5]

- The risk of perinatal psychosis is 0.1–0.25% in the general population, but is about 50% in women with a history of bipolar disorder.
- During the month after childbirth there is a 20-fold increase in the relative risk of psychosis.
- The risk of post-partum psychosis in patients with a history of post-partum psychosis is 50–90%.

The risks of not treating psychosis include:

- harm to the mother through poor self-care, lack of obstetric care, poor judgement or impulsive acts
- harm to the foetus or neonate (ranging from neglect to infanticide)

The mental health of the mother influences foetal well-being, obstetric outcome and child development.

Treatment with antipsychotics

It has long been established that people with schizophrenia are more likely to have minor physical anomalies than the general population[6]. Some of these anomalies may be apparent at birth, while others are more subtle and may not be obvious until later in life. This background risk complicates the assessment of antipsychotic drug risk. Data relating to antipsychotics and pregnancy are poor: Cochrane suggests that the risk of harm remains unknown[7].

Older, conventional antipsychotics are generally considered to have minimal risk of teratogenicity, although data are less than convincing, as might be expected[8,9]. It remains uncertain whether conventional antipsychotics are entirely without risk to the foetus or to later development – an association with malformation has been suggested[10] and neonatal dyskinesia reported[11]. However, this uncertainty and the wide use of these drugs over several decades suggest that any risk is small – an assumption borne out by most studies[12].

Data relating to atypical antipsychotics are now appearing. The use of clozapine appears to present no increased risk of malformation, although gestational diabetes and neonatal seizures may be more likely to occur[13] and stillbirth has been reported[14]. Similarly, limited data suggest that olanzapine is not associated with teratogenicity, but may increase the risk of gestational diabetes[8,13,15]. Not all authorities agree that olanzapine is likely to be free of risk of teratogenicity[16]. Still more limited data tentatively suggest that neither risperidone[17] nor quetiapine[18,19] is teratogenic in humans. There are virtually no published data relating to other atypicals.

Overall, these data do not allow an assessment of relative risks associated with different agents and certainly do not confirm absolutely the safety of any particular drug. Older, conventional drugs may still be preferred in pregnancy, but, considering data now available on some atypical drugs, it may not now be appropriate always to switch to these conventional drugs, should continued treatment be necessary. As with other drugs, decisions must be based on the latest available information and an individualised assessment of probable risks and benefits. If possible, specialist advice should be sought and primary reference sources consulted.

Recommendations – psychosis in pregnancy

- Patients with a history of psychosis who are maintained on antipsychotic medication should be advised to discuss a planned pregnancy as early as possible.
- Such patients, particularly if they have suffered repeated relapses, are best maintained on antipsychotics during and after pregnancy. This may minimise foetal exposure by avoiding the need for higher doses should relapse occur.
- There is most experience with **chlorpromazine** (constipation and sedation can be a problem), **trifluoperazine, olanzapine** and **clozapine** (gestational diabetes may be a problem with both atypicals). If the patient is established on another antipsychotic, the most up-to-date advice should always be obtained. Experience with other drugs is growing and a change in treatment may not be necessary or wise. Olanzapine is widely used by perinatal services in the UK.
- A few authorities recommend discontinuation of antipsychotics 5–10 days before anticipated delivery to minimise the chances of neonatal EPSEs. This may, however, put mother and infant at risk and needs to be considered carefully. Antipsychotic discontinuation symptoms can occur in the neonate (e.g. crying, agitation, increased suckling). With atypical drugs, discontinuation may not be necessary or desirable. Consult specialist services for the latest advice on pre-delivery prescribing.

Risk of depression during pregnancy and postpartum[4,19,20]

- Approximately 10% of pregnant women develop a depressive illness and a further 16% a self-limiting depressive reaction.
- There is a significant increase in new psychiatric episodes in the first 3 months after delivery. At least 80% are mood disorders, primarily depression.
- Women who have had a previous episode of depressive illness (postpartum or not) are at higher risk of further episodes post-partum.
- The risk is highest in women with bipolar illness.

The risks of not treating depression include:

- harm to the mother through poor self-care, lack of obstetric care or self-harm
- harm to the foetus or neonate (ranging from neglect to infanticide).

The mental health of the mother influences foetal well-being, obstetric outcome and child development.

Treatment with antidepressants

Tricyclic antidepressants have been widely used throughout pregnancy without apparent detriment to the foetus[9,21] and have for many years been agents of choice in pregnancy. Some authorities recommend the use of nortriptyline and desipramine (not available in the UK) because these drugs are less anticholinergic and hypotensive than amitriptyline and imipramine (respectively, their tertiary amine parent molecules). Note that use of tricyclics in the third trimester is well known to produce neonatal withdrawal effects (agitation, irritability, seizures)[22]. In addition, little is known of the developmental effects of prenatal exposure to tricyclics, although one small study detected no adverse consequences[23].

SSRIs also appear not to be teratogenic, with most data supporting the safety of fluoxetine[21-25]. They have, however, been associated with both decreased gestational age (mean 1 week) and birth weight (mean 175 g)[24-26]. (Note that depression itself carries an increased risk of early birth and of obstetric complications so evaluating these findings is difficult.) Sertraline appears to result in the least placental exposure[27]. Third-trimester exposure has been associated with reduced early APGAR scores[24]. Third-trimester use of paroxetine may give rise to neonatal complications, presumably related to abrupt withdrawal[28]. Other SSRIs may have similar effects[29]. Rather more scarce data suggest the absence of terotogenic potential with mocobemide[30], reboxetine[31] and venlafaxine (although neonatal withdrawal may occur)[25,32], but none of these drugs can be specifically recommended at the time of writing. Similarly, trazodone, bupropion (amfebutamone) and mirtazapine cannot be recommended because there are few data supporting their safety[9,21,25,33,34].

MAOIs should be avoided in pregnancy because of a suspected increased risk of congenital malformation and because of the risk of hypertensive crisis[35].

There is no evidence to suggest that ECT causes harm to either the mother or foetus during pregnancy[36].

Recommendations – depression in pregnancy

- Patients who are already receiving antidepressants and are at high risk of relapse are best maintained on antidepressants during and after pregnancy.
- Those who develop a depressive illness during pregnancy should be treated with antidepressant drugs if psychological management has failed or is not available.
- There is most experience with **amitriptyline, imipramine** (constipation and sedation can be a problem with both) and **fluoxetine** (increased chance of earlier delivery and reduced birth weight). If the patient is established on another antidepressant, always obtain the most up-to-date advice. Experience with other drugs is growing and a change in treatment may not be necessary or wise.
- The neonate may experience discontinuation symptoms such as agitation and irritability, or even convulsions (with SSRIs). The risk is assumed to be particularly high with short-half-life drugs such as paroxetine and venlafaxine.

Risks in patients with bipolar illness during pregnancy and postpartum

- The risk of relapse after delivery is hugely increased: up to eight fold in the first month post-partum.

The risks of not treating depression include:

- harm to the mother through poor self-care, lack of obstetric care or self-harm
- harm to the foetus or neonate (ranging from neglect to infanticide).

The mental health of the mother influences foetal well-being, obstetric outcome and child development.

Treatment with mood-stabilisers

Lithium use during pregnancy has a well-known association with the cardiac malformation Ebstein's anomoly[9] (relative risk is 10–20 times more than control, but the absolute risk is low at 1:1000)[37]. The period of maximum risk to the foetus is 2–6 weeks after conception[38], before the majority of women know that they are pregnant. Although the risk of major malformations in the infant has probably been overestimated, lithium should be avoided in pregnancy if possible. Slow discontinuation before conception is the preferred course of action[13,39] because abrupt discontinuation is suspected of worsening the risk of relapse. The relapse rate post-partum may be as high as 70% in women who discontinued lithium before conception[40]. If discontinuation is unsuccessful during pregnancy – restart and continue. If lithium is continued during pregnancy, high-resolution ultrasound and echocardiography should be performed at 6 and 18 weeks of gestation. In the third trimester, the use of lithium may be problematic because of changing pharmacokinetics: an increasing dose of lithium is required to maintain the lithium level during pregnancy as total body water increases, but the requirements return abruptly to prepregnancy levels immediately after delivery. Neonatal goitre and cardiac arrhythmia can occur.

Most data relating to carbamazepine and valproate come from studies in epilepsy, a condition associated with increased neonatal malformation. These data may not be precisely relevant to use in mental illness. Nonetheless, both carbamazepine and valproate have a clear causal link with increased risk of a variety of foetal abnormalities, particularly spina bifida[9,21,41]. Both drugs should be avoided, if possible. Valproate is more dangerous than carbamazepine[42] and probably should be avoided (see page 109). Where continued use is deemed essential, low-dose monotherapy is strongly recommended, as the teratogenic effect is probably dose-related[43]. Ideally, all patients should take folic acid (5 mg daily) for at least a month before conception (this may reduce the risk of neonatal neural tube defects). Note, however, that some authorities recommend a lower dose[44], presumably because of a risk of twin births[45]. Use of carbamazepine in the third trimester may necessitate maternal vitamin K. Early data for lamotrigine suggest a low risk of foetal malformations when used as monotherapy[44,46]. Clearance of lamotrigine seems to increase radically during pregnancy[47].

Recommendations – bipolar disorder in pregnancy

- For women who have had a long period without relapse, the possibility of withdrawing treatment before conception and for at least the first trimester should be considered.
- The risk of relapse both pre- and post-partum is very high if medication is discontinued abruptly.
- Women with severe illness or who are known to relapse quickly after discontinuation of a mood-stabiliser should be advised to continue their medication following discussion of the risks.
- No mood-stabiliser is clearly safe. Women prescribed lithium should undergo level 2 ultrasound of the foetus at 6 and 18 weeks' gestation to screen for Ebstein's anomaly. Those prescribed valproate or carbamazepine (both teratogenic) should receive prophylactic folic acid to reduce the incidence of neural tube defects. Prophylactic vitamin K should be administered to the mother and neonate after delivery.
- Valproate (the most teratogenic) and combinations of mood-stabilisers should be avoided if possible.

Risks in patients with epilepsy during pregnancy and post-partum[48,49]

- There is an increased risk of maternal complications such as severe morning sickness, eclampsia, vaginal bleeding and premature labour. Women should get as much sleep and rest as possible and comply with medication (if prescribed) in order to minimise the risk of seizures.
- The risk of having a child with minor malformations may be increased regardless of treatment with antiepileptic drugs (AEDs).
- The risks of not treating epilepsy are as follows:
  - If seizures are inadequately controlled, there is an increased risk of accidents resulting in foetal injury. Post-partum the mother may be less able to look after herself and her child.
  - The risk of seizures during delivery is 1–2%, potentially worsening maternal and neonatal mortality.

Treatment with anticonvulsant drugs[50–53]

It is established that treatment with anticonvulsant drugs increases the risk of having a child with major congenital malformation to two- to three-fold that seen in the general population. Congential heart defects (1.8%) and facial clefts (1.7%) are the most common congenital malformations. Both carbamazepine and valproate are associated with a hugely increased incidence of spina bifida at 0.5–1% and 1–2%, respectively. The risk of other neural tube defects is also increased. In women with epilepsy, the risk of foetal malformations with carbamazepine is 2.3%; with lamotrigine, 3%; and with vaproate, 7.2%[54]. Higher doses (particularly doses of valproate exeeding 1000 mg/day) and anticonvulsant polypharmacy are particularly problematic. Cognitive deficits have been reported in older children who have been exposed to valproate *in utero*. Those exposed to carta-mazepine may not be similarly disadvantaged[55]. Early data with lamotrigine[46,56] and oxcarbazepine[57] suggest a relatively lower risk of malformation, but confirmation is required.

Pharmacokinetics change during pregnancy. Dosage adjustment may be required to keep the patient seizure-free. Serum levels usually return to prepregnancy levels within a month of delivery often much more rapidly. Doses may need to be reduced at this point.

Best practice guidelines recommend that a woman should receive the lowest possible dose of a single AED.

Recommendations – epilepsy in pregnancy

- For women who have been seizure free for a long period, the possibility of withdrawing treatment before conception and for at least the first trimester should be considered.
- No anticonvulsant is clearly safer. Valproate should be avoided if possible. Women prescribed valproate or carbamazepine should receive prophylactic folic acid to reduce the risk of neural tube defects. Prophylactic vitamin K should be administered to the mother and neonate after delivery.
- Valproate and combinations of anticonvulsants should be avoided if possible.
- All women with epilepsy should have a full discussion with their neurologist to quantify the risks and benefits of continuing anticonvulsant drugs.

Sedatives

First-trimester exposure to benzodiazepines appears to be associated with an increased risk of oral clefts in newborns, although there is debate about the magnitude of this risk[58]. Third-trimester use is commonly associated with neonatal difficulties (floppy baby syndrome)[59]. Benzodiazepines are best avoided in pregnancy.

Promethazine has been used in hyperemesis gravidarum and appears not to be teratogenic, although data are limited.

Recommendations – psychotropics in pregnancy

Psychotropic group	Recommendations
Antidepressants	Nortriptyline Amitriptyline Imipramine Fluoxetine
Antipsychotics	**Conventional drugs** have been widely used, although safety is not fully established. Most experience with **chlorpromazine** and **trifluoperazine**. No clear evidence that **clozapine** and **olanzapine** have teratogenic potential but data are limited
Benzodiazepines	Best avoided
Mood-stabilisers	Avoid unless risks and consequences of relapse outweigh known risk of teratogenesis. Women of childbearing potential taking carbamazepine or valproate should receive prophylactic folic acid. Avoid valproate and combinations where possible
Sedatives	Promethazine is widely used but supporting data are scarce

Special groups

References

1. McElhatton PR. General principles of drug use in pregnancy. *Pharm J* 2003; **270**: 232–234.
2. Oates M. Patients as patents: the risk to children. *Br J Psychiatry* 1997; **170**(Suppl. 32): 22–27.
3. Terp IM, Mortensen PB. Post-partum psychoses. *Br J Psychiatry* 1998; **172**: 521–526.
4. Stein G. Postpartum and related disorders. In: Stein G, Wilkinson G (eds). *Seminars in General Adult Psychiatry.* London: Royal College of Psychiatrists, 1998, pp. 903–953.
5. Spinelli M. A systematic investigation of 16 cases of neonaticide. *Am J Psychiatry* 2001; **158**: 811–813.
6. Ismail B, Cantor-Graae E, McNeil TF *et al.* Minor physical anomalies in schizophrenic patients and their siblings. *Am J Psychiatry* 1998; **155**: 1695–1702.
7. Webb RT, Howard L, Abel KM. Antipsychotic drugs for non-affective psychosis during pregnancy and postpartum. *Cochrane Database Syst Rev* 2004, Issue 2. Art. No.: CD004411.pub2. DOI: 10.1002/14651858.CD004411.pub2.
8. Patton SW, Misri S, Corral MR *et al.* Antipsychotic medication during pregnancy and lactation in women with schizophrenia: evaluating the risk. *Can J Psychiatry* 2002; **47**: 959–965.
9. Cohen LS, Rosenbaum JF. Psychotropic drug use during pregnancy: weighing the risks. *J Clin Psychiatry* 1998; **59**(Suppl. 2): 18–28.
10. Patton SW, Misiri S, Corral MR *et al.* Antipsychotic medication during pregnancy and lactation in women with schizophrenia: evaluating the risk. *Can J Psychiatry* 2003; **47**: 959–965.
11. O'Collins K, Comer JB. Maternal haloperidol therapy associated with dyskinesia in a newborn. *Am J Health Syst Pharm* 2003; **60**: 2253–2255.
12. Trixler M, Tényi T. Antipsychotic use in pregnancy: what are the best treatment options? *Drug Saf* 1997; **16**: 403–410.
13. Ernst CL, Goldberg JF. The reproductive safety profile of mood stabilizers, atypical antipsychotics, and broad-spectrum psychotropics. *J Clin Psychiatry* 2002; **63**:(Suppl. 4): 42–55.
14. Mendhekar DN, Sharma JB, Srivastava PK *et al.* Clozapine and pregnancy (Letter). *J Clin Psychiatry* 2003; **64**: 850.
15. Zyprexa – use in pregnancy. Personal communication. Eli Lilly & Co., 2003.
16. Howard L, Webb R, Abel K. Safety of antipsychotic drugs for pregnant and breastfeeding women with non-affective psychosis. *BMJ* 2004; **329**: 933–934.
17. Ratnayaka T, Libretto SE. No complications with risperidone treatment before and throughout pregnancy and during the nursing period. *J Clin Psychiatry* 2002; **63**: 76–77.
18. Tényi T, Trixler M, Keresztes Z. Quetiapine and pregnancy. *Am J Psychiatry* 2002; **159**: 674.
19. Taylor TM, O'Toole MS, Ohlsen RI *et al.* Safety of quetiapine during pregnancy (Letter). *Am J Psychiatry* 2003; **160**: 588–589.
20. Llewellyn AM, Stowe ZN, Nemeroff CB. Depression during pregnancy and the puerperium. *J Clin Psychiatry* 1997; **58**: 26–32.
21. Altshuler LL, Cohen L, Szuba MP. Pharmacologic management of psychiatric illness during pregnancy: dilemmas and guidelines. *Am J Psychiatry* 1996; **153**: 592–606.
22. Wisner KL, Gelenberg AJ, Leonard H *et al.* Pharmacologic treatment of depression during pregnancy. *JAMA* 1999; **282**: 1264–1268.
23. Nulman I, Rovet J, Stewart DE *et al.* Child development following exposure to tricyclic antidepressants or fluoxetine throughout fetal life: a prospective, controlled study. *Am J Psychiatry* 2002; **159**: 1889–1895.
24. Hallberg P, Sjoblom V. The use of selective serotonin reuptake inhibitors during pregnancy and breast-feeding: a review and clinical aspects. *J Clin Psychopharmacol* 2005; **25**: 59–73.
25. Gentile S. The safety of newer antidepressants in pregnancy and breastfeeding. *Drug Saf* 2005; **28**: 137–152.
26. Simon GE, Cunningham ML, Davis RL. Outcomes of prenatal antidepressant exposure. *Am J Psychiatry* 2002; **159**: 2055–2061.
27. Hendrick V, Stowe ZN, Altshuler LL *et al.* Placental passage of antidepressant medications. *Am J Psychiatry* 2003; **160**: 993–996.
28. Moldovan Costei A, Kozer E, Ho T *et al.* Perinatal outcome following third trimester exposure to paroxetine. *Arch Pediatr Adolesc Med* 2002; **156**: 1129–1132.
29. Koren G. Discontinuation syndrome following late pregnancy exposure to antidepressants. *Arch Pediatr Adolesc Med* 2004; **158**: 307–308.
30. Rybakowski JK. Moclobemide in pregnancy. *Pharmacopsychiatry* 2001; **34**: 82–83.
31. Edronax®: Use in pregnancy, renally and hepatically impaired patients. Personal communication – Pharmacia Ltd, 2003.
32. Einarson A, Fatoye B, Sarkar M. Pregnancy outcome following gestational exposure to venlafaxine: a multicentre prospective controlled study. *Am J Psychiatry* 2001; **158**: 1728–1730.
33. Einarson A, Bonari L, Voyer-Lavigne S *et al.* A multicentre prospective controlled study to determine the safety of trazodone and nefazodone use during pregnancy. *Can J Psychiatry* 2003; **48**: 106–109.
34. Rohde A, Dembinski J, Dorn C. Mirtazapine (Remergil) for treatment resistant hyperemesis gravidarum: rescue of a twin pregnancy. *Arch Gynecol Obstet* 2003; **268**: 219–221.
35. Hendrick V, Altshuler L. Management of major depression during pregnancy. *Am J Psychiatry* 2002; **159**: 1667–1673.
36. Miller LJ. Use of electroconvulsive therapy during pregnancy. *Hosp Community Psychiatry* 1994; **45**: 444–450.
37. Cohen LS, Friedman JM, Jefferson JW *et al.* A re-evaluation of risk of *in utero* exposure to lithium. *JAMA* 1994; **271**: 146–150.
38. Yonkers KA, Little BB, March D. Lithium during pregnancy. *CNS Drugs* 1998; **9**: 261–269.
39. Dodd S, Berk M. The pharmacology of bipolar disorder during pregnancy and breastfeeding. *Expert Opin Drug Saf* 2004; **3**: 221–229.

Special groups

40. Viguera AC, Nonacs R, Cohen LS *et al*. Risk of recurrence of bipolar disorder in pregnant and non-pregnant women after discontinuing lithium maintenance. *Am J Psychiatry* 2000; 157: 179–184.
41. Holmes LB, Harvey EA, Brent A *et al*. The teratogenicity of anticonvulsant drugs. *N Engl J Med* 2001; 344: 1132–1138.
42. Wide K, Winbladh B, Kallen B. Major malformations in infants exposed to antiepileptic drugs *in utero*, with emphasis on carbamazepine and valproic acid: a nation-wide, population-based register study. *Acta Paediatr* 2004; 93: 174–176.
43. Vajda FJ, O'Brien TJ, Hitchcock A *et al*. Critical relationship between sodium valproate dose and human teratogenicity: results of the Australian register of anti-epileptic drugs in pregnancy. *J Clin Neurosci* 2004; 11: 854–858.
44. Management of bipolar disorder during pregnancy and the postpartum period. *Am J Psychiatry* 2004; 161: 608–620.
45. Czeizel AE. Folic acid and the prevention of neural-tube defects. *N Engl J Med* 2004; 350: 2209–2211.
46. Sabers A, Dam M, Rogvi-Hansen A *et al*. Epilepsy and pregnancy: lamotrigine as main drug used. *Acta Neurol Scand* 2004; 109: 9–13.
47. De Haan GJ, Edelbroek P, Segers J *et al*. Gestation-induced changes in lamotrigine pharmacokinetics: a monotherapy study. *Neurology* 2004; 63: 571–573.
48. Shorvon S. Antiepileptic drug therapy during pregnancy: the neurologist's perspective. *J Med Genet* 2002; 39: 248–250.
49. Cleland PG. Risk-benefit assessment of anticonvulsants in women of child-bearing potential. *Drug Saf* 1991; 6: 70–81.
50. Dolk H, McElhatton P. Assessing epidemiological evidence for the teratogenic effects of anticonvulsant medication. *J Med Genet* 2002; 39: 243–244.
51. Holmes LB. The teratogenicity of anticonvulsant drugs: a progress report. *J Med Genet* 2002; 39: 245–247.
52. Adab N, Tudur Smith C, Vinten J *et al*. Common antiepileptic drugs in pregnancy in women with epilepsy. *Cochrane Database Syst Rev* 2004; Issue 3. Art No.: CD004848. DOI: 10.1002/14651858.CD004848.
53. Iqbal MM, Sohhan T, Mahmud SZ. The effects of lithium, valproic acid and carbamazepine during pregnancy and lactation. *Clin Toxicol* 2001; 39: 381–392.
54. National Institute for Clinical Excellence. Newer drugs for epilepsy in adults. Health Technology Appraisal No 76, 2004. www.nice.org.uk.
55. Gaily E, Kantola-Sorsa E, Hiilesmaa V *et al*. Normal intelligence in children with prenatal exposure to carbamazepine. *Neurology* 2004; 62: 28–32.
56. Vajda FJ, O'Brien TJ, Hitchcock A *et al*. The Australian registry of anti-epileptic drugs in pregnancy: experience after 30 months. *J Clin Neurosci* 2003; 10: 543–549.
57. Meischenguisher R, D'Giano CH, Ferraro SM. Oxcarbazepine in pregnancy: clinical experience in Argentina. *Epilepsy Behav* 2004; 5: 163–167.
58. Dolovich LR, Addis A, Vaillancourt JMR *et al*. Benzodiazepine use in pregnancy and major malformations or oral cleft: meta-analysis of cohort and case-control studies. *BMJ* 1998; 317: 839–843.
59. McElhatton PR. A review of the effects of benzodiazepine use during pregnancy and lactation. *Reprod Toxicol* 1994; 8: 461–475.

Further reading

Einarson A, Selby P, Koren G. Abrupt discontinuation of psychotropic drugs during pregnancy: fear of teratogenic risk and impact of counselling. *J Psychiatry Neurosci* 2001; 26: 44–48.

Gentile S. Clinical utilization of atypical antipsychotics in pregnancy and lactation. *Ann Pharmacother* 2004; 38: 1265–1271.

Sanz EJ, De las Cuevas C, Kiuru A *et al*. Selective serotonin reuptake inhibitors in pregnant women and neonatal withdrawal syndrome: a database analysis. *Lancet* 2005; 365: 482–487.

Ruchkin V, Martin A. SSRIs and the developing brain. *Lancet* 2005; 365: 451–453.

Wisner KL, Zarin DA, Holmboe C *et al*. Risk-benefit decision making for treatment of depression during pregnancy. *Am J Psychiatry* 2000; 157: 1933–1940.

Special groups

Breast-feeding guidelines

The data on the safety of psychotropic medication in breast-feeding are largely derived from small studies or case reports and case series. With the majority of data, only acute adverse effects (or absence of) are reported. Long-term safety cannot therefore be guaranteed for the psychotropics mentioned. The information presented must be interpreted with caution with respect to the limited data from which it is derived and the need for such information to be regularly updated.

General principles of prescribing psychotropics in breast-feeding

- In each case, the benefits of breast-feeding to the mother and infant must be weighed against the risk of drug exposure in the infant.
- Premature infants and infants with renal, hepatic, cardiac or neurological impairment are at a greater risk from exposure to drugs.
- The infants should be monitored for any specific adverse effects of the drugs as well as for feeding patterns and growth and development.
- It is usually inappropriate to withhold treatment to allow breast-feeding. Treatment of maternal illness is the highest priority.

Wherever possible:
- use the lowest effective dose
- avoid polypharmacy
- time the feeds to avoid peak drug levels in the milk or express milk to give later.

Summary of recommendations (see full review below for details)

Drug group	Recommended drugs
Antidepressants	Paroxetine or sertraline
Antipsychotics	Sulpiride; olanzapine
Mood-stabilisers	Avoid if possible; valproate if essential
Sedatives	Lorazepam for anxiety; zolpidem for sleep

Antidepressants in breast-feeding

Drug	Comment
Tricyclic anti-depressants (TCAs)[1-5]	All TCAs are excreted in human breast milk. Infant serum levels range from undetectable to low. Adverse effects have not been reported in infants exposed to amitriptyline, nortriptyline, clomipramine, imipramine, dothiepin (dosulepin) and desipramine. There are two case reports of doxepin exposure during breast-feeding leading to adverse effects in the infant. In one, an 8-week-old infant experienced respiratory depression, which resolved 24 hours after stopping nursing. In the other, poor suckling, muscle hypotonia and drowsiness were observed in a newborn, again resolving 24 hours after removing doxepin exposure. Data on TCAs not mentioned in this section were not available and their use can therefore not be recommended unless used during pregnancy.
Citalopram[1,6-11]	Citalopram is excreted in breast milk. Infant serum levels appear to be low or undetectable, although higher than reported with fluvoxamine, sertaline and paroxetine. Breast milk peak levels have been observed 3–9 hours after maternal dose. There is one case report of uneasy sleep in an infant exposed to citalopram while breast-feeding. This resolved on halving the mother's dose. In a study of 31 infants exposed to citalopram via breast milk, one case each of colic, decreased feeding, and irritability/restlessness was reported.
Fluvoxamine[1,12 17]	Fluvoxamine is excreted in breast milk. The levels detected in infants exposed to fluvoxamine while breast-feeding vary from undetectable to up to half the maternal serum level. No adverse effects were noted in these infants. Peak drug levels in breast milk have been observed 4 hours after maternal dose.
Fluoxetine[1,18-23]	Of the SSRIs, most data relate to fluoxetine. Fluoxetine is excreted into breast milk. Infant serum levels appear to be low, although higher than reported with paroxetine, fluvoxamine and sertraline, and close to those reported for citalopram. Adverse effects have not been reported for the majority of fluoxetine-exposed infants. However, in two infants, reported adverse effects included excessive crying, decreased sleep, diarrhoea and vomiting in one and somnolence, decreased feeding, hypotonia, moaning, grunting and fever in the other. In another, seizure activity at 3 weeks, 4 months and then 5 months was reported. The mother was taking a combination of fluoxetine and carbamazepine. A retrospective study found the growth curves of breast-fed infants of mothers taking fluoxetine to be significantly below those of infants receiving breast milk free of fluoxetine. However, in another study of 11 infants exposed to fluoxetine during pregnancy and lactation, neurological developments and weight gain were found to be normal. No developmental abnormalities were noted in another four infants exposed to fluoxetine during breast-feeding.
Paroxetine[1,12,22,24-29]	Paroxetine is excreted in breast milk. Infant serum levels vary from low to undetectable. No adverse effects were noted in these infants. Breast-fed infants of 27 women taking paroxetine reached the usual developmental milestones at 3, 6 and 12 months, similar to a control group.
Sertraline[22,28,30]	Sertraline is excreted in breast milk. Infant serum levels appear to be low. Peak drug levels in breast milk have been observed 7–10 hours after the maternal dose. No adverse effects were noted in these infants. Withdrawal symptoms (agitation, restlessness, insomnia and an enhanced startle reaction) developed in a breast-fed neonate, after abrupt withdrawal of maternal sertraline. The neonate was exposed to sertraline *in utero*.

Antidepressants in breast-feeding – continued

Drug	Comment
Nefazodone[31,32]	From the three published case reports available, it appears that nefazodone is excreted into breast milk. Recorded infant serum levels are low. In one infant, drowsiness and poor feeding were reported. These symptoms resolved over a 72-hour period after breast-feeding ceased. Peak breast milk levels were seen 1–3 hours after the maternal dose.
Venlafaxine[22,28]	Venlafaxine is excreted in breast milk. Infant serum levels were found to be low. Although not directly compared, these levels appear to be higher than those seen with fluvoxamine, sertraline and paroxetine. No adverse effects were seen in these infants.
MAOIs	There are no published data available.
Moclobemide[33,34]	Moclobemide is excreted in breast milk. Infant serum levels appear to be low. No adverse effects were detected in these infants. Peak drug levels in breast milk were seen at 3 hours.
Mirtazapine[35]	Psychomotor development in an infant exposed to mirtazapine in breast milk was found to be normal after 6 weeks of exposure. No sedation or abnormal weight gain was noted in the infant.
Trazodone[36]	Trazodone is excreted into breast milk in small quantities based on assessments after a single maternal dose.

Antipsychotics in breast-feeding

Drug	Comment
Butyrophenones[1,2,22,37,38]	Haloperidol is excreted in breast milk. The extent appears variable. Normal development was noted in one infant. However, delayed development was noted in three infants exposed to a combination of haloperidol and chlorpromazine in breast milk. Data on butyrophenones not mentioned in this section were not available.
Phenothiazines[1,2,37,38]	Most of the data relate to chlorpromazine. Chlorpromazine is excreted in breast milk. There is a wide variation in the breast milk concentrations quoted. Similarly, infant serum levels vary greatly. Lethargy was reported in one infant whose mother was taking chlorpromazine while breast-feeding. In another case, however, an infant exposed to much higher levels showed no signs of lethargy. There is a report of delayed development in three infants exposed to a combination of chlorpromazine and haloperidol while breast-feeding. In the one case of perphenazine exposure and two cases of trifluoperazine exposure, no adverse effects were noted in the infants. Data on phenothiazines not mentioned in this section were not available.
Thioxanthenes[1,39]	There is one case of infant exposure to flupentixol and one to zuclopenthixol. The amount excreted in breast milk of both drugs is low. No adverse effects or developmental abnormalities were noted in the infant exposed to flupentixol. The clinical status of the other infant was not reported.
Sulpiride[40–44]	There are a number of small studies in which sulpiride has been shown to improve lactation in nursing mothers. The amounts excreted in breast milk were low. No adverse effects were noted in the nursing infants.

Special groups

Antipsychotics in breast-feeding – continued

Drug	Comment
Amisulpride	There are no published data available.
Aripiprazole	There are no published data available.
Clozapine[1,2,22,38]	Clozapine is excreted in breast milk. In a study of four infants exposed to clozapine in breast milk, sedation was noted in one and another developed agranulocytosis, which resolved on stopping clozapine. No adverse effects were noted in the other two. Decreased sucking reflex, irritability, seizures and cardiovascular instability have also been reported in nursing infants exposed to clozapine. Because of the risk of neutropenia and seizures, it is advisable to avoid breast-feeding while on clozapine until more data become available.
Olanzapine[1,22,45–48]	Olanzapine is excreted in breast milk. Estimates of infant serum levels are low. There is one case of an infant developing jaundice and sedation on exposure to olanzapine during breast-feeding. This continued on cessation of breast-feeding. This infant was exposed to olanzapine in utero and had cardiomegaly. No adverse effects were reported in four of seven breast-fed infants of mothers taking olanzapine. Of the rest, one was not assessed, one had a lower developmental age than chronological age (but the mother had also been taking additional psychotropic medication), and drowsiness was noted in another, which resolved on halving the maternal dose. The median maximum concentration in the milk was found at around 5 hours after maternal ingestion.
Quetiapine[49]	Quetiapine is excreted into breast milk. From a single case report the levels were found to be low although the maternal dose was only 200 mg. No adverse effects were noted in the infant.
Risperidone[50,51]	Risperidone is excreted in breast milk. There are two case reports of infant exposure to risperidone. Although no developmental abnormalities were noted in either, the authors advise against breast-feeding.
Sertindole	There are no published data available.
Ziprasidone	There are no published data available.

Mood stabilisers in breast-feeding

Drug	Comment
Carbamazepine[1,52–54]	Carbamazepine is excreted in breast milk. Infant serum levels range from 6% to 65% of maternal serum levels. Adverse effects have been reported in a number of infants exposed to carbamazepine during breast-feeding. These include one case of cholestatic hepatitis, and one of transient hepatic dysfunction with hyperbilirubinaemia and elevated GGT. The adverse effects in the first case resolved after discontinuation of breast-feeding and the second resolved despite continued feeding. Other adverse effects reported include seizure-like activity, drowsiness, irritability and high-pitched crying in one infant whose mother was on multiple agents, hyperexcitability in two infants and poor feeding in another three. In contrast, in a number of infants, no adverse effects were noted.

Mood stabilisers in breast-feeding – continued

Drug	Comment
Lamotrigine[55,56]	Lamotrigine is excreted in breast milk. Infant serum levels range between 25% and 50% of maternal serum levels. No adverse effects have been reported in exposed infants. However, because of the risk of life-threatening rashes, it is advisable to avoid lamotrigine while breast-feeding until more data on its effects become available.
Lithium[52,54,57]	Lithium is excreted in breast milk. Infant serum levels range from 5% to 200% of maternal serum concentrations. Adverse effects have been reported in infants exposed to lithium while breast-feeding. One infant developed cyanosis, lethargy, hypothermia, hypotonia and a heart murmur, all of which resolved within 3 days of stopping breast-feeding. The infant was exposed to lithium *in utero*. Non-specific signs of toxicity have been reported in others. There are also reports of no adverse effects in some infants exposed to lithium while breast-feeding. Opinions on the use of lithium while breast-feeding vary from absolute contraindication to mother's informed choice. Conditions which may alter the infant's electrolyte balance and state of hydration must be borne in mind. If it is used, the infant must be carefully monitored for signs of toxicity.
Valproate[1,52–54,58]	Valproate is excreted into breast milk. Infant serum levels vary from undetectable to 40% of maternal serum levels. Thrombocytopenia and anaemia were reported in a 3-month-old infant exposed to valproate *in utero* and while breast-feeding. This reversed on stopping breast-feeding.

Sedatives in breast-feeding

Drug	Comment
Benzo-diazepines[1,22,59–63]	Diazepam is excreted in breast milk. Infant serum levels vary from undetectable to nearly 14% of the maternal serum levels. In some infants, no adverse effects were noted. In others, reported adverse effects included sedation, lethargy and weight loss. Lorazepam, temazepam and clonazepam are excreted in breast milk in small amounts. Apart from one case report of persistent apnoea in one infant exposed to clonazepam *in utero* and during breast-feeding, no adverse effects were reported. Any infant exposed to benzodiazepines in breast milk should be monitored for CNS depression and apnoea.
Zopiclone, zolpidem and zaleplon[64,65]	All three are excreted into breast milk in small amounts. No adverse effects were noted in exposed infants. Peak concentrations of zolpidem in breast milk were found 4 hours after ingestion of a single 20-mg dose. Zaleplon peak breast milk levels were found 1 hour after the dose and breast milk concentrations were approximately 50% of plasma concentrations.

References

1. Burt VK, Suri R, Alshuler L *et al.* The use of psychotropic medications during breast-feeding. *Am J Psychiatry* 2001; **158**: 1001–1009.
2. Yoshida K, Smith B, Kumar R. Psychotropic drugs in mothers' milk: a comprehensive review of assay methods, pharmacokinetics and of safety of breast-feeding. *J Psychopharmacol* 1999; **13**: 64–80.
3. Misri S, Kostaras X. Benefits and risks to mother and infant of drug treatment for postnatal depression. *Drug Saf* 2002; **25**: 903–911.
4. Yoshida K, Smith B, Craggs M *et al.* Investigation of pharmacokinetics and of possible adverse effects in infants exposed to tricyclic antidepressants in breast-milk. *J Affect Disord* 1997; **43**: 225–237.
5. Frey OR, Scheidt P, von Brenndorff AL. Adverse effects in a newborn infant breast-fed by a mother treated with doxepin. *Ann Pharmacother* 1999; **33**: 690–693.
6. Lee A. Woo J, Ito S. Frequency of infant adverse events that are associated with citalopram use during breast-feeding. *Am J Obstet Gynecol* 2004; **190**: 218–221.
7. Heikkinen T, Ekblad U, Kero P. Citalopram in pregnancy and lactation. *Clin Pharmacol Ther* 2002; **72**: 184–191.
8. Jensen PN, Olesen OV, Bertelsen A *et al.* Citalopram and desmethylcitalopram concentrations in breast milk and in serum of mother and infant. *Ther Drug Monit* 1997; **19**: 236–239.
9. Spigset O, Carleborg L, Öhman R *et al.* Excretion of citalopram in breast milk. *Br J Clin Pharmacol* 1997; **44**: 295–298.
10. Rampono J, Kristensen JH, Hackett LP *et al.* Citalopram and desmethylcitalopram in human milk; distribution, excretion and effects in breast fed infants. *Br J Clin Pharmacol* 2000; **50**: 263–268.
11. Schmidt K, Olesen OV, Jensen PN. Citalopram and breast-feeding: serum concentration and side effects in the infant. *Biol Psychiatry* 2000; **47**: 164–165.
12. Hendrick V, Fukuchi A, Altshuler L *et al.* Use of sertraline, paroxetine and fluvoxamine by nursing women. *Br J Psychiatry* 2001; **179**: 163–166.
13. Piontek CM, Wisner KL, Perel JM *et al.* Serum fluvoxamine levels in breastfed infants. *J Clin Psychiatry* 2001; **62**: 111–113.
14. Yoshida K, Smith B, Channi Kumar R. Fluvoxamine in breast-milk and infant development. *Br J Clin Pharmacol* 1997; **44**: 209–213.
15. Hägg S, Granberg K, Carleborg L. Excretion of fluvoxamine into breast milk. *Br J Clin Pharmacol* 2000; **49**: 283–288.
16. Arnold LM, Suckow RF, Lichtenstein PK. Fluvoxamine concentrations in breast milk and in maternal and infant sera. *J Clin Psychopharmacol* 2000; **20**: 491–492.
17. Kristensen JH, Hackett P, Kohan R *et al.* The amount of fluvoxamine in milk is unlikely to be a cause of adverse effects in breastfed infants. *J Hum Lactation* 2002; **18**: 139–143.
18. Yoshida K, Smith B, Craggs M *et al.* Fluoxetine in breast-milk and developmental outcome of breast-fed infants. *Br J Psychiatry* 1998; **172**: 175–179.
19. Lester BM, Cucca J, Andreozzi L *et al.* Possible association between fluoxetine hydrochloride and colic in an infant. *J Am Acad Child Adolesc Psychiatry* 1993; **32**: 6.
20. Hendrick V, Stowe ZN, Altshuler LL *et al.* Fluoxetine and norfluoxetine concentrations in nursing infants and breast milk. *Biol Psychiatry* 2001; **50**: 775–782.
21. Hale TW, Shum S, Grossberg M. Fluoxetine toxicity in a breastfed infant. *Clin Pediatr* 2001; **40**: 681–684.
22. Malone K, Papagni K, Ramini S *et al.* Antidepressants, antipsychotics, benzodiazepines and the breastfeeding dyad. *Perspect Psychiatr Care* 2004; **40**: 73–85.
23. Heikkinen T, Ekblad U, Palo P *et al.* Pharmacokinetics of fluoxetine and norfluoxetine in pregnancy and lactation. *Clin Pharmacol Ther* 2003; **73**: 330–337.
24. Begg EJ, Duffull SB, Saunders DA *et al.* Paroxetine in human milk. *Br J Clin Pharmacol* 1999; **48**: 142–147.
25. Stowe ZN, Cohen LS, Hostetter A *et al.* Paroxetine in human breast milk and nursing infants. *Am J Psychiatry* 2000; **157**: 185–189.
26. Misri S, Kim J, Riggs KW *et al.* Paroxetine levels in postpartum depressed women, breast milk, and infant serum. *J Clin Psychiatry* 2000; **61**: 828–832.
27. Öhman R, Hägg S, Carleborg L *et al.* Excretion of paroxetine into breast milk. *J Clin Psychiatry* 1999; **60**: 519–523.
28. Berle OJ, Steen VM, Aamo TO *et al.* Breastfeeding during maternal antidepressant treatment with serotonin reuptake inhibitors: infant exposure, clinical symptoms and cytochrome P450 genotypes. *J Clin Psychiatry* 2004; **65**: 1228–1234.
29. Merlob P, Stahl B, Sulkes J. Paroxetine during breast-feeding: infant weight gain and maternal adherence to counsel. *Eur J Pediatr* 2004; **163**: 135–139.
30. Llewellyn A, Stowe ZN. Psychotropic medication in lactation. *J Clin Psychiatry* 1998; **59**(suppl 2): 41–52.
31. Yapp P, Ilett KF, Kristensen JH *et al.* Drowsiness and poor feeding in a breast-fed infant: association with nefazodone and its metabolites. *Ann Pharmacother* 2000; **34**: 1269–1272.
32. Dodd S, Maguire KP, Burrows GD *et al.* Nefazodone in the breast milk of nursing mothers: a report of two patients. *J Clin Psychopharmacol* 2000; **20**: 717–718.
33. Pons G, Schoerlin MP, Tam YK. Moclobemide excretion in human breast milk. *Br J Clin Pharmacol* 1990; **29**: 27–31.
34. Buist A, Dennerstein L, Maguire KP *et al.* Plasma and human milk concentrations of moclobemide in nursing mothers. *Hum Psychopharmacol Clin Exp* 1998; **13**: 579–582.
35. Aichhorn W, Whitworth AB, Weiss U *et al.* Mirtazapine and breast-feeding. *Am J Psychiatry* 2004; **161**: 2325.
36. Verbeeck RK, Ross SG, McKenna EA. Excretion of trazodone in breast milk. *Br J Clin Pharmacol* 1986; **22**: 367–370.
37. Yoshsida K, Kumar R. Breast feeding and psychotropic drugs. *Int Rev Psychiatry* 1996; **8**: 117–124.

Special groups

38. Patton SW, Misri S, Corral MR *et al*. Antipsychotic medication during pregnancy and lactation in women with schizophrenia: evaluating the risk. *Can J Psychiatry* 2002; **47**: 959–965.

39. Matheson I, Skjeraasen J. Milk concentrations of flupenthixol, nortriptyline and zuclopenthixol and between-breast differences in two patients. *Eur J Clin Pharmacol* 1988; **35**: 217–220.

40. Ylikorkala O, Kauppila A, Kivinen S *et al*. Treatment of inadequate lactation with oral sulpiride and buccal oxytocin. *Obstet Gynecol* 1984; **63**: 57–60.

41. Aono T, Shioji T, Aki T *et al*. Augmentation of puerperal lactation by oral administration of sulpiride. *J Clin Endocrinol Metab* 1979; **48**: 478–482.

42. Ylikorkala O, Kauppila A, Kivinen S *et al*. Sulpiride improves inadequate lactation. *BMJ* 1982; **285**: 249–251.

43. Aono T, Aki T, Koike K *et al*. Effect of sulpiride on poor puerperal lactation. *Am J Obstet Gynecol* 1982; **143**: 927–932.

44. Polatti F. Sulpiride isomers and milk secretion in puerperium. *Clin Exp Obstet Gynecol* 1982; **3**: 144–147.

45. Goldstein DJ, Corbin LA, Fung MC. Olanzapine-exposed pregnancies and lactation: early experience. *J Clin Psychopharmacol* 2000; **20**: 399–403.

46. Croke S, Buist A, Hackett LP *et al*. Olanzapine excretion in human breast milk: estimation of infant exposure. *Int J Neuropsychopharmacol* 2002; **5**: 243–247.

47. Gardiner SJ, Kristensen JH, Begg EJ *et al*. Transfer of olanzapine into breast milk, calculation of infant dose, and effect on breast-fed infants. *Am J Psychiatry* 2003; **160**; 1428–1431.

48. Ambresin G, Berney P, Schulz P *et al*. Olanzapine excretion into breast milk: a case report. *J Clin Psychopharmacol* 2004; **24**: 93–95.

49. Lee A, Giesbrecht E, Dunn E *et al*. Excretion of quetiapine in breast milk. *Am J Psychiatry* 2004; **161**: 1715–1716.

50. Ratnayake T, Libretto SE. No complications with risperidone treatment before and throughout pregnancy and during the nursing period. *J Clin Psychiatry* 2002; **63**: 76–77.

51. Hill RC, McIvor RJ, Wojnar-Horton RE *et al*. Risperidone distribution and excretion into human milk: case report and estimated infant exposure during breast-feeding. *J Clin Psychopharmacol* 2000; **20**: 285–286.

52. Chaudron LH, Jefferson JW. Mood stabilizers during breastfeeding: a review. *J Clin Psychiatry* 2000; **61**: 79–90.

53. Wisner KL, Perel JM. Serum levels of valproate and carbamazepine in breastfeeding mother–infant pairs. *J Clin Psychopharmacol* 1998; **18**: 167–169.

54. Ernst CL, Goldberg JF. The reproductive safety profile of mood stabilizers, atypical antipsychotics, and broad-spectrum psychotropics. *J Clin Psychiatry* 2002; **63**(Suppl. 4): 42–55.

55. Ohman I, Vitols S, Tomson T. Lamotrigine in pregnancy: pharmacokinetics during delivery, in the neonate, and during lactation. *Epilepsia* 2000; **41**: 709–713.

56. Liporace J, Kao A, D'Abreu A. Concerns regarding lamotrigine and breast-feeding. *Epilepsy Behav* 2004; **5**: 102–105.

57. Moretti ME, Koren G, Verjee Z *et al*. Monitoring lithium in breast milk: an individualized approach for breast-feeding mothers. *Ther Drug Monit* 2003; **25**: 364–366.

58. Piontek CM, Baab S, Peindl KS *et al*. Serum valproate levels in 6 breastfeeding mother–infant pairs. *J Clin Psychiatry* 2000; **61**: 170–172.

59. Spigset O, Hägg S. Excretion of psychotropic drugs into breast milk: pharmacokinetic overview and therapeutic implications. *CNS Drugs* 1998; **9**: 111–134.

60. Hägg S, Spigset O. Anticonvulsant use during lactation. *Drug Saf* 2000; **22**: 425–440.

61. Masud Iqbal M, Sobhan T, Ryals T. Effects of commonly used benzodiazepines on the fetus, the neonate, and the nursing infant. *Psychiatr Serv* 2002; **53**: 39–49.

62. Buist A, Norman TR, Dennerstein L. Breastfeeding and the use of psychotropic medication: a review. *J Affect Disord* 1990; **19**: 197–206.

63. Fisher JB, Edgren BE, Mammel MC *et al*. Neonatal apnoea associated with maternal clonazepam therapy: a case report. *J Obstet Gynecol* 1985; **66**: 345–355.

64. Darwish M, Martin PT, Cevallos WH *et al*. Rapid disappearance of zaleplon from breast milk after oral administration to lactating women. *J Clin Pharmacol* 1999; **39**: 670–674.

65. Pons G, Rey E, Matheson I. Excretion of psychoactive drugs into breast milk; pharmacokinetic principles and recommendations. *Clin Pharmacokinet* 1994; **27**(4): 270–289.

Special groups

Renal impairment

- Using drugs in patients with renal impairment can be difficult. This is because some drugs are nephrotoxic and also because the pharmacokinetics (absorption, distribution, metabolism, excretion) of drugs is altered in renal impairment.
- Essentially, **patients with renal impairment have a reduced capacity to excrete drugs** and their metabolites.

Prescribing in renal impairment – general principles

1. **Estimate the excretory capacity of the kidney** by calculating the glomerular filtration rate (GFR). GFR can also be more accurately measured by collection of urine over 24 hours. GFR in *adults* can be estimated by calculating the creatinine clearance (CrCl) with the Cockroft and Gault equation*:

$$\text{CrCl (ml/min)} = \frac{F\,(140 - \text{age}) \times \text{ideal body weight (kg)}}{\text{plasma creatinine (}\mu\text{mol/l)}}$$

F = 1.23 (men) and 1.04 (women)
For men, ideal body weight (kg) = 50 kg + 2.3 kg per inch over 5 feet
For women, ideal body weight (kg) = 45.5 kg + 2.3 kg per inch over 5 feet

* This equation is not accurate if plasma creatinine is unstable, in pregnant women or children or in diseases causing production of abnormal amounts of creatinine. Creatinine clearance is less representative of GFR in severe renal failure.

2. **Grade the severity of renal impairment** as below:

Grade	GFR	Approx. serum creatinine
Mild	20–50 ml/min	150–300 μmol/l
Moderate	10–20 ml/min	300–700 μmol/l
Severe	<10 ml/min	>700 μmol/l

In severe renal impairment, most patients require dialysis.

3. **Note that elderly patients are assumed to have mild renal impairment.** Their creatinine may not be raised because they have a smaller muscle mass.

4. **Avoid drugs that are nephrotoxic** (e.g. lithium) in moderate or severe renal failure.

5. **Choose a drug that is safer to use in renal impairment** (see tables below).

6. **Be cautious when using drugs that are extensively renally cleared** (e.g. sulpiride, amisulpride, lithium).

7. **Start at a low dose and increase slowly** because, in renal impairment, the half-life of a drug and the time for it to reach steady state are often prolonged. Plasma level monitoring may be useful for some drugs.

8. **Avoid long-acting drugs** (e.g. depot preparations). Their dose and frequency cannot be easily adjusted should renal function change.

9. **Prescribe as few drugs as possible.** Patients with renal failure take many medications requiring regular review. Interactions and side-effects can be avoided if fewer drugs are used.

10. **Monitor patient for adverse effects.** Patients with renal impairment are more likely to experience side-effects and these may take longer to develop than in healthy patients. Adverse effects such as sedation, confusion and postural hypotension can be more common.

11. **Be cautious when using drugs with anticholinergic effects,** since they may cause urinary retention.

12. There are **few clinical studies** of the use of psychotropic drugs in people with renal impairment. Advice about drug use in renal impairment is often based on knowledge of the drug's pharmacokinetics in healthy patients.

13. **The effect of renal replacement therapies on drugs is difficult to predict.** Dosing advice is available from tables and data on each drug's volume of distribution and protein-binding affinity. Seek specialist advice.

Table	Antipsychotics in renal impairment
Drug	**Comments**
Aripiprazole[1,2]	Less than 1% of unchanged aripiprazole renally excreted. Manufacturer states no dose adjustment required in renal failure; however, no published studies in patients with renal disease.
Amisulpride[1–4]	Primarily renally excreted, 50% excreted unchanged in urine. Limited experience in renal disease; manufacturer states no data with doses >50 mg, but recommends following dosing: 50% of dose if GFR 30–60 ml/min; 33% of dose if GFR is 10–30 ml/min; no recommendations for GFR <10 ml/min so best avoided in severe renal impairment.
Chlorpromazine[1,2,4–6]	Less than 1% excreted unchanged in urine. Manufacturer advises avoiding in renal dysfunction. Dosing: GFR 10–50 ml/min, dose as in normal renal function; GFR <10 ml/min, start with a small dose because of an increased risk of anticholinergic, sedative and hypotensive side-effects. Monitor carefully.
Clozapine[2,6–9]	Only trace amounts of unchanged clozapine excreted in urine; however, there are rare cases of interstitial nephritis and acute renal failure. Nocturnal enuresis and urinary retention are common side-effects. Contraindicated by manufacturer in severe renal disease. Anticholinergic, sedative and hypotensive side-effects are common and may occur more frequently in patients with renal disease.
Flupentixol[1,7]	Negligible renal excretion of unchanged flupentixol. Dose adjustment may not be necessary in renal impairment. Manufacturer recommends caution in renal failure.
Fluphenazine[2]	Little information available; manufacturer cautions in renal impairment and contraindicates in renal failure.
Haloperidol[1,2,4,6,10]	Less than 1% excreted unchanged in urine. Manufacturer advises caution in renal failure. Dosing: GFR 10–50 ml/min dose as in normal renal function; GFR <10 ml/min start with lower dose. A case report of haloperidol use in renal failure suggests starting at a low dose and increasing slowly.
Olanzapine[1,2,4]	57% of olanzapine is excreted unchanged in urine mainly as metabolites. No dose adjustment needed in renal impairment; however, a single-dose study of olanzapine in severe renal impairment used 5 mg, so start at this dose and increase as necessary.
Pimozide[1,2,4]	Less than 1% of pimozide is excreted unchanged in the urine; dose reductions not usually needed in renal impairment. Dosing: GFR 10–50 ml/min, dose as in normal renal function; GFR <10 ml/min start with 50% of normal dose. Manufacturer advises caution in renal dysfunction.
Quetiapine[1,2,4,11]	Less than 5% of quetiapine excreted unchanged in the urine. Plasma clearance reduced by an average of 25% in patients with a GFR <30 ml/min. In patients with GFR of <50 ml/min start at 25 mg/day and increase in daily increments of 25–50 mg to an effective dose.
Risperidone[1,2,4,12]	Clearance of the active metabolite of oral risperidone is reduced by 60% in patients with renal disease. Dosing: GRF < 50 ml/min 0.5 mg twice daily increasing by 0.5 mg twice daily to 1–2 mg twice daily. The manufacturer advises caution when using risperidone in renal impairment. The long-acting injection should be used only after titration with oral risperidone as described above. If 2 mg orally is tolerated, 25 mg intramuscularly every two weeks can be administered.

Table Antipsychotics in renal impairment *continued*

Drug	Comments
Sertindole[1,2,13]	Less than 1% of sertindole is excreted into urine. A single-dose study of sertindole found no dose adjustment needed in mild, moderate or severe renal impairment.
Sulpiride [1,2,4,14]	Almost totally renally excreted with 95% excreted in urine and faeces as unchanged sulpiride. Dosing regimen: GFR 30–60 ml/min, give 70% of normal dose; GFR 10–30 ml/min, give 50% of normal dose; GFR < 10 ml/min, give 30% of normal dose. Probably best avoided in renal impairment.
Trifluoperazine[4]	Less than 1% excreted unchanged in the urine; dose as for normal renal function.
Ziprasidone[1,15]	<1% is renally excreted unchanged. No dose adjustment needed for GFR >10 ml/min but care needed when using the injectable form, as it contains a renally eliminated excipient (cyclodextrin sodium).
Zotepine[1,2,4]	<0.1% is excreted as unchanged zotepine in urine. Patients with renal dysfunction have higher plasma levels than healthy patients, so start low, gradually titrate and reduce the maximum daily dose. The manufacturer suggests a starting dose of 25 mg twice daily, gradually titrating to a maximum of 75 mg twice daily in patients with a GFR < 50 ml/min.

Table Antidepressants in renal impairment

Drug	Comments
Amitriptyline[1,2,4,6,16]	<10% excreted unchanged in urine; no dose adjustment needed in renal failure. Dose as in normal renal function but start at a low dose and increase slowly. Monitor patient for urinary retention, confusion, sedation and postural hypotension.
Bupropion[1,2,4,6] (amfebutamone)	0.5% excreted unchanged in the urine. No studies of buproprion in renal impairment so use with caution. Dosing: GFR < 50 ml/min, 150 mg once daily.
Citalopram[1,2,4,17–19]	<13% of citalopram is excreted unchanged in the urine. Single-dose studies in mild and moderate renal impairment show no change in the pharmacokinetics of citalopram. Dosing is as for normal renal function; however, use with caution if GFR <10 ml/min due to reduced clearance. The manufacturer does not advise use if GFR <20 ml/min. Renal failure has been reported with citalopram overdose.
Clomipramine[1,2,4,6]	2% of unchanged clomipramine is excreted in the urine. Dosing: GFR 20–50 ml/min, dose as for normal renal function; GFR <20 ml/min, effects unknown, start at a low dose and monitor patient for urinary retention, confusion, sedation and postural hypotension.
Dosulepin[1,4,20] (dothiepin)	56% of mainly active metabolites renally excreted. They have a long half-life and may accumulate, resulting in excessive sedation. Dosing: GFR 20–50 ml/min, dose as for normal renal function; GFR <20 ml/min, start with 25 mg at night and monitor patient for urinary retention, confusion, sedation and postural hypotension.
Doxepin[1,2,4]	<1% excreted unchanged in urine. Dose as in normal renal function but monitor patient for urinary retention, confusion, sedation and postural hypotension. Manufacturer advises using with caution.

Table Antidepressants in renal impairment *continued*	
Drug	**Comments**
Duloxetine[1,2]	Manufacturer states no dose adjustment is necessary for GFR >30 ml/min; however, starting at a low dose and increasing slowly is advised. Duloxetine is contraindicated in patients with a GFR <30 ml/min.
Fluvoxamine[1,2]	Little information on its use in renal impairment. Dose as for normal renal function but start on a low dose and monitor carefully.
Fluoxetine[1,2,4,6,21,22]	2.5–5% of fluoxetine and 10% of the active metabolite norfluoxetine are excreted unchanged in the urine. Dosing: GFR 20–50 ml/min dose as normal renal function; GFR <20 ml/min dose as normal renal function or alternate days.
Imipramine[1,2,4,6,16]	<5% excreted unchanged in the urine. No specific dose adjustment necessary in renal impairment. Monitor patient for urinary retention, confusion, sedation and postural hypotension. Renal impairment with imipramine has been reported and manufacturer advises caution in severe renal impairment.
Lofepramine[1,2,23]	There is little information about the use of lofepramine in renal impairment. Most lofepramine is excreted in the urine along with some as the active metabolite desipramine. Desipramine has a long half-life (12–24 hours) and can accumulate, so avoid in renal impairment. Manufacturer advises caution in patients with impaired renal function.
Mirtazapine[1,2,4,24]	75% excreted unchanged in the urine. Clearance is reduced by 30% in patients with a GFR of 11–39 ml/min and by 50% in patients with a GFR <10 ml/min. Dosing advice: GFR 20–50 ml/min, dose as for normal renal function; GFR <10 ml/min, start at a low dose and monitor closely. Mirtazapine has been used to treat pruritis caused by renal failure.
Moclobemide[1,2,25,26]	<1% of parent drug excreted unchanged in the urine. However, an active metabolite was found to be raised in patients with renal impairment but was not thought to affect dosing. Dose adjustments are not required in renal impairment.
Nortriptyline[1,4,16,27]	If GFR 10–50 ml/min, dose as in normal renal function; if GFR <10 ml/min, start at a low dose. Plasma level monitoring recommended at doses of >100 mg/day, as plasma concentrations of active metabolites are raised in renal impairment. Worsening of GFR in elderly patients has also been reported.
Paroxetine[1,2,4,6,28,29]	Less than 2% of oral dose is excreted unchanged in the urine. Single-dose studies show increased plasma concentrations of paroxetine when GFR <30 ml/min. Dosing start at 10 mg/day if GFR <30 ml/min and increase dose according to response.
Phenelzine[1,4]	Approximately 1% excreted unchanged in the urine. No dose adjustment required in renal failure.
Reboxetine[1,2,4,30,31]	Approximately 10% of unchanged drug is excreted unchanged in the urine. Dosing: GFR < 20 ml/min, 2 mg twice daily, adjusting dose according to response. Half-life is prolonged as renal function decreases.
Sertraline[1,2,4,6,32]	<0.2% of unchanged sertraline excreted in urine. Pharmacokinetics in renal impairment is unchanged in single-dose studies but no published data on multiple dosing. Dosing is as for normal renal function. Sertraline has been used to treat dialysis-associated hypotension.

Table Antidepressants in renal impairment *continued*

Drug	Comments
Trazodone[1,2,4,6,33]	<5% excreted unchanged in urine but care needed, as approximately 70% of active metabolite also excreted. Dosing: GFR 20–50 ml/min, dose as normal renal function; GFR 10–20 ml/min, dose as normal renal function but start with small dose and increase gradually; GFR <10 ml/min, avoid or use half the dose or half frequency.
Trimipramine[1,6,16,34,35]	No dose reduction required in renal impairment; however, elevated urea and interstitial nephritis have been reported. As with all tricyclic antidepressants, monitor patient for urinary retention, confusion, sedation and postural hypotension, as patients with renal impairment are at increased risk of having these side-effects.
Venlafaxine[1,2,6,36]	1–10% is excreted unchanged in the urine (30% as the active metabolite). Clearance is decreased and half-life prolonged in renal impairment. Dosing advice differs: GFR 30–50 ml/min, dose as in normal renal function or reduce by 50%; GFR 10–30 ml/min, reduce dose by 50% and give once daily; GFR <10 ml/min, reduce dose by 50% and give once daily; however, manufacturer advises avoiding use in these patients. Avoid using the XL preparation if GFR < 30 ml/min.

Table Mood stabilisers in renal impairment

Drug	Comments
Carbamazepine[1,2,4,37–42]	2–3% of the dose is excreted unchanged in urine. Dose reduction not necessary in renal disease, although cases of renal failure, tubular necrosis and tubulointerstitial nephritis have been reported rarely.
Lamotrigine[1,2,4,43–46]	<10% of lamotrigine is excreted unchanged in the urine. Single-dose studies in renal failure show pharmacokinetics is little affected; however, inactive metabolites can accumulate (effects unknown) and half-life can be prolonged. Renal failure and interstitial nephritis have also been reported. Dosing: GFR <10–50 ml/min, use cautiously, start with a low dose, increase slowly and monitor closely.
Lithium[1,2,4,6,47]	Lithium is nephrotoxic and contraindicated in severe renal impairment; 95% is excreted unchanged in the urine. Long-term treatment may result in impaired renal function and both reversible and irreversible kidney damage. If lithium is used in renal impairment, toxicity is more likely. The manufacturer contraindicates lithium in renal impairment. Dosing: GFR 10–50 ml/min, avoid or reduce dose (50–75% of normal dose) and monitor levels; GFR <10 ml/min, avoid if possible; however, if used, it is essential to reduce dose (25–50% of normal dose). Renal damage is more likely with chronic toxicity than acute.
Valproate[1,2,4,48–52]	Approximately 2% excreted unchanged as valproate. Dose adjustment usually not required in renal impairment; however, free valproate levels may be increased. Renal impairment, interstitial nephritis, Fanconi's syndrome, renal tubular acidosis and renal failure have been reported. Dose as in normal renal function; however, in severe impairment it may be necessary to alter doses according to free (unbound) valproate levels.

Table Anxiolytics and hypnotics in renal impairment

Drug	Comments
Buspirone[1,2,4,6]	Less than 1% is excreted unchanged; however, active metabolite is renally excreted. Dosing advice contradictory; suggest: GFR 10–50 ml/min, dose as normal; GFR <10 ml/min, avoid if possible due to accumulation of active metabolites; if essential, reduce dose by 25–50% if patient is anuric.
Clomethiazole[1,2,4,53] (chlormethiazole)	0.1–5% of unchanged drug excreted unchanged in urine. Dose as in normal renal function but monitor for excessive sedation. Manufacturer recommends caution in renal disease.
Chlordiazepoxide[2,4,6]	<5% excreted unchanged but chlordiazepoxide has a long-acting active metabolite that can accumulate. Dosing: GFR 10–50 ml/min, dose as normal renal function; GFR<10 ml/min, reduce dose by 50%. Monitor for excessive sedation.
Clonazepam[1,2,4,6]	<1% of clonazepam excreted unchanged in urine. Dose adjustment not required in impaired renal function, however with long-term administration active metabolites may accumulate so lower doses may be needed. Monitor for excessive sedation.
Diazepam[1,4,6,54]	Less than 1% is excreted unchanged. Dosing: GFR 20–50 ml/min, dose as in normal renal function; GFR <20 ml/min, use small doses and titrate to response. Long-acting active metabolites accumulate in renal impairment; monitor patients for excessive sedation and encephalopathy. One case of interstitial nephritis with diazepam has been reported in a patient with chronic renal failure.
Lorazepam[1,2,4,6,55–58]	<5% excreted unchanged in urine, dose as in normal renal function but carefully according to response as some may need lower doses. Monitor for excessive sedation. Impaired elimination reported in two patients with severe renal impairment and also reports of propylene glycol in lorazepam injection causing renal impairment and acute tubular necrosis.
Nitrazepam[2,4]	Less than 5% excreted unchanged in the urine. Dosing GFR 10–50 ml/min as per normal renal function; GFR <10 ml/min, start with small dose and increase slowly. Manufactuurer advises halving dose in renal impairment. Monitor patient for sedation.
Oxazepam[1,4,6,59]	Less than 1% excreted unchanged in the urine. Dose adjustment needed in severe renal impairment. Oxazepam may take longer to reach steady state in patients with renal impairment. Dosing: GFR 10–50 ml/min, dose as in normal renal function; GFR <10 ml/min, 10–20 mg three or four times a day. Monitor for excessive sedation.
Promethazine[1,2,4,6]	Dose reduction usually not necessary; however, promethazine has a long half-life so monitor for excessive sedative effects in patients with renal impairment. Manufacturer advises caution in renal impairment.
Temazepam[1,2,4,6]	<2% excreted unchanged in urine. In renal impairment the inactive metabolite can accumulate. Monitor for excessive sedative effects. Dosing: GFR 20–50 ml/min, dose as normal renal function; GFR 10–20 ml/min, start with small doses, maximum 20 mg/day; GFR <10 ml/min, start with small doses, maxmium 10 mg daily.
Zaleplon[1,2,60,61]	<0.1% excreted unchanged in the urine. In renal impairment inactive metabolites accumulate. No dose adjustment appears to be necessary in patients with GFR >20 ml/min. Zaleplon is not recommended if GFR <20 ml/min; however, it has been used in patients on haemodialysis.
Zolpidem[1,2,4,60]	Clearance moderately reduced in renal impairment. No dose adjustment required in renal impairment; however, there are no published studies of zolpidem in severe renal impairment.
Zopiclone[1,2,4,61,62]	5–11% excreted unchanged in urine. Manufacturer states no accumulation of zopiclone in renal impairment but suggests starting at 3.75 mg in those with GFR <10 ml/min.

Summary – psychotropics in renal impairment

Drug group	Recommended drugs
Antipsychotics	No agent clearly preferred to another, however: • avoid sulpiride and amisulpride • avoid highly anticholinergic agents because they may cause urinary retention • typical antipsychotic – suggest **haloperidol** 2–6 mg/day • atypical antipsychotic – suggest **olanzapine** 5 mg/day
Antidepressants	No agent clearly preferred to another; however: • **citalopram** and **sertraline** are suggested as reasonable choices
Mood-stabilisers	No agent clearly preferred to another, however: • avoid lithium • suggest start one of the following at a low dose and increase slowly, monitoring for adverse effects: **valproate**, **carbamazepine** or **lamotrigine**
Anxiolytics and hypnotics	No agent clearly preferred to another; however: • excessive sedation is more likely to occur in patients with renal impairment, so monitor all patients carefully • **lorazepam** and **zopiclone** are suggested as reasonable choices

References

1. Drugdex® System, Micromedex Inc., Englewood, Colorado. First quarter, 2005.
2. Electronic Medicines Compendium; http://emc. medicines.org.uk/.
3. Noble S, Benfield P. Amisulpride. A review of its clinical potential in dysthymia. *CNS Drugs* 1999; **12**: 471–483.
4. Moorhead J, Bunn R, Ashley C. *The Renal Drug Handbook*, 2nd edn. Oxford: Radcliffe Medical Press, 2004.
5. Fabre J, De Freudenreich J, Duckert A *et al.* Influence of renal insufficiency on the excretion of chloroquine, phenobarbital, phenothiazines and methacycline. *Helv Med Acta* 1966; **4**: 307–316.
6. Aronoff GR, Berns JS, Brier ME *et al. Drug Prescribing in Renal Failure – Dosing Guidelines for Adults,* 4th edn. Philadelphia: American College of Physicians, 1999.
7. Fraser D, Jibani M. An unexpected and serious complication of treatment with the atypical antipsychotic drug clozapine. *Clin Nephrol* 2000; **43**: 78–80.
8. Elias TJ, Bannister KM, Clarkson AR *et al.* Clozapine-induced acute interstitial nephritis. *Lancet* 1999; **354**: 1801–1811.
9. Au AF, Luthra V, Stern R. Clozapine-induced acute interstitial nephritis. *Am J Psychiatry* 2004; **161**: 1501.
10. Lobeck F, Jethanandani V, Evans RL *et al.* Haloperidol concentrations in an elderly patient with moderate chronic renal failure. *J Geriatr Drug Ther* 1986; **1**: 91–97.
11. Thyrum PT, Wong YWJ, Yeh C. Single-dose pharmacokinetics of quetiapine in subjects with renal or hepatic impairment. *Prog Neuropsychopharmacol Biol Psychiatry* 2000; **24**: 521–533.
12. Snoeck E, Van Peer A, Sack M *et al.* Influence of age, renal and liver impairment on the pharmacokinetics of risperidone in man. *Psychopharmacology* 1995; **122**: 223–229.
13. Wong SL, Menacherry S, Mulford D *et al.* Pharmacokinetics of sertindole and dehydrosertindole in volunteers with normal or impaired renal function. *Eur J Clin Pharmacol* 1997; **52**: 223–227.
14. Bressolle F, Bres J, Mourad G. Pharmacokinetics of sulpiride after intravenous administration in patients with impaired renal function. *Clin Pharmacokinet* 1989; **17**: 367–373.
15. Aweeka F, Jayesekara D, Horton M *et al.* The pharmacokinetics of ziprasidone in subjects with normal and impaired renal function. *Br J Clin Pharmacol* 2000; **49**(S1): 27S–33S.
16. Lieberman JA Cooper TB, Suckow RF *et al.* Tricyclic antidepressants and metabolite levels in chronic renal failure. *Clin Pharmacol Ther* 1985; **37**: 301–307.
17. Spigset O, Hagg S, Stergmayr B *et al.* Citalopram pharmacokinetics in patients with chronic renal failure and the effect of haemodialysis. *Eur J Clin Pharmacol* 2000; **56**: 699–703.
18. Joffe P, Larsen FS, Pedersen V *et al.* Single-dose pharmacokinetics of citalopram in patients with moderate renal insufficiency or hepatic cirrhosis compared with healthy subjects. *Eur J Clin Pharmacol* 1998; **54**: 237–242.
19. Kelly CA, Upex A, Spencer EP *et al.* Adult respiratory distress syndome and renal failure associated with citalopram overdose. *Hum Exp Toxicol* 2003; **22**: 103–105.

20. Rees JA. Clinical interpretation of pharmacokinetic data on dothiepin hydrochloride (dosulepin, prothiaden). *J Int Med Res* 1981; 9: 98–102.
21. Blumenfield M, Levy NB, Spinowitz B *et al.* Fluoxetine in depressed patients on dialysis. *Int J Psychiatry Med* 1997; 27: 71–80.
22. Bergstrom RF, Beasley CM, Levy NB *et al.* The effects of renal and hepatic disease on the pharmacokinetics, renal tolerance and risk-benefit profile of fluoxetine. *Int Clin Psychopharmacol* 1993; 8: 261–266.
23. Lancaster SG, Gonzalez JP. Lofepramine. A review of its pharmacodynamic and pharmacokinetic properties and therapeutic efficacy in depressive illness. *Drugs* 1989; 37: 123–140.
24. Davis MP, Frandsen JL, Walsh D *et al.* Mirtazapine for puritus. *J Pain Symptom Manage* 2003; 25: 288–291.
25. Schoerlin MP, Horber FF, Frey FJ *et al.* Disposition kinetics of moclobemide, a new MAO-A inhibitor, in subjects with impaired renal function. *J Clin Pharmacol* 1990; 30: 272–274.
26. Stoeckel K, Pfefen JP, Mayersohn M *et al.* Absorption and disposition of moclobemide in patients with advanced age or reduced liver or kidney function. *Acta Psychiatr Scand* 1990; 360(S): 94–97.
27. Pollock BG, Perel JM, Paradis CF *et al.* Metabolic and physiologic consequences of nortriptyline treatment in the elderly. *Psychopharmacol Bull* 1994; 30: 145–150.
28. Doyle GD, Laher M, Kelly JG *et al.* The pharmacokinetics of paroxetine in renal impairment. *Acta Psychiatr Scand* 1989; 80(S350): 89–90.
29. Kaye CM, Haddock RE, Langely PF *et al.* A review of the metabolism and pharmacokinetics of paroxetine in man. *Acta Psychiatr Scand* 1989; 80(S350): 60–75.
30. Coulomb F, Ducret F, Laneury JP *et al.* Pharmacokinetics of single dose reboxetine in volunteers with renal insufficiency. *J Clin Pharmacol* 2000; 40: 482–487.
31. Dostert P, Benedetti MS, Poggesi I. Review of the pharmacokinetics and metabolism of reboxetine, a selective noradrenaline reuptake inhibitor. *Eur Neuropsychopharmacol* 1997; 7(S1): S23–S35.
32. Brewster UC, Ciampi MA, Abu-Alfa AK *et al.* Addition of sertraline to other therapies to reduce dialysis associated hypotension. *Nephrology* 2003; 8: 296–301.
33. Catanese B, Dionisio A, Barillari G *et al.* A comparative study of trazodone serum concentrations in patients with normal or impaired renal function. *Boll Chim Farm* 1978; 117: 424–427.
34. Simpson GM, Blair JH, Igbal J *et al.* A preliminary study of trimipramine in chronic schizophrenia *Curr Ther Res* 1966; 99: 248.
35. Leighton JD, Walker RJ, Lynn KL. Trimipramine induced acute renal failure (Letter). *N Z Med J* 1986; 99: 248.
36. Troy SM, Schulz RW, Parker VD *et al.* The effect of renal disease on the disposition of venlafaxine. *Clin Pharmacol Ther* 1994; 56: 14–21.
37. Verrotti A, Greco R, Pascarella R *et al.* Renal tubular function in patients receiving anticonvulsant therapy: a long term study. *Epilepsia* 2000; 41: 1432–1435.
38. Hogg RJ, Sawyer M, Hecox K *et al.* Carbamazepine-induced acute tubulointerstitial nephritis. *J Pediatr* 1981; 98: 830–831.
39. Hegarty J, Picton M, Agarwal G *et al.* Carbamazepine-induced acute granulomatous interstitial nephritis. *Clin Nephrol* 2002; 57: 310–313.
40. Nicholls DP, Yasin M. Acute renal failure from carbamazepine (Letter). *BMJ* 1972; 4: 490.
41. Jubert P, Almirall J, Casanovas A *et al.* Carbamazepine-induced acute renal failure. *Nephron* 1994; 66: 121.
42. Imai H, Nakamoto Y, Hirokawa M *et al.* Carbamazepine-induced granulomatous necrotizing angiitis with acute renal failure. *Nephron* 1989; 51: 405–408.
43. Fillasatre JP, Taburet AM, Failaire A *et al.* Pharmacokinetics of lamotrigine in patients with renal impairment – influence of hemodialysis. *Drugs Exp Clin Res* 1993; 19: 25–32.
44. Wootton R, Soul-Lawton J, Rolan PE *et al.* Comparison of the pharmacokinetics of lamotrigine in patients with chronic renal failure and healthy volunteers. *Br J Clin Pharmacol* 1997; 43: 23–27.
45. Schaub JEM, Williamson PJ, Barnes EW *et al.* Multisystem adverse reaction to lamotrigine. *Lancet* 1994; 344: 481.
46. Fervenza FC, Kanakiriya S, Kunau RT *et al.* Acute granulomatous interstitial nephritis and colitis in anticonvulsant hypersensitivity syndrome associated with lamotrigine treatment. *Am J Kidney Dis* 2000; 36: 1034–1040.
47. Gitlin M. Lithium and the kidney, an updated review. *Drug Saf* 1999; 20: 231–243.
48. Smith GC, Balfe JW, Kooh SW. Anticonvulsants as a cause of Fanconi syndrome. *Nephrol Dial Transplant* 1995; 10: 543–545.
49. Fukuda Y, Watanabe H, Ohtomo Y *et al.* Immunologically mediated chronic tubulo-interstitial nephritis caused by valproate therapy. *Nephron* 1996; 72: 328–329.
50. Zaki EL, Springate JE. Renal injury from valproic acid: case report and literature review. *Pediatr Neurol* 2002; 27: 318–319.
51. Tanaka H, Onodera N, Ryosuke I *et al.* Distal type of renal tubular acidosis after anti-epileptic therapy in a girl with infantile spasms. *Clin Exp Nephrol* 1999; 3: 311–313.
52. Knorr M, Schaper J, Harjes M *et al.* Fanconi syndrome caused by antiepileptic therapy with valproic acid. *Epilepsia* 2004; 45: 868–871.
53. Pentikainen PJ, Neuvonen PJ, Jostell KG. Pharmacokinetics of chlormethiazole in healthy volunteers and patients with cirrhosis of the liver. *Eur J Clin Pharmacol* 1980; 17: 275–284.
54. Sadjadi SA, McLaughlin K, Shah RM. Allergic interstitial nephritis due to diazepam. *Arch Intern Med* 1987; 147: 579.
55. Verbeeck RK, Tjandramaga TB, de Schepper PJ *et al.* Impaired elimination of lorazepam following subchronic administration to two patients with renal failure. *Br J Clin Pharmacol* 1981; 12: 749–751.
56. Reynolds HN, Teiken P, Regan ME *et al.* Hyperlactinemia, increased osmolar gap and renal dysfunction during continuous lorazepam infusion. *Crit Care Med* 2000; 28: 1631–1634.

Special groups

57. Yaucher NE, Fish JT, Smith HW *et al*. Propylene glycol-associated renal toxicity from lorazepam infusion. *Pharmacotherapy* 2003; **23**: 1094–1099.
58. Hayman M, Seidl EC, Ali M *et al*. Acute tubular necrosis associated with propylene glycol from concomitant administration of intravenous lorazepam and trimethoprim-sulfamethoxazole. *Pharmacotherapy* 2003; **23**: 1190–1194.
59. Murray TG, Chiang ST, Koepke HH *et al*. Renal disease, age and oxazepam kinetics. *Clin Pharmacol Ther* 1981; **30**: 805–809.
60. Drover DR. Comparative pharmacokinetics and pharmcodynamics of short-acting hypnosedatives. *Clin Pharmacokinet* 2004; **43**: 227–238.
61. Sabbatini M, Crispo A, Pisani A *et al*. Zaleplon improves sleep quality in maintenance hemodialysis patients. *Nephron Clin Pract* 2003; **94**: c99–c103.
62. Goa KL, Heel RC. Zopiclone. A review of its pharmacodynamic and pharmacokinetic properties and therapeutic efficacy as a hypnotic. *Drugs* 1986; **32**: 48–65.

Special groups

Hepatic impairment

Patients with hepatic impairment may have:

- **reduced capacity to metabolise** biological waste products, dietary proteins and foreign substances such as drugs. Clinical consequences include hepatic encephalopathy and increased dose-related side-effects from drugs.

- **reduced ability to synthesise** plasma proteins and vitamin K-dependent clotting factors. Clinical consequences include hypoalbuminaemia, leading in extreme cases to ascites. Increased toxicity from highly protein-bound drugs should be anticipated. There is also an increased risk of bleeding from GI irritant drugs and perhaps with SSRIs.

- **reduced hepatic blood flow.** Clinical consequences include oesophageal varices.

General principles

Liver function tests (LFTs) are a poor marker of hepatic metabolising capacity, as the hepatic reserve is large. There are few clinical studies relating to the use of psychotropic drugs in people with hepatic disease. The following principles should be adhered to:

1. Prescribe as **few drugs** as possible.

2. Use **lower starting doses**, particularly of drugs that are highly protein bound. TCAs, SSRIs (except citalopram), trazodone and antipsychotics may have increased free plasma levels, at least initially. This will not be reflected in measured (total) plasma levels. Use lower doses of drugs known to be subject to extensive first pass metabolism. Examples include TCAs and haloperidol.

3. Be **cautious with drugs that are extensively hepatically metabolised** (most psychotropic drugs). Lower doses may be required. Exceptions are sulpiride, amisulpride, lithium and gabapentin, which all undergo no or minimal hepatic metabolism.

4. **Leave longer intervals between dosage increases.** Remember that the half-life of most drugs is prolonged in hepatic impairment, so it will take longer for plasma levels to reach steady state.

5. Always **monitor carefully for side-effects**, which may be delayed.

6. **Avoid drugs that are very sedative** because of the risk of precipitating hepatic encephalopathy.

7. **Avoid drugs that are very constipating** because of the risk of precipitating hepatic encephalopathy.

8. **Avoid drugs that are known to be hepatotoxic** in their own right (e.g. MAOIs, chlorpromazine).

9. **Choose a low-risk drug** (see tables below) and **monitor LFTs** weekly, at least initially. If LFTs deteriorate after a new drug is introduced, consider switching to another drug.

These rules should always be observed in severe liver disease (low albumin, increased clotting time, ascites, jaundice, encephalopathy, etc.). Many patients with chronic liver disease are asymptomatic or have fluctuating clinical symptoms. The information above, and on the following pages, should be interpreted in the context of the patient's clinical presentation.

Special groups

Table Antipsychotics in hepatic impairment

Drug	Comments
Amisulpride[1,2]	Predominantly renally excreted, so dosage reduction should not be necessary as long as renal function is normal *but* there are no clinical studies in people with hepatic impairment and little clinical experience. Caution required
Aripiprazole[1]	Extensively hepatically metabolised. Limited data that hepatic impairment has minimal effect on pharmacokinetics but no clinical experience. Best avoided
Clozapine[1–5]	Very sedative and constipating. Contraindicated in active liver disease associated with nausea, anorexia or jaundice, progressive liver disease or hepatic failure. In less severe disease, start with 12.5 mg and increase slowly, using plasma levels to gauge metabolising capacity and guide dosage adjustment Transient elevations in AST, ALT and GGT to over twice the normal range occur in over 10% of physically healthy people. Clozapine-induced hepatitis, jaundice, cholestasis and liver failure have been reported
Flupentixol/ zuclopenthixol[1,2,6,7]	Both are extensively hepatically metabolised. Small, transient elevations in transaminases have been reported in some patients treated with zuclopenthixol. No other literature reports of use or harm. Both drugs have been in use for many years. Depot preparations are best avoided, as altered pharmacokinetics will make dosage adjustment difficult and side-effects from dosage accumulation more likely
Haloperidol[1]	Drug of choice in clinical practice and no problems reported although UK SPC states 'caution in liver disease'
Olanzapine[1,2,8–11]	Although extensively hepatically metabolised, the pharmacokinetics of olanzapine seems to change little in severe hepatic impairment. It is sedative and anticholinergic (can cause constipation) so caution is advised. Consider using plasma levels to guide dosage (aim for 20–40 µg/l). Dose-related, transient, asymptomatic elevations in ALT and AST reported in physically healthy adults. People with liver disease may be at increased risk. Rare cases of hepatitis in the literature
Phenothiazines[1,2,12–14]	All cause sedation and constipation. Associated with cholestasis and some reports of fulminant hepatic cirrhosis. Best avoided completely in hepatic impairment. Chlorpromazine is particularly hepatotoxic
Quetiapine[1,2,15–18]	Extensively hepatically metabolised but short half-life. One single-dose, kinetic study suggests that no change in starting dose is required. Clearance reduced by a mean of 30% in hepatic impairment so small dosage adjustments may be required. Can cause sedation and constipation. Little clinical experience in hepatic impairment so caution recommended. One case of fatal hepatic failure reported in the literature
Risperidone[1,2,19–22]	Highly protein bound. Manufacturers recommend a maximum dose of 4 mg in hepatic impairment. Transient, asymptomatic elevations in LFTs, cholestatic hepatitis and rare cases of hepatic failure have been reported. Steatohepatitis may arise as a result of weight gain. Clinical experience limited in hepatic impairment so caution recommended
Sulpiride[1,2,23,24]	Almost completely renally excreted with a low potential to cause sedation or constipation. Dosage reduction should not be required. Some clinical experience in hepatic impairment with few problems. Fairly old established drug. Isolated case reports of cholestatic jaundice and primary biliary cirrhosis

Table	Antidepressants in hepatic impairment
Drug	**Comments**
Fluoxetine[1,2,25–29]	Extensively hepatically metabolised with a long half-life. Kinetic studies demonstrate accumulation in compensated cirrhosis. Although dosage reduction (of at least 50%) or alternate day dosing could be used, it would take many weeks to reach steady-state serum levels, making fluoxetine complex to use. Asymptomatic increases in LFTs found in 0.5% of healthy adults. Rare cases of hepatitis reported
Other SSRIs[1,2,29–37]	All are hepatically metabolised and accumulate on chronic dosing. Dosage reduction may be required. Raised LFTs and rare cases of hepatitis, including chronic active hepatitis, have been reported with paroxetine. Sertraline and fluvoxamine have also been associated with hepatitis. Citalopram has minimal effects on hepatic enzymes and may be the SSRI of choice although clinical experience is limited and occasional hepatotoxicity has been reported. Paroxetine is used by some specialised liver units with few apparent problems
Tricyclics[1,2,38]	All are hepatically metabolised, highly protein bound and will accumulate. They vary in their propensity to cause sedation and constipation. All are associated with raised LFTs and rare cases of hepatitis. There is most clinical experience with imipramine. Sedative TCAs such as trimipramine, dothiepin (dosulepin) and amitriptyline are best avoided. Lofepramine is possibly the most hepatotoxic and should be avoided completely
Venlafaxine[1,2,39]	Dosage reduction of 50% advised in moderate hepatic impairment. Little clinical experience. Rare cases of hepatitis reported. Caution advised
MAOIs[1,2,40,41]	People with hepatic impairment reported to be more sensitive to the side-effects of MAOIs. MAOIs are also more hepatotoxic than other antidepressants, so best avoided completely
Moclobemide[1,2,42,43]	Clinical experience limited but probably safer than the irreversible MAOIs. 50% reduction in dose advised by manufacturers. Rare cases of hepatotoxicity reported. Caution advised
Reboxetine[1,2,44]	50% reduction in starting dose recommended. Clinical experience limited. Does not seem to be associated with hepatotoxicity. Caution advised
Mirtazapine[1,2]	Hepatically metabolised and sedative. 50% dose reduction recommended based on kinetic data, but clinical experience limited. Mild, asymptomatic increases in LFTs seen in healthy adults. Caution advised
Duloxetine[1,2]	Hepatically metabolised. Clearance markedly reduced even in mild impairment. Limited experience. Best avoided

Special groups

295

Table Mood stabilisers in hepatic impairment

Drug	Comments
Carbamazepine[1,2,45–47]	Extensively hepatically metabolised and potent inducer of CYP450 enzymes. Contraindicated in acute liver disease. In chronic stable disease, caution advised. Reduce starting dose by 50%, and titrate up slowly, using plasma levels to guide dosage. Stop if LFTs deteriorate. Associated with hepatitis, cholangitis, cholestatic and hepatocellular jaundice, and hepatic failure (rare). Adverse hepatic effects are most common in the first month of treatment
Lamotrigine[1,2,48]	Manufacturers recommend 50% reduction in initial dose, dose escalation and maintenance dose in moderate hepatic impairment and 75% in severe lamotrigine-induced rash (which can be serious). Extreme caution advised, particularly if co-prescribed with valproate. Elevated LFTs and hepatitis reported
Lithium[1,2,49,50]	Not metabolised so dosage reduction not required as long as renal function is normal. Use serum levels to guide dosage and monitor more frequently if ascites status changes (volume of distribution will change). One case of ascites and one of hyperbilirubinaemia reported over many decades of lithium use worldwide
Valproate[1,2,51–53]	Highly protein bound and hepatically metabolised. Dosage reduction with close monitoring of LFTs in moderate hepatic impairment. Use plasma levels (free levels if possible) to guide dosage. Caution advised. Contraindicated in severe and/or active hepatic impairment. Associated with elevated LFTs and serious hepatotoxicity including fulminant hepatic failure. Mitochondrial disease may be a risk factor. Particularly hepatotoxic in children

Summary – psychotropics in hepatic impairment

Drug group	Recommended drugs
Antipsychotics	**Haloperidol**: low dose or **Sulpiride/amisulpride**: no dosage reduction required if renal function is normal
Antidepressants	**Imipramine**: start with 25 mg/day and titrate slowly (weekly at most) if required or **Paroxetine** or **citalopram**: start at 10 mg if severe hepatic impairment. Titrate slowly (if required) as above
Mood-stablisers	**Lithium**: use plasma levels to guide dosage. Care needed if ascites status changes
Sedatives	**Lorazepam, oxazepam, temazepam**: as short half-life with no active metabolites Use low doses with caution, as sedative drugs can precipitate hepatic encephalopathy **Zopiclone**: 3.75 mg with care in moderate hepatic impairment

References

1. Electronic Medicines Compendium at http//:emc.medicines.org.uk.
2. Drugdex® System. Micromedex Inc., Englewood, Colorado, 2005.
3. Hummer M, Kurz M, Kurzthaler I *et al.* Hepatotoxicity of clozapine. *J Psychopharmacol* 1997; **17**: 314–317.
4. Kellner CH. Toxic hepatitis by clozapine treatment. *Am J Psychiatry* 1993; **150**: 985–986.
5. Thatcher GW. Clozapine induced toxic hepatitis. *Am J Psychiatry* 1995; **152**: 296–297.
6. Amdisen A, Nielsen MS, Dencker SJ *et al.* Zuclopenthixol acetate in viscoleo. *Acta Psychiatr Scand* 1987; **75**: 99–107.
7. Wistedt B, Koskinen T, Thelander S *et al.* Zuclopenthixol decanoate and haloperidol decanoate in chronic schizophrenia: a double-blind multicentre study. *Acta Psychiatr Scand* 1991; **84**: 14–16.
8. Beasley CM, Tollefson GD, Tran PV. Safety of olanzapine. *J Clin Psychiatry* 1997; **58**(Suppl. 10): 13–17.
9. Kolpe M, Ravasia S. Effect of olanzapine on the liver transaminases (Letter). *Can J Psychiatry* 2003; **48**: 210.
10. Jadallah KA, Limauro DI, Colarella AM. Acute hepatocellular-cholestatic liver injury after olanzapine therapy (Letter). *Ann Intern Med* 2003; **138**: 357–358.
11. Tchernichovsky E, Sirota P. Hepatotoxicity, leucopenia and neutropenia associated with olanzapine therapy. *Int J Psychiatry Clin Pract* 2004; **8**: 173–177.
12. Regal R, Billi JE, Glazer HM. Phenothiazine-induced cholestatic jaundice. *Clin Pharm* 1987; **6**: 787–794.
13. Zimmerman HJ, Lewis JH. Drug induced cholestasis. *Med Toxicol* 1987; **2**: 112–160.
14. de Abajo FJ, Montero D, Madurga M *et al.* Acute and clinically relevant drug-induced liver injury: a population based case-control study. *Br J Clin Pharmacol* 2004; **58**: 71–80.
15. Thyrum PT, Wong YW, Yeh C. Single dose pharmacokinetics of quetiapine in subjects with renal or hepatic impairment. *Prog Neuropsychopharmacol Biol Psychiatry* 2000; **24**: 521–533.
16. Nemeroff CB, Kinkead B, Goldstein J. Quetiapine: preclinical studies, pharmacokinetics, drug interactions and dosing. *J Clin Psychiatry* 2002; **63**(Suppl. 13): 5–11.
17. Green B. Focus on quetiapine. *Curr Med Res Opin* 1999; **15**: 145–151.
18. El Hajj I, Sharara AI, Rockey DC. Subfulminant liver failure associated with quetiapine. *Eur J Gastroenterol Hepatol* 2004; **16**: 1415–1418.
19. Cordeiro Q, Elkis H. Pancreatitis and cholestatic hepatitis induced by risperidone. *J Clin Psychopharmacol* 2001; **21**: 529–530.
20. Phillips EJ, Liu BA, Knowles SR. Rapid onset of risperidone induced hepatotoxicity. *Ann Pharmacother* 1998; **32**: 843.
21. Whitworth AB, Liensberger D, Gleischhacker WW. Transient increase of liver enzymes induced by risperidone: two case reports. *J Clin Psychopharmacol* 1999; **19**: 475–476.
22. Holtmann M, Kopf D, Mayer M *et al.* Risperidone-associated steatohepatitis and excessive weight-gain. *Pharmacopsychiatry* 2003; **36**: 206–207.
23. Melzer E, Knobel B. Severe cholestatic jaundice due to sulpiride. *Isr J Med Sci* 1987; **23**: 1259–1260.
24. Ohmoto K, Yamamoto S, Hirokawa M. Symptomatic primary biliary cirrhosis triggered by administration of sulpiride. *Am J Gastroenterol* 1999; **94**: 3660–3661.
25. Schenker S, Bergstrom RF, Wolen RL *et al.* Fluoxetine disposition and elimination in cirrhosis. *Clin Pharm Therapeutics* 1998; **44**: 353–359.
26. Cai Q, Benson MA, Talbot TJ *et al.* Acute hepatitis due to fluoxetine therapy. *Mayo Clin Proc* 1999; **74**: 692–694.
27. Friedenberg FK, Rothstein KD. Hepatitis due to fluoxetine treatment. *Am J Psychiatry* 1996; **153**: 580.
28. Johnston DE, Wheeler DE. Chronic hepatitis related to use of fluoxetine. *Am J Gastroenterol* 1997; **92**: 1225–1226.
29. Hale AS. New antidepressants: use in high-risk patients. *J Clin Psychiatry* 1993; **54**(Suppl. 8): 61–70.
30. Benbow SJ, Gill G. Paroxetine and hepatotoxicity. *BMJ* 1997; **314**: 1387.
31. Odeh M, Misselevech I, Boss JH *et al.* Severe hepatotoxicity with jaundice associated with paroxetine. *Am J Gastroenterol* 2001; **96**: 2494–2496.
32. Dunbar GC. An interim overview of the safety and tolerability of paroxetine. *Acta Psychiatr Scand* 1989; **80**(Suppl. 350): 135–137.
33. Kuhs H, Rudolf GAE. A double blind study of the comparative antidepressant effect of paroxetine and amitriptyline. *Acta Psychiatr Scand* 1989; **80**(Suppl. 350): 145–146.
34. DeBree H, Van der Schoot JB, Post LC. Fluvoxamine maleate: disposition in man. *Eur J Drug Metab Pharmacokinet* 1983; **8**: 175–179.
35. Green BH. Fluvoxamine and hepatic function. *Br J Psychiatry* 1998; **153**: 130–131.
36. Milne RJ, Goa KL. Citalopram: a review of its pharmacodynamic and pharmacokinetic properties, and therapeutic potential in depressive illness. *Drugs* 1991; **41**: 450–477.
37. Lopez-Torres E, Lucena MI, Seoane J *et al.* Hepatotoxicity related to citalopram (Letter). *Am J Psychiatry* 2004; **161**: 923–924.
38. Committee on Safety of Medicines. Lofepramine (Gamanil) and abnormal blood tests of liver function. *Curr Probl* 1988; **23**: 2.
39. Cardona X, Avila A, Castellanos P. Venlafaxine-associated hepatitis. *Ann Intern Med* 2000; **132**: 417.
40. Gomez GE, Salmeron JM, Mas A. Phenelzine induced fulminant hepatic failure. *Ann Intern Med* 1996; **124**: 692–693.
41. Bonkovsky HL, Blanchette PL, Schned AR. Severe liver injury due to phenelzine with unique hepatic deposition of extracellular material. *Am J Med* 1986; **80**: 689–692.
42. Stoeckel K, Pfefen JP, Mayersohn M *et al.* Absorption and disposition of moclobemide in patients with advanced age or reduced liver or kidney function. *Acta Psychiatr Scand* 1990; **360**: 94–97.

Special groups

43. Timmings P, Lamont D. Intrahepatic cholestasis associated with moclobemide leading to death. *Lancet* 1996; **347**: 762–763.
44. Tran A, Laneury JP, Duchene P *et al.* Pharmacokinetics of reboxetine in patients with hepatic impairment. *Clin Drug Invest* 2000; **9**: 473–477.
45. El-Serag HB, Johnston DE. Carbamazepine-associated severe bile duct injury. *Am J Gastroenterol* 1999; **92**: 526–527.
46. Forbes GM, Jeffrey GP, Shilkin KB *et al.* Carbamazepine hepatotoxicity: another cause of vanishing bile duct syndrome. *Gastroenterology* 1992; **102**: 1385–1388.
47. Morales-Diaz M, Pinilla-Roa E, Ruiz I. Suspected carbamazepine-induced hepatotoxicity. *Pharmacotherapy* 1999; **19**: 252–255.
48. Sauve G, Bresson-Hadni S, Prost P *et al.* Acute hepatitis after lamotrigine administration. *Dig Dis Sci* 2000; **45**: 1874–1877.
49. Cohen LS, Cohen DE. Lithium-induced hyperbilirubinemia in an adolescent. *J Clin Psychopharmacol* 1991; **11**: 274–275.
50. Hazelwood RE. Ascites: a side effect of lithium? *Am J Psychiatry* 1981; **138**: 257.
51. Krahenbuhl S, Brandner S, Kleinle S *et al.* Mitochondrial diseases represent a risk factor for valproate-induced fulminant liver failure. *Liver* 2000; **20**: 346–348.
52. Klotz U, Rapp T, Muller WA *et al.* Disposition of valproate acid in patients with liver disease. *Eur J Clin Pharmacol* 1978; **13**: 550–560.
53. Pinkston R, Walker LA. Multiorgan system failure caused by valproic acid toxicity. *Am J Emerg Med* 1997; **15**: 504–506.

Special groups

Prescribing in the elderly

General principles

The pharmacokinetics and pharmacodynamics of most drugs are altered to an important extent in the elderly. These changes in drug action must be taken into account if treatment is to be effective and adverse effects minimised. The elderly often have a number of concurrent illnesses and may require treatment with several drugs. This leads to a greater chance of problems arising because of drug interactions and to a higher rate of drug-induced problems in general[1]. It is reasonable to assume that all drugs are more likely to cause adverse effects in the elderly than in younger patients.

How drugs affect the ageing body (altered pharmacodynamics)

As we age, control over reflex actions such as blood pressure and temperature regulation is reduced. Receptors may become more sensitive. This results in an increased incidence and severity of side-effects. For example, drugs that decrease gut motility are more likely to cause constipation (e.g. TCAs and opioids) and drugs that affect blood pressure are more likely to cause falls (e.g. TCAs and diuretics). The elderly are more sensitive to the effects of benzodiazepines than younger adults. Therapeutic response can also be delayed; the elderly may take longer to respond to antidepressants than younger adults[2].

How the ageing body affects drug therapy (altered pharmacokinetics)[3]

ABSORPTION
Gut motility decreases with age, as does secretion of gastric acid. This leads to drugs being absorbed more slowly, resulting in a slower onset of action. The same *amount* of drug is absorbed as in a younger adult.

DISTRIBUTION
The elderly have more body fat, less body water and less albumin than younger adults. This leads to an increased volume of distribution and a longer duration of action for some fat-soluble drugs (e.g. diazepam), higher concentrations of some drugs at the site of action (e.g. digoxin) and a reduction in the amount of drug bound to albumin (increased amounts of active 'free drug'; e.g. warfarin, phenytoin).

METABOLISM
The majority of drugs are hepatically metabolised. Liver size is reduced in the elderly, but in the absence of hepatic disease or significantly reduced hepatic blood flow, there is no significant reduction in metabolic capacity. The magnitude of pharmacokinetic interactions is unlikely to be altered but the pharmacodynamic consequences of these interactions may be amplified.

EXCRETION
Renal function declines with age: 35% of function is lost by the age of 65 years and 50% by the age of 80.

More is lost if there are concurrent medical problems such as heart disease, diabetes or hypertension. Measurement of serum creatinine or urea can be misleading in the elderly because muscle mass is reduced, so less creatinine is produced. Creatinine clearance is the only accurate measure of renal function in this age group. It is best to assume that all elderly patients have at most two-thirds of normal renal function.

Most drugs are eventually excreted by the kidney. A few do not undergo biotransformation first. Lithium and sulpiride are important examples. Drugs primarily excreted via the kidney will accumulate in the elderly, leading to toxicity and side-effects. Dosage reduction is likely to be required (see page 217 *et seq.* for full review of renal effects of psychotropics).

Drug interactions

Some drugs have a narrow therapeutic index (a small increase in dose can cause toxicity and a small reduction in dose can cause a loss of therapeutic action). The most commonly prescribed ones are: digoxin, warfarin, theophylline, phenytoin and lithium. Changes in the way these drugs are handled in the elderly and the greater chance of interaction with other drugs mean that toxicity and therapeutic failure are more likely. These drugs can be used safely but extra care must be taken and blood levels should be measured where possible.

Some drugs inhibit or induce hepatic metabolising enzymes. Important examples include the SSRIs, erythromycin and carbamazepine (see page 154 for further information). This may lead to the metabolism of another drug being altered. Many drug interactions occur through this mechanism. Details of individual interactions and their consequences can be found in Appendix 1 of the *BNF*. Most can be predicted by a sound knowledge of pharmacology.

Reducing drug-related risk

Adherence to the following principles will reduce drug-related morbidity and mortality:

- Use drugs only when absolutely necessary.
- Avoid, if possible, drugs that block α_1 adrenoceptors, have anticholinergic side-effects, are very sedative, have a long half-life or are potent inhibitors of hepatic metabolising enzymes.
- Start with a low dose and increase slowly but do not undertreat. Some drugs still require the full adult dose.
- Try not to treat the side-effects of one drug with another drug. Find a better-tolerated alternative.
- Keep therapy simple; that is, once daily administration whenever possible.

Administering medicines in foodstuffs[4,5]

Sometimes patients may refuse treatment with medicines, even when such treatment is thought to be in their best interests. Where the patient has a mental illness or has capacity, the Mental Health Act should be used, but if the patient lacks capacity, this option may not be desirable. Medicines should never be administered covertly to elderly patients with dementia without a full discussion with the MDT and the patient's relatives. The outcome of this discussion should be clearly documented in the patient's clinical notes. Medicine should be administered covertly only if the clear and express purpose is to reduce suffering for the patient.

References

1. Royal College of Physicians. Medication for older people. Summary and recommendations of a report of a working party of the Royal College of Physicians. *J R Coll Physicians Lond* 1997; 3: 254–257.
2. Paykel ES, Raman R, Cooper Z *et al.* Residual symptoms after partial remission: an important outcome in depression. *Psychol Med* 1995; 25: 1171–1180.
3. Mayersohn M. Special pharmacokinetic considerations in the elderly. In: Evans WE, Schentag JJ, Jusko WJ (eds). *Applied Therapeutics: principles of therapeutic drug monitoring.* Spokane, WA: Applied Therapeutics, 1986, pp. 229–293.
4. Treloar A, Philpot M, Beats B. Concealing medication in patients' food. *Lancet* 2001; 357: 62–64.
5. Treloar A, Beck S, Paton C. Administering medicines to patients with dementia and other organic cognitive syndromes. *Adv Psychiatr Treat* 2001; 7: 444–450.

Further reading

National Service Framework for Older People. London: Department of Health, 2001.

Alzheimer's disease

Acetylcholinesterase (AChE) inhibitors

Four inhibitors of AChE are currently licensed in the UK for the treatment of Alzheimer's disease: tacrine, donepezil, rivastigmine and galantamine. Tacrine is very poorly tolerated and has been superseded by the other three drugs. Cholinesterase inhibitors differ in pharmacological action: donepezil and galantamine are selective inhibitors of AChE; rivastigmine affects both AChE and butyrylcholinesterase (BuChE); donepezil and rivastigmine are relatively selective for AChE in the brain; and galantamine also affects nicotinic receptors[1]. To date, these differences have not been shown to result in differences in efficacy or tolerability.

All three drugs seem to have broadly similar clinical effects, as measured with the Mini Mental State Examination (MMSE), a 30-point basic evaluation of cognitive function and the Alzheimer's Disease Assessment Scale – cognitive subscale (ADAS-cog), a 70 point evaluation largely of cognitive dysfunction. Major trials of donepezil[2–4] suggest an advantage over placebo of 2.5–3.1 points on the ADAS-cog scale. For rivastigmine[5,6], the advantage is 2.6–4.9 points and for galantamine[7–9] 2.9–3.9. Estimates of the number needed to treat (NNT) (improvement of >4 points ADAS cog) range from 4 to 12. Direct comparisons of anticholinesterases have given equivocal results – a Pfizer-sponsored study suggested the superiority of donepezil to galantamine[10]; a Janssen-sponsored study suggested the converse[11].

All the above results need to be interpreted with caution, especially as so few head-to-head studies have been published. Alzheimer's disease is usually characterised by inexorable cognitive decline, which is generally well quantified by tests such as ADAS-cog and MMSE. The average rate of decline is 4–6 points on the ADAS-cog over 1 year, but the range is large. It is therefore difficult to accurately assess treatment effect in individual patients. The effect of anticholinesterases is, on average, to improve modestly cognitive function for several months (scores return to baseline after about 9–12 months)[4,8].

This average incorporates and to some extent conceals three groups of patients: 'non-responders', who continue to decline at the anticipated rate; 'non-decliners', who neither improve significantly nor decline; and 'improvers', who improve to a clinically relevant extent. This last group is usually defined as those who show a >4 point improvement on ADAS-cog. In trials of around 6 months, approximately 25–35% of those on anticholinesterases will be classified as 'improvers' compared with around 15–25% on placebo. Around 55–70% of patients treated with anticholinesterases will show no cognitive decline during a 5–6-month trial[6,8] – about 20% more patients in absolute terms than those on placebo. Note that, for the most part, results of trials so far conducted relate only to patients with mild-to-moderate Alzheimer's disease (those giving a score of 10–26 on MMSE), although data on those with more severe illness are encouraging[12].

Taking into account trial differences and all assessments made, available anticholinesterases can be said to have broadly similar efficacy against cognitive symptoms in clinical trials. Any minor differences observed may be accounted for by differences in trial design or patient characteristics. In the absence of sufficient 'head-to-head' studies, the available drugs should be assumed to have equal efficacy. Overall, in a cohort of patients given anticholinesterases at optimal doses under clinical trial conditions, approximately one-third would be expected to improve over 6 months and around another third would be expected not to deteriorate. These observations appear to be broadly reflected in practice.

Other effects

Anticholinesterases may also affect non-cognitive aspects of Alzheimer's disease. For example, they seem to have useful psychotropic activity against neuropsychiatric symptoms[13–15]. These drugs may also lower caregiver burden[16] and improve patients' abilities with daily activities[17]. Differential effects for different drugs have yet to be demonstrated. However, anticholinesterases appear to have minimal effects on time to institutionalisation or progression of disability[18].

Special groups

Tolerability

Drug tolerability may differ between anticholinesterases, but, again, in the absence of sufficient direct comparisons, it is difficult to draw cogent conclusions. Overall tolerability can be broadly evaluated by reference to the numbers withdrawing from clinical trials. Withdrawal rates in trials of donepezil[2,3] ranged from 4% to 16% (placebo 1–7%). With rivastigmine[5,6], rates ranged from 7% to 29% (placebo 7%) and with galantamine[7–9] from 7% to 23% (placebo 7–9%). (All figures relate to withdrawals specifically associated with adverse effects.)

Tolerability seems to be affected by speed of titration and, perhaps less clearly, by dose. Most adverse effects occurred in trials during titration, and slower titration schedules are recommended in clinical use. This may mean that these drugs are equally well tolerated in practice.

Dosing

Different titration schedules do, to some extent, differentiate anticholinesterases. **Donepezil** is perhaps easiest to use, starting at 5 mg/day and increasing 'if necessary' (however this might be determined) to 10 mg after a month. **Rivastigmine** is taken twice daily, starting at 1.5 mg b.d. and increasing to 3 mg b.d. after 2 weeks or more and then to 4.5 mg b.d. after a further 2 weeks (maximum 6 mg b.d.). With **galantamine**, the starting dose is 4 mg twice daily, increasing to 8 mg twice daily after 4 weeks and then to 12 mg b.d., if necessary, 4 weeks later. Thus, both rivastigmine and galantamine need to be given twice daily and have prolonged titration schedules. These factors may be important to prescribers, patients and carers.

Interactions

Potential for interaction may also differentiate currently available cholinesterase inhibitors. Donepezil[19] and galantamine[20] are metabolised by cytochromes 2D6 and 3A4 and so drug levels may be altered by other drugs affecting the function of these enzymes. Anticholinesterases themselves may also interfere with the metabolism of other drugs, although this is perhaps a theoretical consideration. Rivastigmine has almost no potential for interaction since it is metabolised at the site of action and does not affect hepatic cytochromes. Overall, rivastigmine appears to be least likely to cause problematic drug interactions, a factor that may be important in an elderly population subject to polypharmacy.

Adverse effects

When adverse effects occur, they are largely predictable: excess cholinergic stimulation leads to nausea, vomiting, dizziness, insomnia and diarrhoea[21]. Urinary incontinence has also been reported[22]. There appear to be no important differences between drugs in respect to type or frequency of adverse events, although clinical trials do suggest a relatively lower frequency of adverse events for donepezil. This may simply be a reflection of the aggressive titration schedules used in trials of other drugs.

NICE recommendations[23]

Using a protocol like that suggested by NICE (below) may mean that, of a cohort of patients referred for treatment, only three-quarters may be considered suitable for treatment, and only one-third of these may continue treatment for a year or more[24]. In contrast, in the artificial environment of a clinical trial, nearly half of patients continued for 2 years or more[25]. (Note that long-term, double-blind trials may underestimate real-life benefits of treatment because non-responders or poor responders are continued on drug treatment[18].)

Summary of NICE guidance on anticholinesterases

- Anticholinesterase drugs may be prescribed for those with Alzheimer's disease with a MMSE score of >12 points. *Note that Alzheimer's disease is difficult to diagnose accurately during life. Mixed cause dementias are common and there is no evidence that the modest benefits offered by AChE inhibitors are specific to Alzheimer's disease.*
- Diagnosis must be made in a specialist clinic.
- Assessments of cognitive functioning and activities of daily living should be made before starting drug treatment.
- Only specialists should initiate treatment.
- Only those likely to comply with drug treatment should be considered.
- Further assessments should be made 2–4 months after starting treatment. If MMSE scores indicate no deterioration or improvement and there is evidence of global or functional improvement, treatment should continue.
- Those remaining on drug treatment should thereafter be assessed at 6-monthly intervals. Anticholinesterases should not normally be used in patients where MMSE scores fall before 12 points. (Note, however, that abrupt discontinuation of AChE inhibitors in patients whose MMSE score drops below this level is not advised – a careful trial of graduated discontinuation is preferred.)

Memantine

Memantine is licensed in the UK for the treatment of moderately severe to severe Alzheimer's disease. It acts as an antagonist at *N*-methyl-D-aspartate (NMDA) receptors, an action which, in theory, may be neuroprotective and thus disease modifying[26]. Memantine appears to be well tolerated[27,28] and clinical experience is encouraging. Trials in severe dementia[29] and vascular dementia[30] suggest an advantage over placebo of around 2 points on the ADAS-cog scale and NNTs (improvement) of 3–8[31]. Improvement was also seen in other domains of functioning.

Early data suggest memantine is effective in mild to moderate Alzheimer's disease with an advantage over placebo of 1.9 points on ADAS-cog[32].

Ginkgo biloba

Ginkgo biloba has been widely touted as a cognitive enhancer and there are some experimental data to suggest that it has neuroprotective effects[33]. There are also well-controlled human trial data which suggest that *G. biloba* is effective in mild to moderate Alzheimer's disease with an advantage over placebo of around 1.4 points on ADAS-cog[34]. The drug is widely used in Germany but less so elsewhere.

Combination treatment

A wide range of drug combinations have been evaluated but few have involved more modern treatments such as anticholinestrases and memantine[35], perhaps the most obvious combination to use. None the less, a combination of memantine and donepezil has been shown to be more effective than donepezil in patients with moderate to severe Alzhemier's disease[36]. The combination appears to be well tolerated[36,37].

Special groups

Vascular dementia

None of the currently avaliable drugs are formally licensed in the UK for vascular dementia. There is growing evidence that donepezil[38,39], rivastigmine[40], galantamine[41,42] and memantine[43] are effective in vascular dementia. Overall effect seems to be similar or slightly less than that seen in Alzheimer's disease. Note, however, that it is impossible to diagnose with certainty vascular or Alzheimer's dementia and much dementia has mixed causation.

Table Summary – anticholinesterases in Alzheimer's disease

Drug	Starting dose	Usual treatment dose	Adverse effects	Costs (1-month treatment) at usual dose
Donepezil	5 mg daily	10 mg daily	Nausea Vomiting Insomnia Diarrhoea	£103
Rivastigmine	1.5 mg b.d.	6 mg b.d.	Nausea Vomiting Insomnia Diarrhoea	£73
Galantamine	4 mg b.d.	12 mg b.d.	Nausea Vomiting Insomnia Diarrhoea	£90
Memantine	5 mg daily	20 mg daily	Hallucinations Dizziness Confusion	£79

References

1. Weinstock M. Selectivity of cholinesterase inhibition: clinical implications for the treatment of Alzheimer's disease. *CNS Drugs* 1999; **12**: 307–323.
2. Rogers SL, Doody RS, Mohs RC *et al.* Donepezil improves cognition and global function in Alzheimer disease: a 15-week, double-blind, placebo-controlled study. *Arch Intern Med* 1998; **158**: 1021–1031.
3. Rogers SL, Farlow MR, Doody RS *et al.* A 24-week, double-blind, placebo-controlled trial of donepezil in patients with Alzheimer's disease. *Neurology* 1998; **50**: 136–145.
4. Rogers SL, Friedhoff LT. Long-term efficacy and safety of donepezil in the treatment of Alzheimer's disease: an interim analysis of the results of a US multicentre open label extension study. *Eur Neuropsychopharmacol* 1998; **8**: 67–75.
5. Corey-Bloom J, Anand R, Veach J. A randomized trial evaluating the efficacy and safety of ENA 713 (rivastigmine tartrate), a new acetylcholinesterase inhibitor, in patients with mild to moderately severe Alzheimer's disease. *Int J Geriatr Psychopharmacol* 1998; **1**: 55–65.
6. Rösler M, Anand R, Cicin-Sain A *et al.* Efficacy and safety of rivastigmine in patients with Alzheimer's disease: international randomised controlled trial. *BMJ* 1999; **318**: 633–640.
7. Tariot PN, Solomon PR, Morris JC *et al.* A 5-month, randomized, placebo-controlled trial of galantamine in AD. *Neurology* 2000; **54**: 2269–2276.
8. Raskind MA, Peskind ER, Wessel T *et al.* 6-month randomized, placebo-controlled trial with a 6-month extension. *Neurology* 2000; **54**: 2261–2268.
9. Wilcock GK, Lilienfeld S, Gaens E. Efficacy and safety of galantamine in patients with mild to moderate Alzheimer's disease: multicentre randomised controlled trial. *BMJ* 2000; **321**: 1445–1449.
10. Jones RW, Soininen H, Hager K *et al.* A multinational, randomised, 12-week study comparing the effects of donepezil and galantamine in patients with mild to moderate Alzheimer's disease. *Int J Geriatr Psychiatry* 2004; **19**: 58–67.
11. Wilcock G, Howe I, Coles H *et al.* A long-term comparison of galantamine and donepezil in the treatment of Alzheimer's disease. *Drugs Aging* 2003; **20**: 777–789.
12. Birks JS, Harvey R. Donepezil for dementia due to Alzheimer's disease. *Cochrane Database Syst Rev*, 2003, Issue 3. Art. No.: CD001190. DOI: 10.1002/14651858.CD001190.

Special groups

13. Cummings JL, Askin-Edgar S. Evidence for psychotropic effects of acetylcholinesterase inhibitors. *CNS Drugs* 2000; **13**: 385–395.
14. Weiner MF, Martin-Cook K, Foster BM *et al.* Effects of donepezil on emotional/behavioral symptoms in Alzheimer's disease patients. *J Clin Psychiatry* 2000; **61**: 487–492.
15. Blesa R. Galantamine: therapeutic effects beyond cognition. *Dement Geriatr Cogn Disord* 2000; **11**(Suppl. 1): 28–34.
16. Gauthier S, Lussier I and the TriAD™ Study Group. An open-label trial to assess the effectiveness of donepezil treatment on caregiver burden in Alzheimer's disease – an interim report. Poster presented at the Ninth Congress of the International Psychogeriatric Association, 15–20 August, Vancouver, Canada, 1999.
17. Winblad B, Engedal K, Soininen H *et al.* Donepezil enhances global function, cognition and activities of daily living compared with placebo in a one-year, double-blind trial in patients with mild to moderate Alzheimer's disease. Poster presented at the Ninth Congress of the International Psychogeriatric Association, 15–20 August, 1, Vancouver, Canada, 1999.
18. AD2000 Collaborative Group. Long-term donepezil treatment in 565 patients with Alzheimer's disease (AD2000): randomised double-blind trial. *Lancet* 2004; **363**: 2105–2115.
19. Dooley M, Lamb H. Donepezil. *Drugs Aging* 2000; **16**: 199–226.
20. Scott LJ, Goa KL. Galantamine: a review of its use in Alzheimer's disease. *Drugs* 2000; **60**: 1095–1122.
21. Dunn NR, Pearce GL, Shakir SAW. Adverse effects associated with the use of donepezil in general practice in England. *J Psychopharmacol* 2000; **14**: 406–408.
22. Hashimoto M, Imamura T, Tanimukai S *et al.* Urinary incontinence: an unrecognised adverse effect with donepezil. *Lancet* 2000; **356**: 568.
23. National Institute for Clinical Excellence. Guidance on the use of donepezil, rivastigmine and galantamine for the treatment of Alzheimer's disease. Technology Appraisal Guidance No. 19, 2001.
24. Matthews HP, Korbey J, Wilkinson DG *et al.* Donepezil in Alzheimer's disease: eighteen month results from Southampton Memory Clinic. *Int J Geriatr Psychiatry* 2000; **15**: 713–720.
25. Ieni JR, Perdomo CA, Pratt RD. Safety of donepezil in extended treatment of Alzheimer's disease. *Eur Neuropsychopharmacol* 1999; **9**(Suppl. 5): S328.
26. Danysz W, Parsons CG, Möbius J-J *et al.* Neuroprotective and symptomatological action of memantine relevant for Alzheimer's disease – a unified glutamatergic hypothesis on the mechanism of action. *Neurotox Res* 1999; **2**: 85–97.
27. Parsons CG, Danysz W, Quack G. Memantine is a clinically well tolerated N-methyl-D-aspartate (NMDA) receptor antagonist – a review of preclinical data. *Neuropharmacology* 1999; **38**: 735–767.
28. Reisberg B, Doody R, Stöffler A *et al.* Memantine in moderate-to-severe Alzheimer's disease. *N Engl J Med* 2003; **348**: 1333–1341.
29. Winblad B, Poritis N. Memantine in severe dementia: results of the 9M-Best study (benefit and efficacy in severely demented patients during treatment with memantine). *Int J Geriatr Psychiatry* 1999; **14**: 135–146.
30. Orgogozo J-M, Rigaud A-S, Stöffler A *et al.* Efficacy and safety of memantine in patients with mild to moderate vascular dementia: a randomized, placebo-controlled trial (MMM 300). *Stroke* 2002; **33**: 1834–1839.
31. Livingston G, Katona C. The place of memantine in the treatment of Alzheimer's disease: a number needed to treat analysis. *Int J Geriatr Psychiatry* 2004; **19**: 919–925.
32. Peskind ER, Potkin SG, Pomara N *et al.* Memantine monotherapy is effective and safe for the treatment of mild to moderate Alzheimer's disease: a randomized controlled trial. Presented at the 17th Congress of the European College of Neuropsychopharmacology, 9–13 October 2004, Stockholm, Sweden.
33. Ahlemeyer B, Krieglstein J. Pharmacological studies supporting the therapeutic use of *Ginkgo biloba* extract for Alzheimer's disease. *Pharmacopsychiatry* 2003; **36**: S8–S14.
34. Kanowski S, Hoerr R. *Ginkgo biloba* extract Egb 761 in dementia: intent-to-treat analyses of a 24-week, multi-center, double-blind, placebo-controlled, randomized trial. *Pharmacopsychiatry* 2003; **36**: 297–303.
35. Schnitt B, Bernhardt T, Moeller HJ *et al.* Combination therapy in Alzheimer's disease. *CNS Drugs* 2004; **18**: 827–844.
36. Tariot PN, Farlow MR, Grossberg GT *et al.* Memantine treatment in patients with moderate to severe Alzheimer disease already receiving donepezil: a randomized controlled trial. *JAMA* 2004; **291**: 317–324.
37. Hartmann S, Mobius HJ. Tolerability of memantine in combination with cholinesterase inhibitors in dementia therapy. *Int Clin Psychopharmacol* 2003; **18**: 81–85.
38. Black S, Roman GC, Geldmacher DS *et al.* Efficacy and tolerability of donepezil in vascular dementia positive results of a 24-week, multicenter, international, randomized, placebo-controlled clinical trial. *Stroke* 2003; **34**: 2323–2332.
39. Wilkinson D, Helme R, Taubman K *et al.* Donepezil in vascular dementia: a randomized, placebo-controlled study. *Neurology* 2003; **61**: 479–486.
40. Moretti R, Torre P, Antonello RM *et al.* Rivastigmine superior to aspirin plus nimodipine in subcortical vascular dementia. An open, 16-month, comparative study. *J Clin Pract* 2004; **58**: 346–353.
41. Small G, Erkinjunitti T, Kurz A *et al.* Galantamine in the treatment of cognitive decline in patients with vascular dementia or Alzheimer's disease with cerebrovascular disease. *CNS Drugs* 2003; **17**: 905–914.
42. Kurz AF, Erkinjunitti T, Small GW *et al.* Long-term safety and cognitive effects of galantamine in the treatment of probable vascular dementia or Alzheimer's disease with cerebrovascular disease. *Eur J Neurol* 2003; **10**: 633–640.
43. Wilcock G, Mobius HJ, Stoffler A. A double-blind, placebo-controlled multicentre study of memantine in mild to moderate vascular dementia (MMM500). *Int Clin Psychopharmacol* 2002; **17**: 297–305.

Special groups

Further reading

Areosa Sastre A, Sherriff F. Memantine for dementia. In: *The Cochrane Library*, Issue 1. Oxford: Update Software, 2003.
Loy C, Schneider L. Galantamine for Alzheimer's disease. *Cochrane Database of Syst Rev*, 2004, Issue 4. Art. No.: CD001747. DOI: 10.1002/14651858.CD001747.pub2.

Behavioural disturbance in dementia

Behavioural symptoms are common in patients with dementia but, for a variety of reasons, treatment is not well informed by properly conducted studies.

Antipsychotics

It has been strongly suggested that neither risperidone nor olanzapine should be used to treat behavioural symptoms in dementia[1]. Both have been linked to an increased rate of cerebrovascular events compared with placebo. These observations need to be considered carefully: there are no similar data for other drugs, and comparisons with such drugs suggest no increased risk with olanzapine or risperidone[2,3] and perhaps a lower risk than with haloperidol[4]. Conventional antipsychotics may also worsen cognitive decline in dementia[5].

In general, antipsychotics are effective for behavioural symptoms of dementia[6-9], and atypicals are preferred[10] despite rather weak evidence in their favour[11]. Since restrictions were imposed on the use of risperidone and olanzapine, quetiapine has become widely used at a dose of 50–100 mg daily. However, evidence to support quetiapine's efficacy in dementia[9] is much weaker than that for risperidone or olanzapine.

Others

Donepezil[12,13], rivastigmime[14,15] and galantamine[16] all seem to be effective in reducing behavioural disturbance in dementia. Their effect seems apparent only after several weeks of treatment. Anecdotal evidence suggests memantine has a similar effect.

Benzodiazepines and trazodone[17] are widely used but poorly supported. SSRIs are of doubtful efficacy[18,19]. Mood-stabilisers have also been used[20,21]. One RCT of valproate that included an open-label extension found valproate to be ineffective in controlling symptoms. Seven of the 39 patients enrolled died during the 12-week extension phase[22].

Summary

The evidence base available to guide treatment in this area is insufficient to allow specific recommendations on drug choice. Whichever drug is chosen, the '3T' approach should be followed:

Target symptoms requiring treatment.

Titrate drug dose from a low starting dose.

Time-limit prescriptions so that ineffective treatment is not unnecessarily continued.

Special groups

References

1. www.mhra.gov.uk.
2. Herrmann N, Mamdani M, Lanctot KL. Atypical antipsychotics and risk of cerebrovascular accidents. *Am J Psychiatry* 2004; **161**: 1113–1115.
3. Gill SS, Rochon PA, Herrman N *et al.* Atypical antipsychotic drugs and risk of ischaemic stroke: population based retrospective cohort study. *Br Med J* 2005; **330**: 445–448.
4. Nasrallah HA, White T, Nasrallah A. Lower mortality in geriatric patients receiving risperidone and olanzapine versus haloperidol preliminary analysis of retrospective data. *Am J Geriatr Psychiatry* 2004; **12**: 437–439.

5. McShane R, Keene J, Gedling K et al. Do neuroleptic drugs hasten cognitive decline in dementia? Prospective study with necropsy follow up. BMJ 1997; 314: 266–270.

6. Bhana N, Spencer CM. Risperidone: a review of its use in the management of the behavioural and psychological symptoms of dementia. Drugs Aging 2000; 16: 451–471.

7. Street JS, Clark WS, Gannon KS et al. Olanzapine treatment of psychotic and behavioural symptoms in patients with Alzheimer's disease in nursing care facilities. Arch Gen Psychiatry 2000; 57: 968–976.

8. Devanand DP, Marder K, Michaels KS et al. A randomized, placebo-controlled dose-comparison trial of haloperidol for psychosis and disruptive behaviours in Alzheimer's disease. Am J Psychiatry 1998; 155: 1512–1520.

9. McManus DQ, Arvanitis LA, Kowalcyk BB. Quetiapine, a novel antipsychotic: experience in elderly patients with psychotic disorders. J Clin Psychiatry 1999; 60: 292–298.

10. Alexopoulos GS, Streim J, Carpenter D et al. The expert consensus guideline series using antipsychotic agents in older patients. J Clin Psychiatry 2004; 65: Suppl. 2.

11. Lee PE, Gill SS, Freedman M et al. Atypical antipsychotic drugs in the treatment of behavioural and psychological symptoms of dementia: systematic review. BMJ 2004; 329(7457): 75–79.

12. Terao T, Shimomura T, Nakamura J. Can donepezil be considered a mild antipsychotic in dementia treatment? A report of donepezil use in 6 patients. J Clin Psychiatry 2003; 64: 1392–1393.

13. Weiner MF, Martin-Cook K, Foster BM et al. Effects of donepezil on emotional/behavioural symptoms in Alzheimer's disease patients. J Clin Psychiatry 2000; 61: 487–492.

14. Finkel SI. Effects of rivastigmine on behavioural and psychological symptoms of dementia in Alzheimer's disease. Clin Ther 2004; 26: 980–990.

15. Rosler M, Retz W, Retz-Juninger PR et al. Effects of two-year treatment with the cholinesterase inhibitor rivastigmine on behavioural symptoms in Alzheimer's disease. Behav Neurol 1998/1999; 11: 211–216.

16. Cummings JL, Schneider L, Tariot PN et al. Reduction of behavioural disturbances and caregiver distress by galantamine in patients with Alzheimer's disease. Am J Psychiatry 2004; 161: 532–538.

17. Martinon-Torres G, Fioravanti M, Grimley EJ. Trazodone for agitation in dementia. Cochrane Database Syst Rev 2004; (4): CD004990.

18. Deakin JB, Rahman S, Nestor PJ et al. Paroxetine does not improve symptoms and impairs cognition in frontotemporal dementia: a double-blind randomized controlled trial. Psychopharmacology 2004; 172. 400–408.

19. Finkel SI, Mintzer JE, Dysken M et al. A randomized, placebo-controlled study of the efficacy and safety of sertraline in the treatment of the behavioural manifestations of Alzheimer's disease in outpatients treated with donepezil. Int J Geriatr Psychiatry 2004; 19: 9–18.

20. Lonergan ET, Cameron M, Luxenberg J. Valproic acid for agitation in dementia. Cochrane Database Syst Rev 2004; (2): CD003945.

21. Tariot PN, Erb R, Podgorski CA et al. Efficacy and tolerability of carbamazepine for agitation and aggression in dementia. Am J Psychiatry 1998; 155: 54–61.

22. Sival RC, Duivenvoorden HJ, Jansen PAF et al. Sodium valproate in aggressive behaviour in dementia: a 12 week open label follow-up study. Int J Geriatr Psychiatry 2004; 19: 203–312.

Further reading

Ballard C, Margallo-Lana M, Juszczak E et al. Quetiapine and rivastigmine and cognitive decline in Alzheimer's disease: randomised double-blind placebo controlled trial. BMJ 2005; doi: 10.1136/bmj.38369.459988.8F.

Royal College of Psychiatrists. Atypical antipsychotics and BPSD. Atypical Antipsychotics Prescribing Update v4C at www.rcpsych.ac.uk/college/faculty/oap.

Special groups

Parkinson's disease

Parkinson's disease is a progressive, degenerative neurological disorder characterised by resting tremor, cogwheel rigidity, bradykinesia and postural instability. The prevalence of co-morbid psychiatric disorders is high. Approximately 25% will suffer from major depression at some point during the course of their illness, a further 25% from milder forms of depression, 25% from anxiety spectrum disorders, 25% from psychosis and 25–40% will develop dementia[1]. While depression and anxiety can occur at any time, psychosis, dementia and also delirium are more prevalent in the later stages of the illness. Close co-operation between the psychiatrist and neurologist is required to optimise treatment for this group of patients.

Depression

Depression in Parkinson's disease predicts greater cognitive decline, deterioration in functioning and progression of motor symptoms[2]. Pre-existing dementia is an established risk factor for the development of depression.

| **Recommendations for treatment**	
Step	**Intervention**
1	Exclude/treat organic causes such as hypothyroidism (the prevalence of which is higher in Parkinson's disease[2]).
2	**SSRI**s are considered to be first-line treatment. Some patients may experience a worsening of motor symptoms although the absolute risk is low[3]. Care must be taken when combining SSRIs with selegiline, as the risk of serotonin syndrome is increased[2]. TCAs are generally poorly tolerated because of their anticholinergic (can worsen cognitive problems; constipation) and alpha-blocking effects (can worsen symptoms of autonomic dysfunction).
3	Consider **ECT**. Depression and motor symptoms generally respond well[2] but the risk of inducing delirium is high[4], particularly in patients with pre-existing cognitive impairment.
4	Consider augmentation with dopamine agonists/releasers such as amantadine[5] or pramiprexole[2].
5	Follow the algorithm for treatment-resistant depression (see page 150) from this point. Be aware of the increased propensity for side-effects and drug interactions in this patient group.

Psychosis

Psychosis in Parkinson's disease is often characterised by visual hallucinations. Auditory hallucinations and delusions occur far less frequently[6]. Psychosis and dementia frequently co-exist. Having one predicts the development of the other[7]. Sleep disorders are also an established risk factor for the development of psychosis[1].

Abnormalities in dopamine, serotonin and acetylcholine neurotransmission have all been implicated, but the exact aetiology of Parkinson's disease psychosis is poorly understood. In the majority

308

of patients, psychotic symptoms are thought to be secondary to dopaminergic medication rather than part of Parkinson's disease itself. From the limited data available, anticholinergics and dopamine agonists seem to be associated with a higher risk of inducing psychosis than levodopa or COMT inhibitors[6]. Psychosis is a major contributor to caregiver distress and a risk factor for institutionalisation and early death[7].

Recommendations for treatment

Step	Intervention
1	Exclude organic causes (delirium).
2	Optimise the environment to maximise orientation and minimise problems due to poor caregiver–patient interactions.
3	If the patient has insight and hallucinations are infrequent and not troubling, do not treat.
4	Consider reducing or stopping anticholinergics and dopamine agonists. Monitor for signs of motor deterioration. Be prepared to restart/increase the dose of these drugs again to achieve the best balance between psychosis and mobility.
5	Try an atypical antipsychotic. **Quetiapine** (start at 12.5 mg – usual dose 75 mg, but higher doses may be required) is effective and well tolerated[8], although EPSEs[9] and stereotypical movements[10] can occur. Higher doses have been used successfully in the treatment of levodopa-induced dyskinesia[11] although motor function may worsen[12]. Olanzapine[13-15] and risperidone[16,18] tend to be less well tolerated. Aripiprazole has been reported to worsen motor function[19,20]. Data for ziprasidone are sparse. Typical antipsychotics should be avoided completely.
6	Consider a **cholinesterase inhibitor**, particularly if the patient has co-morbid dementia[21-23].
7	Try **clozapine**. Start at 6.25 mg – usual dose 25 mg/day[24,25]. Monitor as for clozapine (see page 31). The elderly are more prone to develop serious blood dyscrasia. A case of aplastic anaemia has been reported[26].
8	Consider **ECT**[27]. Psychotic and motor symptoms usually respond well[28] but the risk of inducing delirium is high[4], particularly in patients with pre-existing cognitive impairment.

Dementia

Cholinesterase inhibitors have been shown to improve cognition, delusions and hallucinations in patients with Lewy body dementia (which has some similarities to Parkinson's disease). Motor function may deteriorate[29].

References

1. Reich SG, Marsh L. The most commonly asked questions about the psychiatric aspects of Parkinson's disease. *Neurologist* 2003; 9: 50–56.
2. McDonald WM, Richard IH, DeLong MR. Prevalence, etiology and treatment of depression in Parkinson's disease. *Biol Psychiatry* 2003; 54: 363–375.
3. Gony M, Lapeyre-Mestre M, Montastruc JL *et al.* Risk of serious extrapyramidal symptoms in patients with Parkinson's disease receiving antidepressant drugs: a pharmacoepidemiologic study comparing serotonin reuptake inhibitors and other antidepressant drugs. *Clin Neuropharmacol* 2003; 26: 142–145.
4. Fiegel GS, Hassen MA, Zorumski C *et al.* ECT-induced delirium in depressed patients with Parkinson's disease. *J Neuropsychiatry Clin Neurosci* 1991; 3: 405–411.
5. Huber TJ, Dietrich DE, Emrich HM. Possible use of amantadine in depression. *Pharmacopsychiatry* 1999; 32: 47–55.

6. Ismail MS, Richard IH. A reality test: how well do we understand psychosis in Parkinson's disease. *J Neuropsychiatry Clin Neurosci* 2004; **16**: 8–18.
7. Factor SA, Feustel PJ, Friedman JH *et al.* Longitudinal outcome of Parkinson's disease patients with psychosis. *Neurology* 2003; **60**: 1756–1761.
8. Fernandez HH, Trieschmann ME, Burke MA *et al.* Long-term outcome of quetiapine use for psychosis among Parkinsonian patients. *Mov Dis* 2003; **18**: 510–514.
9. Prueter C, Habermeyer B, Norra C *et al.* Akathisia as a side effect of antipsychotic treatment with quetiapine in a patient with Parkinson's disease. *Mov Dis* 2003; **6**: 712–713.
10. Miwa H, Morita S, Nakanishi I. Stereotyped behaviours or punding after quetiapine administration in Parkinson's disease. *Parkinsonism Relat Disord* 2004; **10**: 177–180.
11. Baron M, Dalton WB. Quetiapine as treatment for dopaminergic induced dyskinesias in Parkinson's disease. *Mov Dis* 2003; **18**: 1208–1209.
12. Morgante L, Epifanio A, Spina E. Quetiapine versus clozapine: a preliminary report of comparative effects on dopaminergic psychosis in patients with Parkinson's disease. *Neurol Sci* 2002; **23**: 89–90.
13. Friedman JH, Goldstein S. Olanzapine in the treatment of dopaminomimetic psychosis in patients with Parkinson's disease. *Neurology* 1998; **50**: 1195–1196.
14. Friedman JH, Goldstein SM, Jacques C. Substituting clozapine for olanzapine in psychiatrically stable Parkinson's disease patients: results of an open label pilot trial. *Clin Neuropharmacol* 1998; **21**: 285–288.
15. Goetz CG, Blasucci LM, Leurgans S *et al.* Olanzapine and clozapine: comparative effects on motor function in hallucinating Parkinson's disease patients. *Neurology* 2000; **55**: 789–794.
16. Ford B, Lynch T, Greene P. Risperidone and Parkinson's disease. *Lancet* 1994; **344**: 681.
17. Rich SS, Friedman JH, Ott BR. Risperidone versus clozapine in the treatment of psychosis in six patients with Parkinson's disease and other akinetic rigid syndromes. *J Clin Psychiatry* 1995; **56**: 556–559.
18. Factor SA, Friedman JH. Risperidone and Parkinson's disease. *Mov Dis* 2001; **17**: 221–225.
19. Fernandez HH, Trieschmann ME, Friedman JH. Aripiprazole for drug-induced psychosis in Parkinson disease: preliminary experience. *Clin Neuropharmacol* 2004; **27**: 4–5.
20. Schonfeldt-Lecuona C, Connemann BJ. Aripiprazole and Parkinson's disease psychosis. *Am J Psychiatry* 2004; **161**: 373–374.
21. Shea C, MacKnight C, Rockwood K. Donepezil for treatment of dementia with Lewy bodies: a case series of 9 patients. *Int Psychogeriatr* 1998; **10**: 229–238.
22. McKeith I, Delser T, Spano P *et al.* Efficacy of rivastigmine in dementia with Lewy bodies: a randomised, double blind, placebo-controlled international study. *Lancet* 2000; **356**: 2031–2036.
23. Fernandez HH, Trieschmann ME, Friedman JH. Treatment of psychosis in Parkinson's disease. *Drug Saf* 2003; **26**: 643–659.
24. Parkinson Study Group. Low-dose clozapine for the treatment of drug induced psychosis in Parkinson's disease. *N Engl J Med* 1999; **340**: 757–763.
25. Parkinson Study Group. Clozapine for the treatment of psychosis in Parkinson's disease: results of 12 week open label extension in the PSYCLOPS trial. *Mov Dis* 2001; **16**: 135–139.
26. Ziegenbein M, Steinbrecher A. Clozapine-induced aplastic anaemia in a patient with Parkinson's disease. *Can J Psychiatry* 2003; **48**: 352.
27. Factor SA, Molho ES, Brown DL. Combined clozapine and electroconvulsive therapy for the treatment of drug induced psychosis in Parkinson's disease. *J Neuropsychiatry* 1998; **7**: 304–307.
28. Martin BA. ECT for Parkinson's? *CMAJ* 2003; **168**: 1391–1392.
29. Richard IH, Justus AW, Greig N *et al.* Rivastigmine-induced worsening of motor function and mood in a patient with Parkinson's disease. *Mov Dis* 2001; **16**: 33–34.

Multiple sclerosis and depression

Depression is a common feature of multiple sclerosis (MS) with a point prevalence of around 14–27% and a lifetime prevalence of up to 50%[1]. Rapid mood swings and suicidality are also commonly encountered[2]. Depression in MS may be associated with fatigue – a symptom reported by the large majority of patients with MS[3].

Depression in MS may result from the psychological impact of the MS diagnosis and likely prognosis, pathological changes in neurone and brain structure, and exposure to various treatments for MS (corticosteroids and beta-interferon)[1,4]. Reversal of depression in MS may partly explain the apparent efficacy of the 'Cari Loder regime', which consists of lofepramine, L-phenylalanine and vitamin B_{12}[5,6].

Treatment of depression in MS is not well informed by published trials. Cognitive behavioural therapy is probably effective[7] and it is assumed that antidepressants have similar effects to those in non-MS patients. Tricyclics seem to be poorly tolerated and adverse effects are dose-limiting[8]. Limited data suggest that moclobemide is effective and well tolerated[9,10]. SSRIs also seem effective[11–13] and are widely used[14]. Effective treatment of depression is associated with improved compliance with beta interferon[15] and improvement in fatigue[16]. The role of beta interferon in the aetiology of MS depression is somewhat controversial, but readers should note that antidepressants seem to be effective treatments and prophylaxis in depression induced by interferons (mainly alpha interferon)[17–19].

Depression in MS – Summary of recommendations

CBT

SSRIs

Moclobemide

References

1. Patten S, Metz L. Depression in multiple sclerosis. *Psychother Psychosom* 1997; **66**: 286–292.
2. Scott T, Allen D, Price T *et al.* Characterisation of major depression symptoms in multiple sclerosis patients. *Neuropsychiatry Clin Neurosci* 1996; **8**: 318–323.
3. Bakshi R, Shaikh Z, Miletich R *et al.* Fatigue in multiple sclerosis and its relationship to depression and neurologic disability. *Mult Scler* 2000; **6**: 181–185.
4. Noseworthy J. Management of multiple sclerosis: current trials and future options. *Curr Opin Neurol* 2003; **16**: 289–297.
5. Loder C, Allawi J, Horrobin D. Treatment of multiple sclerosis with lofepramine, L-phenylalanine and vitamin B_{12}: mechanism of action and clinical importance: roles of the locus coeruleus and central noradrenergic systems. *Med Hypotheses* 2002; **59**: 594–602.
6. Wade D, Young C, Chaudhuri K *et al.* A randomised placebo controlled exploratory study of vitamin B-12, lofepramine, and L-phenylalanine (the 'Cari Loder regime') in the treatment of multiple sclerosis. *J Neurol Neurosurg Psychiatry* 2002; **73**: 246–249.
7. Larcombe N, Wilson P. An evaluation of cognitive-behaviour therapy for depression in patients with multiple sclerosis. *Br J Psychiatry* 1984; **145**: 366–371.
8. Schiffer R, Wineman N. Antidepressant pharmacotherapy of depression associated with multiple sclerosis. *Am J Psychiatry* 1990; **147**: 1493–1497.
9. Barak Y, Erel U, Achiron A. Moclobemide treatment in multiple sclerosis patients with comorbid depression: an open-label safety trial. *J Neuropsychiatry Clin Neurosci* 1999; **11**: 271–273.
10. Bergh F, Kumpfel T, Grasser A *et al.* Combined treatment with corticosteroids and moclobemide favors normalisation of hypothalamo-pituitary-adrenal axis dysregulation in relapsing-remitting multiple sclerosis: a randomised, double blind trial. *J Clin Endocrinol Metab* 2001; **86**: 1610–1615.

Special groups

11. Scott T, Nussbaum P, McConnell H *et al.* Measurement of treatment response to sertraline in depressed multiple sclerosis patients using the Carroll scale. *Neurol Res* 1995; **17**: 421–422.

12. Shafey H. The effect of fluoxetine in depression associated with multiple sclerosis. *Can J Psychiatry* 2004; **37**: 147–148.

13. Benedetti F, Campori E, Colombo C *et al.* Fluvoxamine treatment of major depression associated with multiple sclerosis. *J Neuropsychiatry Clin Neurosci* 2004; **16**: 364–366.

14. Tremlett H, Luscombe D, Wiles C. Prescribing for multiple sclerosis patients in general practice: a case-control study. *J Clin Pharm Ther* 2001; **26**: 437–444.

15. Mohr D, Goodkin D, Likosky W *et al.* Treatment of depression improves adherence to interferon beta-1b therapy for multiple sclerosis. *Arch Neurol* 1997; **54**: 531–533.

16. Mohr D, Hart S, Goldberg A. Effects of treatment for depression on fatigue in multiple sclerosis. *Psychosom Med* 2003; **65**: 542–547.

17. Maddock C, Baita A, Orru M *et al.* Psychopharmacological treatment of depression, anxiety, irritability and insomnia in patients receiving interferon-α: a prospective case series and a discussion of biological mechanisms. *J Psychopharmacol* 2004; **18**: 41–46.

18. Musselman D, Lawson D, Gumnick J *et al.* Paroxetine for the prevention of depression induced by high-dose interferon alfa. *N Engl J Med* 2001; **344**: 961–966.

19. Russo S, Boon J, Korf J *et al.* Mirtazapine for the treatment of interferon-induced psychopathology. *Gen Hosp Psychiatry* 2003; **25**: 497.

Special groups

Acutely disturbed or violent behaviour

Acute behavioural disturbance can occur in the context of psychiatric illness, physical illness, substance abuse or personality disorder. Psychotic symptoms are common and the patient may be aggressive towards others secondary to persecutory delusions or auditory, visual or tactile hallucinations.

The common clinical practice of rapid tranquillisation (RT) is used when appropriate psychological and behavioural approaches have failed to de-escalate acutely disturbed behaviour. It is, essentially, a treatment of last resort. RT is not underpinned by a strong evidence base. Patients who require RT are often too disturbed to give informed consent and therefore cannot participate in randomised controlled trials (RCTs). Recommendations are therefore based partly on research data, partly on theoretical considerations and partly on clinical experience.

Several studies supporting the efficacy of oral risperidone[1-4] and one observational study supporting the efficacy of quetiapine[5] have been published. The level of behavioural disturbance exhibited by the patients in these studies was moderate at most, and all of them accepted oral treatment (this degree of compliance would be unusual in clinical practice).

Larger, placebo-controlled RCTs support the efficacy of IM olanzapine[6,7], ziprasidone[8] and aripiprazole[9]. Again, the level of behavioural disturbance in these studies was moderate at most.

Two large RCTs (the TREC studies[10,11]) have investigated the efficacy of a benzodiazepine versus an antipsychotic/sedative combination (all administered IM) in 'real-life' acutely disturbed patients. TREC 1[10] found midazolam 7.5–15 mg to be more rapidly sedating than a combination of haloperidol 5–10 mg and promethazine 50 mg. TREC 2[11] found haloperidol 10 mg combined with promethazine 25–50 mg to be more rapidly sedating than lorazepam 4 mg. Although these studies are undoubtedly the best available to date, UK psychiatrists rarely prescribe IM midazolam or promethazine, and have been increasingly reluctant to prescribe IM haloperidol due to its ability to cause EPSEs. Acute EPSEs may adversely affect longer-term compliance[12]. Lorazepam IM is an established treatment and TREC 2[11] supports its efficacy.

Plans for the management of individual patients should ideally be made in advance. The aim is to prevent disturbed behaviour and reduce risk of violence. Nursing interventions (de-escalation, time out), increased nursing levels, transfer of the patient to a psychiatric intensive care unit (PICU) and pharmacological management are options that may be employed. Care should be taken to avoid combinations and high cumulative doses of antipsychotic drugs. The monitoring of routine physical observations after RT is essential. Note that RT is often viewed as punitive by patients.

The aims of RT are threefold:

1. To reduce suffering for the patient: psychological or physical (through self-harm or accidents).

2. To reduce risk of harm to others by maintaining a safe environment.

3. To do no harm (by prescribing safe regimes and monitoring physical health).

Special groups

313

In an emergency situation (NB: *read attached notes carefully*)

Step	Intervention		
1	De-escalation, time out, placement, etc., as appropriate		
2[a,b]	Offer **oral treatment**	**Haloperidol** 5 mg or **Olanzapine** 10 mg or **Risperidone**[1-4] 1–2 mg	with or without lorazepam 1–2 mg. Repeat every 45–60 min. Go to step 3 if three doses fail
3[b-f]	Consider **IM treatment**	**Lorazepam** 1–2 mg[11,g] or **Midazolam** 7.5–15 mg[10] or **Haloperidol** 5 mg[10,11] or **Olanzapine** 5–10 mg[7,h] or **Ziprasidone** 10–20 mg[8,i] or **Aripiprazole** 10 mg[9]	Olanzapine should not be combined with a benzodiazepine[13]. The safety of other atypicals combined with a benzodiazepine is unknown.
		Repeat up to two times at 30–60 min intervals, if insufficient effect. **Promethazine**[j] 50 mg IM is an alternative in benzodiazepine-tolerant patients.	
4	Consider **IV treatment**	**Diazepam**[k-m] 10 mg over at least 5 min Repeat after 5–10 min if insufficient effect (up to three times)	
5	**Seek expert advice.** Amylobarbitone[n] 250 mg IM or paraldehyde[o] 5–10 ml IM are options. Very, very few episodes of RT should reach this point		

Notes

a. Choice depends on current treatment. If the patient is established on antipsychotics, lorazepam may be used alone. If the patient uses street drugs or is already receiving benzodiazepines regularly, an antipsychotic may be used alone. For the majority of patients, the best response will be obtained with a combination of an antipsychotic and lorazepam.

b. Ensure that parenteral anticholinergics are available. Procyclidine 5–10 mg IM or benzatropine 1–2 mg IM may be required to reverse acute dystonic reactions (most likely with haloperidol).

c. Either an antipsychotic or benzodiazepine can be used alone as in (a), but for the majority of patients the best response will be obtained with a combination of an antipsychotic and lorazepam.

d. Have flumazenil available to reverse the effects of lorazepam or midazolam. (Monitor respiratory rate – give flumazenil if rate falls below 10/min.)

e. From this point onwards, review the patient's legal status. The requirement for enforced IM medication in informal patients should prompt the use of the Mental Health Act.

f. From this point onwards, consider consulting a senior colleague.

g. Mix lorazepam 1:1 with water for injections before injecting. Some centres use 2–4 mg.

h. Recommended by NICE only for moderate behavioural disturbance.

i. Ziprasidone is unlikely to be licensed in the UK, but is available in the USA and other countries.

j. Promethazine has a slow onset of action but is often an effective sedative. Dilution is not required before IM injection. May be repeated up to a maximum of 100 mg/day. Wait 1–2 hours after injection to assess response. Note that promethazine alone has been reported to cause NMS[14] although it is an extremely weak dopamine antagonist.

k. Use Diazemuls to avoid injection site reactions. IV therapy may be used instead of IM when a very rapid effect is required. IV therapy also ensures near immediate delivery of the drug to its site of action and effectively avoids the danger of inadvertent accumulation of slowly absorbed IM doses. Note also that IV doses can be repeated after only 5–10 min if no effect is observed.

l. Have flumazenil available to reverse the effects of diazepam. (Monitor respiratory rate – give flumazenil if rate falls below 10/min.)

m. Caution in the very young and elderly and those with pre-existing brain damage or impulse control problems, as disinhibition reactions are more likely[15].

n. Amylobarbitone is a powerful respiratory depressant with no pharmacological antagonist. Have facilities for mechanical ventilation available.

o. Paraldehyde is now used extremely rarely and is difficult to obtain. It should only be used when all else has failed. In many cases, ECT may be more appropriate. Note that paraldehyde is associated with a high incidence of tachycardia and tachypnea[16]. IV diazepam may be more effective and is certainly better tolerated[16].

Special groups

References

1. Lejeune J, Larmo I, Chrzanowski W. Oral risperidone plus oral lorazepam versus standard care with intramuscular conventional neuroleptics in the initial phase of treating individuals with acute psychosis. *Int Clin Psychopharmacol* 2004; **19**: 259–269.
2. Currier GW, Chou JC, Feifel D *et al.* Acute treatment of psychotic agitation: a randomised comparison of oral treatment with risperidone and lorazepam versus intramuscular treatment with haloperidol and lorazepam. *J Clin Psychiatry* 2004; **65**: 386–394.
3. Yildiz A, Turgay A, Alpay M *et al.* Observational data on the antiagitation effect of risperidone tablets in emergency settings: a preliminary report. *Int J Psychiatry Clin Pract* 2003; **7**: 217–221.
4. Currier GW, Simpson GM. Risperidone liquid concentrate and oral lorazepam versus intramuscular haloperidol and intramuscular lorazepam for treatment of psychotic agitation. *J Clin Psychiatry* 2001; **62**: 153–157.
5. Bilsker D. Effectiveness of quetiapine for the management of aggressive psychosis in the emergency psychiatric setting: a naturalistic uncontrolled trial. *Int J Psychiatry Clin Pract* (in press).
6. Wright P, Birkett M, David SR *et al.* Double-blind, placebo-controlled comparison of intramuscular olanzapine and intramuscular haloperidol in the treatment of acute agitation in schizophrenia. *Am J Psychiatry* 2001; **158**: 1149–1151.
7. Breier A, Meehan K, Birkett M *et al.* A double-blind, placebo-controlled dose-response comparison of intramuscular olanzapine and haloperidol in the treatment of acute agitation in schizophrenia. *Arch Gen Psychiatry* 2002; **59**: 441–448.
8. Brook S, Lucey JV, Gunn KP. Intramuscular ziprasidone compared with intramuscular haloperidol in the treatment of acute psychosis. *J Clin Psychiatry* 2000; **61**: 933–944.
9. Gismondi R, Daniel D, Stock E *et al.* Intramuscular aripiprazole treatment for acute agitation in patients with psychosis. Poster presented at the Annual Conference of ECNP, Stockholm, Sweden, October, 2004.
10. TREC collaborative group. Rapid tranquillisation for agitated patients in emergency psychiatric rooms: a randomised trial of midazolam versus haloperidol plus promethazine. *BMJ* 2003; **327**: 708–713.
11. Alexander J, Tharyan P, Adams C et al. Rapid tranquillisation of violent or agitated patients in a psychiatric emergency setting. *Br J Psychiatry* 2004; **185**: 63–69.
12. Van Harten PN, Hoek HW, Kahn RS. Acute dystonia induced by drug treatment. *BMJ* 1999; **319**: 623–626.
13. Eli Lilly & Co. Letter to Healthcare Professionals, 2004.
14. Chan-Tack KM. Neuroleptic malignant syndrome due to promethazine. *South Med J* 1999; **92**: 1017–1018.
15. Paton C. Benzodiazepines and disinhibition: a review. *Psychiatr Bull* 2002; **26**: 460–462.
16. Thompson WL, Johnson AD, Maddrey WL. Diazepam and paraldehyde for treatment of severe delirium tremens. A controlled trial. *Ann Intern Med* 1975; **82**: 175–180.

Further reading

McAllister Williams RH, Ferrier IN. Rapid tranquillisation: time for a reappraisal of options for parenteral therapy. *Br J Psychiatry* 2002; **180**: 485–489.

National Institute for Clinical Excellence. Violence – The short-term management of disturbed/violent behaviour in in-patient psychiatric settings and emergency departments. Guideline No 25, 2005. www.nice.org.uk

Pilowsky LS, Ring H, Shine PJ *et al.* Rapid tranquillisation. A survey of emergency prescribing in a general psychiatric hospital. *Br J Psychiatry* 1992; **160**: 831–835.

Rapid tranquillisation – monitoring

After any parenteral drug administration, monitor as follows:

Temperature

Pulse

Blood pressure

Respiratory rate

Every 5–10 min for 1 hour, and then half-hourly until patient is ambulatory.

If the patient is asleep or **unconscious**, the use of pulse oximetry to measure oxygen saturation continuously is desirable. A nurse should remain with patients until they are ambulatory again.

ECG and haematological monitoring are also strongly recommended when parenteral antipsychotics are given, especially when higher doses are used[1,2]. Hypokalaemia, stress and agitation place the patient at risk of cardiac arrhythmia[3] (see page 87).

References

1. Appleby L, Thomas S, Ferrier N *et al.* Sudden unexplained death in psychiatric in-patients. *Br J Psychiatry* 2000; **176**: 405–406.
2. Yap YG, Camm J. Risk of torsade de pointes with non-cardiac drugs. *BMJ* 2000; **320**: 1158–1159.
3. Taylor DM. Antipsychotics and QT prolongation. *Acta Psychiatr Scand* 2003; **107**: 85–95.

Remedial measures in rapid tranquillisation

Problem	Remedial measures
Acute dystonia (including oculogyric crises)	Give **procyclidine** 5–10 mg IM or IV or **benzatropine** 1–2 mg IM
Reduced respiratory rate (<10/min) or oxygen saturation (<90%)	Give oxygen, raise legs, ensure patient is not lying face down. Give **flumazenil** if benzodiazepine-induced respiratory depression suspected (see protocol) If induced by any other sedative agent: **ventilate mechanically**.
Irregular or slow (<50/min) **pulse**	**Refer** to specialist medical care immediately.
Fall in blood pressure (>30 mmHg orthostatic drop or <50 mmHg diastolic)	**Have patient lie flat**, tilt bed towards head. Monitor closely.
Increased temperature	**Withhold antipsychotics:** (risk of NMS and perhaps arrhythmia). Check creatinine kinase urgently.

Special groups

Guidelines for the use of flumazenil

Indication for use	If, after the administration of lorazepam or diazepam, respiratory rate falls below 10/min.
Contraindications	Patients with epilepsy who have been receiving long-term benzodiazepines.
Caution	Dose should be carefully titrated in hepatic impairment.
Dose and route of administration	*Initial:* 200 µg *intravenously* over 15 seconds – if required level of consciousness not achieved after 60 seconds, then, *Subsequent dose:* 100 µg over 10 seconds.
Time before dose can be repeated	60 seconds.
Maximum dose	1 mg in 24 hours (one initial dose and eight subsequent doses).
Side-effects	Patients may become agitated, anxious or fearful on awakening. Seizures may occur in regular benzodiazepine users.
Management	Side-effects usually subside.
Monitoring ● **What to monitor?** ● **How often?**	Respiratory rate Continuously until respiratory rate returns to baseline level. Flumazenil has a short half-life (much shorter than diazepam) and respiratory function may recover and then deteriorate again. *Note: If respiratory rate does not return to normal or patient is not alert after initial doses given, assume that sedation is due to some other cause.*

Guidelines for the use of clopixol acuphase (zuclopenthixol acetate)

Acuphase should be used only after an acutely psychotic patient has required <u>repeated</u> injections of short-acting antipsychotic drugs such as haloperidol or olanzapine, or sedative drugs such as lorazepam.

Acuphase should be given only when enough time has elapsed to assess the full response to previously injected drugs: allow 15 min after IV injections; 60 min after IM.

*Acuphase should **never** be administered:*
- in an attempt to 'hasten' the antipsychotic effect of other antipsychotic therapy
- for rapid tranquillisation
- at the same time as other parenteral antipsychotics or benzodiazepines
- at the same time as depot medication
- as a 'test dose' for zuclopenthixol decanoate depot
- to a patient who is physically resistant (risk of intravasation and oil embolus).

*Acuphase should **never** be used for, or in, the following:*
- patients who accept oral medication
- patients who are neuroleptic naive
- patients who are sensitive to EPSE
- patients who are unconscious
- patients who are pregnant
- those with hepatic or renal impairment
- those with cardiac disease.

Onset and duration of action
Sedative effects usually begin to be seen 2 hours after injection and peak after 12 hours. The effects may last for up to 72 hours. Note: Acuphase has no place in rapid tranquillisation: *its action is not rapid.*

Dose
Acuphase should be given in a dose of 50–150 mg, up to a maximum of 400 mg over a 2-week period. This maximum duration ensures that a treatment plan is put in place. It does not indicate that there are known harmful effects from more prolonged administration, although such use should be very exceptional. There is no such thing as a 'course of Acuphase'. The patient should be assessed before each administration.

Injections should be spaced at least 24 hours apart.

Note: zuclopenthixol acetate is widely misused as a sort of 'chemical straitjacket'. In reality, it is a potentially toxic preparation with very little published information to support its use[1]. It is perhaps best reserved for those few patients who have a prior history of good response to acuphase.

Reference

1. Gibson RC, Fenton M, Coutinho ESF *et al.* Zuclopenthixol acetate in the treatment of acute schizophrenia and similar serious mental illnesses (Review). *Cochrane Database Syst Rev.* Issue 3 2004 Art No CD000525.pub2. DOI: 1002/14651858. CD 000525. Pub2.

Special groups

Chronic behavioural disturbance in learning disability

Behavioural disturbance is common in those with a learning disability. It is often very difficult to determine the aetiology. The following may be useful prompts:

1. Is there or could there be an underlying physical illness? (look for and treat).

2. Could environmental factors be contributing? (consider and alter if possible).

3. Is there an underlying psychiatric illness? (consider and treat if applicable).

Then consider:

4. Does the patient have a history of mood disturbance? (try an antidepressant/mood-stabiliser).

5. Is the disturbance cyclical? (try a mood-stabiliser).

6. Is/might epilepsy (be) a contributing factor? (try an anticonvulsant)

7. Is the patient aggressive? (try carbamazepine or a β-blocker).

8. Are there any signs of adrenergic overactivity, such as tachycardia or tremor? (try a β-blocker).

9. Is the patient impulsive? (try an SSRI).

10. Is the patient self-injurious? (try an antipsychotic, SSRI or naltrexone).

11. Could the behaviour be driven by psychosis? (try an antipsychotic).

Reference

Tyrer P. The use of psychotropic drugs. In: Russell O (ed.). *The Psychiatry of Learning Disabilities*, Ch. 14. London: Royal College of Psychiatrists, 1997.

Special groups

Self-injurious behaviour in learning disability

Repetitive or stereotypical acts that produce self-inflicted injury (self-injurious behaviour (SIB))[1–3]:

- occur in approximately 20% of adults with learning disability (up to 50% in those requiring institutional care)
- most commonly take the form of head-banging, banging other body parts, biting, scratching, pinching, gouging, hair-pulling and pica
- occur more frequently in males; younger adults; those with impairments in hearing, vision, mobility and communication; and those with a diagnosis of autism and epilepsy. As the IQ falls, the prevalence of SIB (and multiple behaviours) increases.

SIB is a major cause of distress to carers and a major cause of institutional care.

Aetiology[4–7]

SIB is best understood as being caused by a combination of organic and environmental factors. Organic factors include rare genetic syndromes (such as Lesch–Nyhan or Smith–Magenis syndrome), developmental brain damage, neurological disorders (such as epilepsy), physical illness, psychiatric illness and communication problems. SIB may be linked to the menstrual cycle in some women. Environmental factors include lack of stimulation/overstimulation, lack of/too much affection, rejection/lack of attention and adverse life events.

Some factors may predispose to SIB (e.g. genetic syndromes), others precipitate it (e.g. depression, dysphoria) and others perpetuate it (e.g. secondary changes in neuroregulatory systems).

The prevalence of mental illness is increased in those with learning disabilities, and non-specific and atypical presentations of mental illness increase in frequency as the IQ falls. Diagnosis often has to be made from observing behaviour rather than directly eliciting symptoms.

Non-drug treatments[8–10]

It is important to try to understand why the patient self-harms (e.g. self-stimulation, relief of dysphoria, attention, social escape through being removed from communal areas, material reward). Psychological/behavioural strategies for dealing with the behaviour can then be put in place. This should always be tried before resorting to drug treatment.

Successfully preventing one form of SIB may lead to the emergence of another form. Staff may perceive SIB to be due to different causes in the same patient and may react with fear, irritation, anger, disgust or despair. Interventions based on individual belief systems will lead to inconsistent care. Effective management and support of staff is essential.

Drug treatment options – SIB in learning disability

Drug	Rationale
Antipsychotics[11,12]	• Supersensitivity of dopamine neurones in nigrostriatal pathways may predispose to SIB. D_1 blockers (such as thioridazine) may be more effective than D_2 blockers. Atypical antipsychotics are poorly evaluated (may have fewer severe side-effects). There is most experience with risperidone. • Dopamine is involved in reward mechanisms (blocking dopamine blocks reward). • Low-dose antipsychotics reduce stereotypies.
Opiate antagonists[4,7]	• SIB leads to the release of endogenous opiates (endorphins), which may lead to a rewarding mood state (positive reinforcement). • Naltrexone (an opiate antagonist) may decrease SIB acutely but is less effective in the long term (?opiate mechanisms are important in the early stages, but SIB is perpetuated via dopamine reward mechanisms).
Anticonvulsants[12]	• The prevalence of epilepsy is high in moderate/severe learning disabilities. • Aggression (to others or self) can be related to seizure activity (pre-ictal, ictal or post-ictal). Note: vigabatrin and topiramate may cause behavioural problems. • Rapid-cycling mood disorders and mixed affective states are more common in learning disabilities and may respond best to carbamazepine or valproate.
SSRIs[4,7] **Lithium**[12,13] **Buspirone**[14]	• Drugs that increase 5HT neurotransmission have been shown to reduce SIB in some patients. • These drugs may act by targeting the behaviour that precipitates SIB (e.g. fear, irritability, anxiety or depression). • Lithium is licensed for 'the control of aggressive behaviour or intentional self-harm.'
Others[7,12,15]	• Other drugs may be useful in some circumstances (e.g. propranolol – probably through reducing anxiety), methylphenidate (when ADHD has been diagnosed), cyproterone (when severely problematic sexual behaviour contributes).

Most data originate from case reports and small open trials, often of heterogeneous patient groups.

Lithium is the only drug licensed for the treatment of SIB.

Prescribing and monitoring[12,16-19]

There is concern that antipsychotic drugs are prescribed excessively and inappropriately in the learning disability population and may cause undue harm. It is unclear if this patient population is more prone to side-effects. It is therefore important to document:

- The rationale for treatment (including some measure of baseline target behaviours), potential risk/benefit and consent in the patient's notes. If the patient is unable to understand the nature, purpose and side-effects of treatment, a relative or carer should be consulted.
- The impact of medication and any side-effects experienced, each time the patient is reviewed.
- Drug interactions. These should always be considered (both kinetic and dynamic) before prescribing, particularly when anticonvulsant drugs are involved.

References

1. Schroeder SR, Oster-Granite ML, Berkson G *et al.* Self-injurious behaviour: gene–brain–behaviour relationships. *Men Retard Dev Disabil Res Rev* 2001; 7: 3–12.
2. Saloviita T. The structure and correlates of self-injurious behaviour in an institutional setting. *Res Dev Disabil* 2000; 21: 501–511.
3. Collacott R, Cooper SA, Branford D *et al.* Epidemiology of self-injurious behaviour in adults with learning disabilities. *Br J Psychiatry* 1998; 173: 428–432.
4. Mikhail AG, King BH. Self-injurious behaviour in mental retardation. *Curr Opin Psychiatry* 2001; 14: 457–461.
5. Moss S, Emerson E, Kiernan C *et al.* Psychiatric symptoms in adults with learning disability and challenging behaviour. *Br J Psychiatry* 2000; 176: 452–456.
6. Deb S. Self-injurious behaviour as part of genetic syndromes. *Br J Psychiatry* 1998; 172: 385–388.
7. Clarke DJ. Psychopharmacology of severe self-injury associated with learning disabilities. *Br J Psychiatry* 1998; 172: 389–394.
8. Xeniditis K, Russell A, Murphy D. Management of people with challenging behaviour. *Adv Psychiatr Treat* 2001; 7: 109–116.
9. Halliday S, Mackrell K. Psychological interventions in self-injurious behaviour. *Br J Psychiatry* 1998; 172: 395–400.
10. Bromley J, Emerson E. Beliefs and emotional reactions of care staff working with people with challenging behaviour. *J Intellect Disabil Res* 1995; 39: 341–352.
11. Branford D. Antipsychotic drugs in learning disabilities (mental handicap). *Pharm J* 1997; 258: 451–456.
12. Einfeld SL. Systematic management approach to pharmacotherapy for people with learning disabilities. *Adv Psychiatr Pract* 2001; 7: 43–49.
13. Craft M, Ismail IA, Krishnamurti D *et al.* Lithium in the treatment of aggression in mentally handicapped patients: a double-blind trial. *Br J Psychiatry* 1987; 150: 685–689.
14. Ratey JJ, Sovner R, Mikkelsen E *et al.* Buspirone therapy for maladaptive behaviour and anxiety in developmentally disabled persons. *J Clin Psychiatry* 1989; 50: 382–384.
15. Aman MG, Marks RE, Turbott SH *et al.* Clinical effects of methylphenidate and thioridazine in intellectually subaverage children. *J Am Acad Child Adolesc Psychiatry* 1991; 30: 246–256.
16. Deb S, Fraser W. The use of psychotropic medication in people with learning disability: towards rational prescribing. *Hum Psychopharmacol* 1994; 9: 259–272.
17. Cooray SE, Tolmac J. Antipsychotic medications in learning disability. *Psychiatr Bull* 1988; 22: 601–604.
18. Miller HEJ, Foster SE. Psychotropic medication in learning disabilities: audit as an alternative to legislation. *Psychiatr Bull* 1997; 21: 286–289.
19. Ahmed Z, Fraser W, Kerr MP *et al.* Reducing antipsychotic medication in people with a learning disability. *Br J Psychiatry* 2000; 176: 42–46.

Further reading

Brylewski J, Duggan L. Antipsychotic medication for challenging behaviour in people with learning disability. *Cochrane Database Syst Rev* 2004, Issue 3. Art No.: CD000377.pub2. DOI: 10.1002/14651858.CD000377.pub2.
Read S. Self-injury and violence in people with severe learning disabilities. *Br J Psychiatry* 1998; 172: 381–384.
Santosh PJ, Baird G. Psychopharmacology in children and adults with intellectual disability. *Lancet* 1999; 354: 233–240.
Thompson C, Read A. Behavioural symptoms among people with severe and profound intellectual disabilities: a 26-year follow-up study. *Br J Psychiatry* 2002; 181: 67–71.

Special groups

Psychotropics and surgery

There are few worthwhile studies of the effects of non-anaesthetic drugs on surgery and the anaesthetic process[1,2]. Practice is therefore largely based on theoretical considerations, case reports, clinical experience and personal opinion. Any guidance given in this area is therefore somewhat speculative.

The decision as to whether or not to continue a drug during surgery and the perioperative period should take into account a number of interacting factors. For example, surgery, especially major procedures, induces profound physiological changes, which include electrolyte disturbances and the release of cortisol and catacholamines. Postoperatively, surgical stress and some agents used in anaesthesia often lead to gastric or gastrointestinal stasis. Oral absorption is therefore likely to be compromised. There is also the risk of drug-to-drug interactions to consider, as well as the risk to the patient of withdrawing psychotropic agents.

For the most part, psychotropic drugs should be continued during the perioperative period, assuming agreement of the anaesthetist concerned. The table below provides some discussion of the merits or otherwise of continuing individual psychotropics during surgery. Note, however, that psychotropic and other drugs are frequently (accidentally and/or unthinkingly) withheld from preoperative patients simply because they are 'nil by mouth'[1]. When one decides to continue a psychotropic, this needs to be explicitly outlined to appropriate medical and nursing staff.

Special groups

Drug or drug group	Considerations	Safe in surgery?
Antipsychotics[3]	• Some antipsychotics widely used in anaesthetic practice. • Increased risk of arrhythmia with most drugs. • α_1 blockade may lead to hypotension and interfere with effects of adrenaline/noradrenaline. • Most drugs lower seizure threshold.	Probably.
Antidepressants – tricyclics[3–5]	• α_1 blockade may lead to hypotension and interfere with effects of adrenaline/noradrenaline. • Danger of serotonin syndrome (clomipramine; amitriptyline) if administered with pethidine, pentazocine or tramadol. • Many drugs prolong QT interval so arrhythmia possibly more likely. • Most drugs lower seizure threshold. • Sympathomimetic agents may give exaggerated response. • Effects persist for several days after cessation.	Probably, but anaesthetic agents need to be carefully chosen.
Antidepressants – SSRIs[3–6]	• Danger of serotonin syndrome if administered with pethidine, pentazocine or tramadol. • Occasional seizures reported. • Cessation may result in withdrawal syndrome.	Probably, but avoid other serotonergic agents.
Antidepressants – MAOIs[3,7–10]	• Dangerous, potentially fatal interaction with pethidine and dextromethorphan[2] (serotonin syndrome or coma/respiratory depression may occur). • Sympathomimetic agents may result in hypertensive crisis. • MAO inhibition lasts for up to 2 weeks: early withdrawal is required. • Switching to moclobemide 2 weeks before surgery allows continued treatment up until day of surgery (do not give moclobemide on the day of surgery).	Probably not, but careful selection of anaesthetic agents may reduce risks if continuation is essential.
Lithium[3,7,8]	• Prolongs the action of both depolarising and non-depolarising muscle relaxants. • Surgery-related electrolyte disturbance and reduced renal function may precipitate lithium toxicity. • Possible increased risk of arrhythmia.	Probably safe in minor surgery but usually discontinued before major procedures and re-started once electrolytes normalise.
Benzodizepines[3,11]	• Reduced requirements for induction and maintenance anaesthetics. • Many have prolonged action (days or weeks), so early withdrawal is necessary.	Probably; usually continued.
Anticonvulsants[3,11]	• CNS depressant activity may reduce anaesthetic requirements.	Probably; usually continued for people with epilepsy.
Methadone[8,11]	• May reduce opiate requirements. • Naloxone may induce withdrawal.	Probably; usually continued.

References

1. Noble DW, Webster J. Interrupting drug therapy in the perioperative period. *Drug Saf* 2002; **7**: 489–495.
2. Noble DW, Kehlet H. Risks of interrupting drug treatment before surgery. *BMJ* 2000; **321**: 719–720.
3. Stafford Smith M, Muir H, Hall R. Perioperative management of drug therapy clinical considerations. *Drugs* 1996; **2**: 238–259.
4. Chui PT, Chung DCW. Medications to withhold or continue in the preoperative consultation. *Curr Anaesth Crit Care* 1998; **9**: 302–306.
5. Kudoh A, Katagai H, Takazawa T. Antidepressant treatment for chronic depressed patients should not be discontinued prior to anaesthesia. *Can J Anesthe* 2002; **49**: 132–136.
6. Spivey KM, Wait CM. Perioperative seizures and fluvoxamine. *Br J Anaesth* 1993; **71**: 321–329.
7. Rahman MH, Beattie J. Medication in the peri-operative period. *Pharma J* 2004; **272**: 287–289.
8. Anon. Drugs in the peri-operative period. I. Stopping or continuing drugs around surgery. *Drug Ther Bull* 1997; **35**: 73–74.
9. Blom-Peters L, Lamy M. Monoamine oxidase inhibitors and anaesthesia: an updated literature review. *Acta Anaesthesiol Bel* 1993; **2**: 57–60.
10. Hill S, Yau K, Whitwam J. MAOIs to RIMAs in anaesthesia – a literature review. *Psychopharmacology* 1992; **106**: S43–S45.
11. Morrow JI, Routledge PA. Essential drugs in the perioperative period. *Curr Pract Surg* 1990; **90**: 106–109.

Special groups

General principles of prescribing in HIV

Individuals with HIV/AIDs may experience symptoms of mental illness either as a direct consequence of (organic origin), a reaction to, or in addition to their underlying infection. In the first scenario, the focus of treatment should be the underlying infection. Where this is not feasible, or the presentation is not of organic origin, psychotropic medication will be the primary treatment.

When prescribing psychotropics, the following principles should be adhered to:

1. Start with a low dose and titrate according to tolerability and response.

2. Select the simplest dosing regime possible.
   (Remember that the patient's drug regime is likely to be complex already.)

3. Select an agent with the fewest side-effects/interactions. Medical co-morbidity and potential drug interactions must be considered.

4. Ensure that management is conducted in close cooperation with the HIV physicians and the rest of the multi-disciplinary team.

Although most psychotropic agents are thought to be safe in HIV-infected individuals, it has been suggested that this group may be more sensitive to higher doses, adverse side-effects and interactions[1]. Patients with low CD4 counts are more likely to have exaggerated adverse reactions to psychotropic medications.

Psychosis

Atypicals are usually used first line. Risperidone is the most widely studied[2] and generally appears to be safe, although idiosyncratic interactions with ritonavir have been reported[3,4]. The use of clozapine is not routinely recommended, although it may be useful in patients with higher CD4 counts who are otherwise medically stable. Although it is not known whether patients with HIV have a greater risk of agranulocytosis, extremely close monitoring of the WCC is recommended. Patients with HIV may be more susceptible to EPSEs[5], NMS[6] and TD[7].

Delirium

Organic causes should be identified and treated. Short-term symptomatic treatment may include low-dose atypicals such as risperidone[8], olanzapine[9], quetiapine[10] or ziprasidone[11]. The concomitant use of low doses of short-acting benzodiazepines such as lorazepam may also be helpful.

Depression

Depression is common in individuals with HIV, and a recent study estimated the prevalence in this population to be as high as 84%[12]. Of note, depression may be a risk factor for HIV[13], and it has been further suggested that much of this depression is either unrecognised or insufficiently managed[14]. First-line agents include SSRIs, especially citalopram[15] (because it does not inhibit

CYP2D6 or CYP3A4), with further treatment as per standard protocols. The risk of serotonin syndrome may be increased[16]. The use of TCAs may be appropriate in some cases, although side-effects may limit efficacy and compliance[17]. MAOIs are not recommended in this population.

Bipolar affective disorder

Mania is a recognised presentation in HIV[18] and individuals with HIV may be more sensitive to the side-effects of mood-stablisers such as lithium[19], especially if they have neurocognitive dysfunction[18]. Conventional agents such as lithium, valproate, lamotrigine and gabapentin may be used cautiously, but carbamazepine should be avoided because of important interactions with anti-retroviral agents as well as the risk of agranulocytosis.

Anxiety disorders

Benzodiazepines have some utility in the treatment of anxiety in individuals with HIV, but caution should be exercised because of the potential for both misuse and multiple and, in rare cases, potentially serious interactions. SSRIs (remember interactions) and other antidepressants may be efficacious, and there is evidence that buspirone may be especially useful[20].

HIV neurocognitive disorders

Individuals with HIV may present with cognitive impairment at any time in the course of their illness, and this may range from mild forgetfulness to severe and debilitating dementia. The mainstay of treatment is combination antiretroviral therapy[21], with judicious, short-term use of an antipsychotic such as risperidone[22] if necessary. Treatment of these individuals is carried out primarily by HIV physicians, with liaison psychiatric input as required.

Important drug interactions

Although the majority of psychotropic agents are deemed safe for co-administration with antiretroviral agents, there are a number of clinically important interactions. These are shown in the following table. It should be noted that data are lacking, and that there is potential for other interactions not listed in the table. Although many of these interactions are not absolute contraindications to co-prescribing, extreme caution is advised. As those receiving HIV treatment may be taking medication for many different medical indications, additional interactions cannot be excluded.

A number of psychotropic agents that are potent enzyme inducers are **contraindicated** for use with antiretroviral agents of all classes, as they can compromise antiretroviral therapy; these include **carbamazepine, phenobarbital, phenytoin, primidone and St John's wort**. Enzyme inhibitors can cause severe exacerbation of side-effects (e.g. SSRIs, benzodiazepines). Caution is advised when the patient is taking ritonavir and lopinavir/ritonavir, as these drugs are potent enzyme inducers that may compromise the efficacy of psychotropic drugs.

In the table below, interactions are both specific and illustrative, but not exhaustive: reported or sample interactions are outlined; many more interactions are possible. Check the latest literature *and* estimate risk of interaction from first principles (i.e. from understanding of CYP involvement).

Table Reported and suspected interactions of antiretrovirals and psychotropics[23–25]

Antiretroviral	Psychotropic	Clinical effect
Amprenavir (CYP3A4 inhibitor)	Alprazolam, diazepam, midazolam, triazolam	↑ Sedation, confusion, respiratory depression
	Carbamazepine	↑ Carbamazepine effect; ↓ Amprenavir effect
	Clozapine	↑ Clozapine effect*
	Lamotrigine	↓ Lamotrigine levels*
	Nefazodone	↑ Nefazodone concentration
	Phenobarbital, phenytoin	↓ Amprenavir effect
	Pimozide	↑ Cardiac arrhythmia
	Primidone	↓ Amprenavir effect
	St John's wort	↓ Amprenavir effect
Delavirdine (inhibitor of CYP3A4, CYP2C9, CYP2C19)	Alprazolam, midalozam, triazolam	↑ Sedation, confusion, respiratory depression
	Carbamazepine	↓ Delavirdine effect
	Fluoxetine	↑ Delavirdine effect*
	Lamotrigine	↓ Lamotrigine levels*
	Nefazodone	↑ Nefazodone concentration
	Phenobarbital, phenytoin	↓ Delavirdine effect
	Pimozide	↑ Cardiac arrhythmia
	Primidone	↓ Amprenavir effect
Efavirenz (inhibitor and inducer of CYP3A4)	Carbamazepine	↓ Carbamazepine effect; ↓ efavirenz effect
	Lamotrigine	↓ Lamotrigine levels*
	Nefazodone	↑ Nefazodone levels
	Phenobarbital	↓ Efavirenz effect
	Phenytoin	↓ Efavirenz effect; ↓ Phenytoin effect
	Pimozide	↑ Cardiac arrhythmia
	Primidone	↓ Amprenavir effect
	St John's wort	↓ Efavirenz effect
Indinavir (inhibitor of CYP3A4)	Carbamazepine	↓ Indinavir effect
	Lamotrigine	↓ Lamotrigine levels*
	Midazolam	↑ Sedation, confusion, respiratory depression
	Nefazodone	↑ Nefazodone levels
	Phenobarbital, phenytoin	↓ Indinavir effect
	Pimozide	↑ Cardiac arrhythmia

Antiretroviral	Psychotropic	Clinical effect
	Primidone	↓ Amprenavir effect
	St John's wort	↓ Indinavir effect; possible indinavir resistance
	Trazodone	↑ Sedation, confusion
Lopinavir + Ritonavir (inhibtor of CYP3A4, CYP2D6) (may induce glucuronidation)	Bupropion	↑ Bupropion levels
	Buspirone	↑ Parkinonism
	Carbamazepine	↓ Lopinavir/ritonavir effect
	Citalopram	↑ Citalopram levels*
	Clozapine	↓ Clozapine levels
	Desipramine	↑ Antimuscarinic effects*
	Fluoxetine	↑ Fluoxetine levels; possible serotonin syndrome
	Lamotrigine	↓ Lamotrigine levels*
	Midazolam, flurazepam, diazepam	↑ Sedation, confusion, respiratory depression
	Mirtazepine	↑ Mirtazapine levels*
	Nefazodone	↑ Nefazodone levels
	Olanzapine	↓ Olanzapine levels
	Phenobarbital, phenytoin	↓ Lopinavir/ritonavir effect
	Pimozide	↑ Cardiac arrhythmia
	Primidone	↓ Amprenavir effect
	Risperidone	Reversible coma/ ↑ EPSE
	St John's wort	↓ Lopinavir/ritonavir effect
	Trazodone	↑ Trazodone levels*
Nelfinavir (inhibitor of CYP3A4, CYP142)	Bupropion	↑ Bupropion levels*
	Carbamazepine	↓ Nelfinavir effect
	Desipramine	↑ Antimuscarinic effects*
	Lamotrigine	↓ Lamotrigine levels*
	Midazolam, triazolam	↑ Sedation, confusion, respiratory depression
	Nefazodone	↑ Nefazodone levels
	Phenobarbital	↓ Nelfinavir effect
	Phenytoin	↓ Phenytoin effect
	Pimozide	↑ Cardiac arrhythmia
	Primidone	↓ Amprenavir effect
	St John's wort	↓ Nelfinavir effect

Special groups

329

Antiretroviral	Psychotropic	Clinical effect
Nevirapine	Methadone	↑ Methadone effect
	Nefazodone	↑ Nefazodone concentration
(CYP3A4, ? effect)	St John's wort	↓ Nevirapine effect
Ritonavir *(may inhibit and induce CYP3A4, inhibits CYP2D6, CYP2C9, CYP2C19)*	Alprazolam, diazepam, midazolam, triazolam	↑ Sedation, confusion, respiratory depression
	Amitriptyline	↑ Antimuscarinic effects*
	Bupropion	↑ Bupropion levels
	Carbamazepine	↓ Ritonavir effect; ↑ carbamazepine effect
	Citalopram	↑ Citalopram levels*
	Clozapine	↓ Clozapine levels
	Desipramine	↑ Antimuscarinic effects*
	Disulphiram	↑ Disulphiram reaction
	Fluoxetine	↑ Fluoxetine levels; possible serotonin syndrome
	Lamotrigine	↓ Lamotrigine levels*
	Mirtazapine	↑ Mirtazapine levels*
	Nefazodone	↑ Nefazodone levels
	Olanzapine	↓ Olanzapine effect*
	Phenytoin	↑ Phenytoin effect
	Pimozide	↑ Cardiac arrhythmia
	Primidone	↓ Amprenavir effect
	Risperidone	↑ Risk of coma*
	St John's wort	↓ Ritonavir effect
	Trazodone	↑ Trazodone levels*
Saquinavir *(inhibits CYP3A4)*	Carbamazepine	↓ Saquinavir effect
	Lamotrigine	↓ Lamotrigine levels*
	Midazolam, triazolam	↑ Sedation, confusion, respiratory depression
	Nefazodone	↑ Nefazodone concentration
	Phenobarbital, phenytoin	↓ Saquinavir effect
	Pimozide	↑ Cardiac arrhythmia
	Primidone	↓ Amprenavir effect
	St John's wort	↓ Saquinavir effect
* Effects of interaction may be reduced/eliminated by reduction in psychotropic dose.		

Note all antiretrovirals are metabolised via CYP3A4; some also utilise additional enzymatic routes such as CYP2D6.

Psychotropic effects of HIV drugs

Psychosis, mania, agitation and suicidal ideation have been associated with antiretroviral treatment (see following table). Any of these conditions can appear *de novo* in HIV-positive individuals. There is, as yet, no conclusive evidence supporting an association between HIV infection and psychosis[26]. Psychosis is associated with efavirenz, zidovudine, nevirapine and, most recently, abacavir treatment[27]. In many of the reported cases, symptoms abated either when the putative offending agent was stopped or prophylactic agents were added to the medication regime.

Although most reports suggest that these changes in mental state occur within a month of commencing antiretroviral therapy, the time frame can be highly variable, ranging from 2 days in the case of efavirenz[28] to 14 months[29] or even longer[30]. Treatment involves cessation of the putative offending agent and initiation of a suitable alternative. Inclusion of an appropriate prophylactic agent or agents can be useful, usually for a short period of time (1–3 months). It should be remembered that other drugs used to treat physical problems (apart from antiretrovirals) may also induce changes in mental state.

Table	Psychotropic effects of antiretrovirals
Diagnosis	**Implicated agent**
Depression	Abacavir[31] Efavirenz[32,33] Indinavir[34] Nevirapine[35]
Mania	Didanosine[36] Efavirenz[29,37,38] Zidovudine[39,41]
Psychosis	Abacavir[27,31] Efavirenz[28,42-44] Nevirapine[35]
PTSD	Efavirenz[45]
Vivid dreams	Abacavir[46] Nevirapine[47] Efavirenz[48]
Suicidal ideation	Abacavir[31] Efavirenz[30,48]
Miscellaneous symptoms	Efavirenz[48]

References

1. Ayuso JL. Use of psychotropic drugs in patients with HIV infection. *Drugs* 1994; 47: 599–610.
2. Singh AN, Catalan J. Risperidone in HIV-related manic psychosis. *Lancet* 1994; 344(8928): 1029–1030.
3. Jover F, Cuadrado JM, Andreu L *et al.* Reversible coma caused by risperidone–ritonavir interaction. *Clin Neuropharmacol* 2002; 25: 251–253.
4. Kelly DV, Beique LC, Bowmer MI. Extrapyramidal symptoms with ritonavir/indinavir plus risperidone. *Ann Pharmacother* 2002; 36: 827–830.
5. Hriso E, Kuhn T, Maslev J. Extrapyramidal symptoms due to dopamine blocking agents in patients with AIDS encephalopathy. *Am J Psychiatry* 1991; 148: 1558–1561.
6. Horwath E, Cournos F. NMS and HIV. *Psychiatr Serv* 1999; 50: 564.
7. Shedlack KJ, Soldato-Couture CS, Swanson CL. Rapidly progressive tardive dyskinesias in AIDS. *Biol Psychiatry* 1994; 35: 147–148.

Special groups

8. Sipahimalini A, Sime RM, Masand PS. Treatment of delirium with risperidone. *Int J Geriatr Psychopharmacol* 1997; **1**: 24–26.
9. Sipahimalini A, Madand PS.Olanzapine in the treatment of delirium. *Psychosomatics* 1998; **39**: 422–430.
10. Schwartz TL, Masand PS. Treatment of delirium with quetiapine. Primary Care Companion. *J Clin Psychiatry* 2000; **2**: 10–12.
11. Leso L, Schwartz TL. Ziprasidone treatment of delirium. *Psychosomatics* 2002; **43**: 61–62.
12. Anon. Depression is common among AIDS patients. Psych consult often is necessary. *AIDS Alert* 2002; **17**:153–154.
13. McDermott BE, Sautter FJ, Winstead DK *et al.* Diagnosis, health beliefs and risk of HIV infection in psychiatric patients. *Hosp Community Psychiatry* 1994; **45**: 580–585.
14. Katz MH, Douglas JM Jr, Bolan GA *et al.* Depression and use of mental health services among HIV-infected men. *AIDS Care* 1996; **8**: 433–442.
15. Currier MB, Molina G, Kato M. Citalopram treatment of major depressive disorder in Hispanic HIV and AIDS patients: a prospective study. *Psychosomatics* 2004; **45**: 210–216.
16. DeSilva KE, Le Flore DB, Marston BJ *et al.* Serotonin syndrome in HIV-infected individuals receiving antiretroviral therapy and fluoxetine. *AIDS* 2001; **15**: 1281–1285.
17. Elliott AJ, Uldall KK, Bergam K *et al.* Randomized, placebo-controlled trial of paroxetine versus imipramine in depressed HIV-positive outpatients. *Am J Psychiatry* 1998; **155**: 367–372.
18. El-Mallakh RS. Mania in AIDS: clinical significance and theoretical considerations. *Int J Psychiatry Med* 1991; **21**: 383–391.
19. Tanquary J. Lithium-induced neurotoxicity at therapeutic levels in an AIDS patient. *J Nerv Ment Dis* 1993; **181**: 518–519.
20. Bakti SL. Buspirone in drug users with AIDS or AIDS-related complex. *J Clin Psychopharmacol* 1990; **10**: 111S–115S.
21. Portegies P, Solod L, Cinque P *et al.* Guidelines for the diagnosis and management of neurological complications of HIV infection. *Eur J Neurol* 2004; **11**: 297–304.
22. Belzie LR. Risperidone for AIDS-associated dementia: a case series. *AIDS Patient Care STDS* 1996; **10**: 246–249.
23. HIV InSite Database of Antiretroviral Drug Interactions (www.hivinsite.com/InSite.jsp?page=ar-00-02).
24. Toronto General Hospital Immunodeficiency Clinic (www.tthhivclinic.com/interact_tables.html).
25. Liverpool Pharmacology Group (www.hiv-druginteractions.org/).
26. Harris MJ, Jeste DV, Gleghorn A *et al.* New-onset psychosis in HIV-infected patients. *J Clin Psychiatry* 1991; **52**: 369–376.
27. Foster R, Olajide D, Everall IP. Antiretroviral therapy-induced psychosis: case report and brief review of the literature. *HIV Med* 2003; **4**: 139–144.
28. De La Garza CL, Paoletti-Duartes S, Garcia-Martin C *et al.* Efavirenz induced psychosis. *AIDS* 2001; **15**: 1911–1912.
29. Maxwell S, Schaftner WA, Kessler HA *et al.* Manic syndrome associated with zivoduvine. *JAMA* 1998; **259**: 3406–3407.
30. Foster R, Everall IP. Long-term neuropsychiatric effects of efavirenz. Case report and review of the literature. In submission.
31. Colebunders R, Hilbrands R, De Roo A *et al.* Neuropsychiatric reaction induced by abacavir. *Am J Med* 2002; **113**: 616.
32. Lang JP, Halleguen O, Picard A *et al.* [Apropos of atypical melancholia with Sustiva (efavirenz)] (Article in French). *Encephale* 2001; **27**: 290–293.
33. Puzantian T. Central nervous system adverse effects with efavirenz: case report and review. *Pharmacotherapy* 2002; **22**: 930–933.
34. Harry TC, Matthews M, Salvary I. Indinavir use: associated reversible hair loss and mood disturbance. *Int J Sex Trans Dis AIDS* 2000; **11**: 474–476.
35. Jan Wise ME, Mistry K, Reid S. Drug points: neuropsychiatric complications of nevirapine treatment. *BMJ* 2002; **324**: 879.
36. Brouillette MJ, Chouinard G, Lalonde R. Didanosine-induced mania in HIV infection. *Am J Psychiatry* 1994; **151**: 1839–1840.
37. Blanch J, Corbella B, Garcia F *et al.* Manic syndrome associated with efavirenz overdose. *Clin Infect Dis* 2001; **33**: 270–271.
38. Shah MD, Balderson K. A manic episode associated with efavirenz therapy for HIV infection. *AIDS* 2003; **17**: 1713–1714.
39. O'Dowd MA, McKegney F. Manic syndrome associated with zidovudine [Letter]. *JAMA* 1988; **259**: 3587.
40. Schaerf FW, Miller R, Pearlson GD *et al.* Manic syndrome associated with zidovudine [letter]. *JAMA* 1988; **260**: 3587–3588.
41. Wright JM, Sachdev PS, Perkins RJ *et al.* Zidovudine-related mania. *Med J Aust* 1989; **150**: 339–341.
42. Sabato S, Wesselingh S, Fuller A *et al.* Efavirenz-indiced catatonia. *AIDS* 2002; **16**: 1841–1842.
43. Poulsen HD, Lublin HK. Efavirenz-induced psychosis leading to involuntary detention. *AIDS* 2003; **17**: 451–453.
44. Peyriere H, Mauboussin JM, Rouanet I *et al.* Management of sudden psychiatric disorders related to efavirenz. *AIDS* 2001; **15**: 1323–1324.
45. Moreno A, Labelle C, Samet JH. Recurrence of post-traumatic stress disorder symptoms after initiation of antiretrovirals including efavirenz: a report of two cases. *HIV Med* 2003; **4**: 302–304.
46. Foster R, Taylor C, Everall IP. More on abacavir-induced neuropsychiatric reactions. *AIDS* 2004; **18**: 2449.
47. Morlese JF, Qazi NA, Gazzard BG *et al.* Nevirapine-induced neuropsychiatric complications, a class effect of non-nucleoside reverse transcriptase inhibitors? *AIDS* 2002; **16**: 1840–1841.
48. Lochet P, Peyriere H, Lotthe A *et al.* Long-term assessment of neuropsychiatric adverse reactions associated with efavirenz. *HIV Med* 2003; **4**: 62–66.

Special groups

Drug treatment of borderline personality disorder

Borderline personality disorder (BPD) is common in psychiatric settings: up to 15% of inpatients meet diagnostic criteria[1]. In BPD, co-morbid depression, anxiety spectrum disorders and bipolar illness occur more frequently than would be expected by chance association alone. The suicide rate in BPD is similar to that seen in affective disorders and schizophrenia[2,3].

Although it is classified as a personality disorder, several 'symptoms' of BPD may intuitively be expected to respond to drug treatment. These include affective instability, transient stress-related psychotic symptoms, suicidal and self-harming behaviours, and impulsivity[4].

Drug treatments are often used during periods of crisis when 'symptoms' can be severe, distressing and potentially life-threatening. By their very nature, these symptoms can be expected to wax and wane[5]. Drug therapy may then be required intermittently. It is easy to see when treatment is required, but much more difficult to decide when modest gains are worthwhile and whether or not continuation is likely to be necessary.

The majority of studies of drug treatment in BPD last for only 6 weeks, and a large number of different outcome measures have been used, making it difficult to evaluate and compare studies. Not all RCTs report attrition data, but where this information is available, less than 50% of subjects tend to complete studies. The placebo response rate in RCTs is uniformly high. Caution is required when evaluating uncontrolled studies or case reports.

Antipsychotics

Open studies have found benefit for conventional antipsychotics[6], risperidone[7] and olanzapine[8] over a wide range of symptoms. In contrast, RCTs generally show only very modest benefits for active drug over placebo[9,10]. The most convincing RCT demonstrated marked reductions in suicidal behaviour with flupentixol 40 mg/month[11]. Open studies report reductions in aggression and self-harming behaviour with clozapine[12,13]. Olanzapine, with or without fluoxetine, also seems to be effective[14].

Dysphoria and depression may develop during treatment with conventional antipsychotics[6,15].

Antidepressants

Several open studies have found that SSRIs reduce impulsivity and aggression in BPD[16–18], but controlled studies show very modest benefits[19,20]. The prevalence of atypical depression is higher in people with BPD than in the general population and such patients may respond well to phenelzine[21]. Tranylcypromine[22] and amitriptyline[23] have not been shown to be effective, and both may cause behavioural disinhibition.

Mood-stabilisers

Up to 50% of people with BPD may also have a bipolar spectrum disorder[24] and mood-stabilisers are commonly prescribed. Valproate semisodium[25,26] and lamotrigine[27] have both been found to reduce anger, aggression and impulsivity in open studies. Valproate has also been subject to RCTs[28,29]. Both studies suggest that valproate may be superior to placebo with respect to reducing interpersonal sensitivity, anger and hostility, but the numbers in these studies were small and the attrition rate high. Larger studies are required. Lithium may reduce mood variation[30], anger and suicidal ideation[31]. Behavioural disinhibition has been reported with carbamazepine[32].

Special groups

333

Benzodiazepines

One case series reported on three patients who responded to alprazolam after multiple treatment failures[33] whereas 7 of 12 patients randomised to alprazolam during a RCT developed severe behavioural disinhibition [34].

Treatment of co-morbid psychiatric illness

A diagnosis of BPD predicts a poorer outcome from treatment of depression with antidepressants[35] and ECT[36]. Symptoms of OCD may be less responsive to clomipramine[37].

References

1. Winston AP. Recent developments in borderline personality disorder. *Adv Psychiatr Treat* 2000; **6**: 211–218.
2. Links PS, Heselgrave R, van Reekum R. Prospective follow-up of borderline personality disorder: prognosis, prediction of outcome and axis 11 co-morbidity. *Can J Psychiatry* 1998; **43**: 265–270.
3. Paris J. Chronic suicidality among patients with borderline persoality disorder. *Psychiatr Serv* 2002; **53**: 738–742.
4. American Psychiatric Association. Practice guideline for the treatment of patients with borderline personality disorder. *Am J Psychiatry* 2001; **158**: 1–52.
5. Links PS, Heselgrave R, van Reekum R. Prospective follow-up of borderline personality disorder: prognosis, prediction of outcome and Axis 11 comorbidity. *Can J Psychiatry* 1998; **43**: 265–270.
6. Teicher MH, Glod CA, Aaronson ST *et al.* Open assessment of the safety and efficacy of thioridazine in the treatment of patients with borderline personality disorder. *Psychopharmacol Bull* 1989; **25**: 535–549.
7. Rocca P, Marchiavo L, Cocuzza E *et al.* Treatment of borderline personality disorder with risperidone. *J Clin Psychiatry* 2002; **63**: 241–244.
8. Schulz SC, Camlin KL, Berry SA *et al.* Olanzapine safety and efficacy in patients with borderline personality disorder and co-morbid dysthymia. *Biol Psychiatry* 1999; **46**: 1429–1435.
9. Soloff PH, Anselm G, Nathan RS *et al.* Progress in pharmacotherapy of borderline disorders: a double-blind study of amitriptyline, haloperidol and placebo. *Arch Gen Psychiatry* 1986; **43**: 691–697.
10. Goldberg SC, Schulz SC, Schulz P *et al.* Borderline and schizotypal personality disorders treated with low-dose thiothixene vs placebo. *Arch Gen Psychiatry* 1986; **43**: 680–686.
11. Montgomery SA, Montgomery D. Pharmacological prevention of suicidal behaviour. *J Affect Disord* 1982; **4**: 291–298.
12. Chengappa KNR, Ebeling T, Kang JS *et al.* Clozapine reduces severe self-mutilation and aggression in psychotic patients with borderline personality disorder. *J Clin Psychiatry* 1999; **60**: 477–484.
13. Benedetti F, Sforzini L, Colombo C *et al.* Low dose clozapine in acute and continuation treatment of severe borderline personality disorder. *J Clin Psychiatry* 1998; **59**: 103–107.
14. Zanarini MC, Frankenburg FR, Parachini EA. A preliminary, randomized trial of fluoxetine, olanzapine, and the olanzapine-fluoxetine combination in women with borderline personality disorder. *J Clin Psychiatry* 2004; **65**: 903–907.
15. Soloff PH, Cornelius J, George A *et al.* Efficacy of phenelzine and haloperidol in borderline personality disorder. *Arch Gen Psychiatry* 1993; **50**: 377–385.
16. Cornelius JR, Soloff PH, Perel JM *et al.* Fluoxetine trial in borderline personality disorder. *Psychopharmacol Bull* 1990; **26**: 151–154.
17. Markovitz PJ, Calabrese JR, Schulz SC *et al.* Fluoxetine in the treatment of borderline and schizotypal personality disorders. *Am J Psychiatry* 1991; **148**: 1064–1067.
18. Kavoussi RJ, Liu J, Coccaro EF. An open trial of sertraline in personality disordered patients with impulsive aggression. *J Clin Psychiatry* 1994; **55**: 137–141.
19. Rinne T, van der Brink W, Wooters L *et al.* SSRI treatment of borderline personality disorder: a randomised, placebo controlled clinical trial for female patients with borderline personality disorder. *Am J Psychiatry* 2002; **159**: 2048–2054.
20. Salzman C, Wolfson AN, Schatzberg A *et al.* Effect of fluoxetine on anger in symptomatic volunteers with borderline personality disorder. *J Clin Psychopharmacol* 1995; **15**: 23–29.
21. Parsons B, Quitkin FM, McGrath PJ *et al.* Phenelzine, imipramine and placebo in borderline patients meeting criteria for atypical depression. *Psychopharmacol Bull* 1989; **25**: 524–534.
22. Cowdry RW, Gardner DL. Pharmacotherapy of borderline personality disorder: alprazolam, carbamazepine, trifluoperazine and tranylcypromine. *Arch Gen Psychiatry* 1988; **45**: 111–119.
23. Soloff PH, George A, Nathan S *et al.* Paradoxical effects of amitriptyline in borderline patients. *Am J Psychiatry* 1986; **143**: 1603–1605.
24. Deltito J, Martin L, Riefkohl B *et al.* Do patients with borderline personality disorder belong to the bipolar spectrum? *J Affect Disord* 2001; **67**: 221–228.
25. Stein DJ, Simeon D, Frenkel M *et al.* An open trial of valproate in borderline personality disorder. *J Clin Psychiatry* 1995; **56**: 506–510.

26. Kavoussi RJ, Coccaro EF. Divalproex sodium for impulsive aggressive behaviour in patients with borderline personality disorder. *J Clin Psychiatry* 1998; **59**: 676–680.
27. Pinto OC, Akiskal HS. Lamotrigine as a promising approach to borderline personality: an open case series without concurrent DSM-IV major mood disorder. *J Affect Disord* 1998; **51**: 333–343.
28. Hollander E, Allen A, Lopez RP *et al.* A preliminary double blind, placebo controlled trial of divalproex sodium in borderline personality disorder. *J Clin Psychiatry* 2001; **62**: 199–203.
29. Frankenburg FR, Zanarini MC. Divalproex sodium treatment of women with borderline personality disorder and bipolar 11 disorder: a double blind, placebo controlled pilot study. *J Clin Psychiatry* 2002; **63**: 442–446.
30. Rifkin A, Quitkin F, Carrillo C *et al.* Lithium carbonate in emotionally unstable character disorder. *Arch Gen Psychiatry* 1972; **27**: 519–523.
31. Links PS, Steiner M, Boiago I *et al.* Lithium therapy for borderline patients: preliminary findings. *J Pers Disord* 1990; **4**: 173–181.
32. De la Fuente JM, Lotstra F. A trial of carbamazepine in borderline personality disorder. *Eur Neuropsychopharmacol* 1994; **4**: 479–486.
33. Faltus FJ. The positive effect of alprazolam in the treatment of three patients with borderline personality disorder. *Am J Psychiatry* 1984; **141**: 802–803.
34. Gardner DL, Cowdry RW. Alprazolam-induced dyscontrol in borderline personality disorder. *Am J Psychiatry* 1985; **142**: 98–100.
35. Shea MT, Pilkonis PA, Beckham E *et al.* Personality disorders and treatment outcome in the NIMH treatment of depression collaborative research program. *Am J Psychiatry* 1990; **147**: 711–718.
36. DeBattista C, Mueller K. Is electroconvulsive therapy effective for the depressed patient with co-morbid borderline personality disorder? *J ECT* 2001; **17**: 91–98.
37. Baer L, Jenike MA, Black DW *et al.* Effect of axis II diagnoses on treatment outcome with clomipramine in 55 patients with obsessive-compulsive disorder. *Arch Gen Psychiatry* 1992; **49**: 862–866.

chapter 8

Miscellaneous conditions and substances

Psychotropics in overdose

Suicide attempts and suicidal gestures are frequently encountered in psychiatric and general practice, and psychotropic drugs are often taken in overdose. This section gives brief details of the toxicity in overdose of commonly used psychotropics. It is intended to help guide drug choice in those thought to be at risk of suicide and to help identify symptoms of overdose. This section gives no information on the treatment of psychotropic overdose and readers are directed to specialist poisons units. In all cases of suspected overdose, urgent referral to acute medical facilities is, of course, strongly advised.

Drug or drug group	Toxicity in overdose	Smallest dose likely to cause death	Signs and symptoms of overdose
Antidepressants Tricyclics[1–4] (not lofepramine)	High	Around 500 mg. Doses over 50 mg/kg usually fatal.	Sedation, coma, tachycardia, arrhythmia (QRS, QT prolongation), hypotension, seizures.
Lofepramine[4–6]	Low	Unclear. Fatality unlikely if lofepramine taken alone.	Sedation, coma, tachycardia, hypotension.
SSRIs[5–7]	Low	Unclear. Probably above 1–2 g. Fatality unlikely if SSRI taken alone.	Vomiting, tremor, drowsiness, tachycardia, ST depression. Seizures and QT prolongation possible.
Venlafaxine[8,9]	Moderate	Probably above 5 g, but seizures may occur after ingestion of 1 g.	Vomiting, sedation, tachycardia, seizures. Very rarely QT prolongation, arrhythmia.
Moclobemide[10,11]	Low	Unclear, but probably more than 8 g. Fatality unlikely if moclobemide taken alone.	Vomiting, sedation, disorientation.
Trazodone[12]	Low	Unclear but probably more than 10 g. Fatality unlikely in overdose of trazodone alone.	Drowsiness, nausea, dizziness. Very rarely arrhythmia.
Nefazodone[8,13]	Low	Unclear but probably more than 10 g. Fatality unlikely in overdose of nefazodone alone.	Drowsiness, nausea, dizziness.
Reboxetine[8,14]	Low	Not known. Fatality unlikely in overdose of reboxetine alone.	Sweating, tachycardia, changes in blood pressure.
Mirtazapine[8,15,16]	Low	Unclear but probably more than 2.25 g. Fatality unlikely if mirtazapine taken alone.	Sedation; even large overdose may be asymptomatic.
Bupropion[8,17]	Moderate	Around 16 g.	Tachycardia, seizures, QT prolongation, arrhythmia.
Mianserin[18]	Low	Unclear but probably more than 1 g. Fatality unlikely if mianserin taken alone.	Sedation, coma, hypertension, tachycardia.
MAOIs (not moclobemide)[1,2,4]	High	Phenelzine – 400 mg Tranylcypromine – 200 mg	Tremor, weakness, confusion, sweating, tachycardia, hypertension.
Antipsychotics Phenothiazines[19–22]	High	Chlorpromazine 5–10 g Thioridazine 2–5 g	Sedation, coma, tachycardia, arrhythmia, pulmonary oedema, hypotension, QT prolongation, seizures, dystonia, NMS.

Drug or drug group	Toxicity in overdose	Smallest dose likely to cause death	Signs and symptoms of overdose
Butyrophenones[21,23,24]	Moderate	Haloperidol – probably above 500 mg. Arrhythmia may occur at 300 mg.	Sedation, coma, dystonia, NMS, QT prolongation, arrhythmia.
Clozapine[25]	Moderate	Around 2 g.	Lethargy, coma, tachycardia, hypotension, hypersalivation, pneumonia, seizures.
Olanzapine[25,26]	Moderate	Unclear. Probably more than 200 mg.	Lethargy, confusion, myoclonus, hypotension, tachycardia, delirium.
Risperidone[25]	Low	Unclear. Fatality rare in those taking risperidone alone.	Lethargy, tachycardia, changes in blood pressure, QT prolongation.
Quetiapine[25,27]	Low	Unclear. Probably more than 5 g.	Lethargy, tachycardia, hypotension, rhabdomyolysis
Mood stabilisers Lithium[28]	Low (acute overdose)	Acute overdose does not normally result in fatality. Insidious, chronic toxicity is more dangerous.	Nausea, diarrhoea, tremor, confusion, weakness, lethargy, seizures, coma, cardiovascular collapse, arrhythmia.
Carbamazepine[29,30]	Moderate	Around 20 g, but seizures may occur at around 5 g.	Somnolence, coma, respiratory depression, ataxia, seizures, tachycardia, arrhythmia, electrolyte disturbance.
Valproate[31–33]	Moderate	Unclear but probably more than 20 g.	Somnolence, coma, cerebral oedema, respiratory depression, blood dyscrasia, hypotension, seizures, electrolyte disturbance.
Others Benzodiazepines[34,35]	Low	Probably more than 100 mg diazepam equivalents. Fatality unusual if taken alone. Alprazolam is most toxic.	Drowsiness, ataxia, dysarthria, nystagmus, respiratory depression, coma.
Zopiclone[34,36,37]	Low	Unclear. Probably above 100 mg. Fatality rare in those taking zopiclone alone.	Ataxia, nausea, diplopia, drowsiness, coma.
Zolpidem[38,39]	Low	Unclear. Probably above 200 mg. Fatality rare in those taking zolpidem alone.	Drowsiness, agitation, respiratory depression, tachycardia, coma.
Methadone[40,41]	High	20–50 mg may be fatal in non-users. Co-ingestion of benzodiazepines increases toxicity.	Drowsiness, nausea, hypotension, respiratory depression, coma, rhabdomyolysis.

High	=	Less than 1 week's supply likely to cause serious toxicity or death
Moderate	=	1–4 weeks' supply likely to cause serious toxicity or death
Low	=	Death or serious toxicity unlikely even if more than 1 month's supply taken

Miscellaneous

References

1. Crome P. Antidepressant overdosage. *Drugs* 1982; 23: 431–461.
2. Henry JA. Epidemiology and relative toxicity of antidepressant drugs in overdose. *Drug Safety* 1997; 16: 374–390.
3. Power BM, Hackett LP, Dusci LJ *et al*. Antidepressant toxicity and the need for identification and concentration monitoring in overdose. *Clin Pharmacokinet* 1995; 29: 154–171.
4. Cassidy S, Henry J. Fatal toxicity of antidepressant drugs in overdose. *BMJ* 1987; 295: 1021–1023.
5. Henry JA, Alexander CA, Sener EK. Relative mortality from overdose of antidepressants. *BMJ* 1995; 310: 221–224.
6. Cheeta S, Schifano F, Oyefso A *et al*. Antidepressant-related deaths and antidepressant prescriptions in England and Wales, 1998–2000. *Br J Psychiatry* 2004; 184: 41–47.
7. Barbey JT, Roose SP. SSRI safety in overdose. *J Clin Psychiatry* 1998; 59(Suppl. 15): 42–48.
8. Buckley NA, Faunce TA. 'Atypical' antidepressants in overdose. *Drug Safety* 2003; 26: 539–551.
9. Whyte IM, Dawson AH, Buckley NA. Relative toxicity of venlafaxine and selective serotonin reuptake inhibitors in overdose compared to tricyclic antidepressants. *Q J Med* 2003; 96: 369–374.
10. Hetzel W. Safety of moclobemide taken in overdose for attempted suicide. *Psychopharmacology* 1992; 106: 127–129.
11. Myrenfors PG, Eriksson T, Sandstedt CS *et al*. Moclobemide overdose. *J Int Med* 1993; 233: 113–115.
12. Gamble DE, Peterson LG. Trazodone overdose: four years of experience from voluntary reports. *J Clin Psychiatry* 1986; 47: 544–546.
13. Lader MH. Tolerability and safety: essentials in antidepressant pharmacotherapy. *J Clin Psychiatry* 1996; 57(Suppl. 2): 39–44.
14. Baldwin DS, Buis C, Carabal E. Tolerability and safety of reboxetine. *Rev Contemp Pharmacother* 2000; 11: 321–330.
15. Montgomery SA. Safety of mirtazapine: a review. *Int Clin Psychopharm* 1995; 10(Suppl. 4): 37–45.
16. Bremner JD, Wingard P, Walshe TA. Safety of mirtazapine in overdose. *J Clin Psychiatry* 1998; 59: 233–235.
17. Paris PA, Saucier JR. ECG conduction delays associated with massive bupropion overdose. *J Toxicol* 1998; 36: 595–598.
18. Chand S, Crome P. One hundred cases of acute intoxication with mianserin hydrochloride. *Pharmacopsychiatry* 1981; 14: 15–17.
19. Anon. Phenothiazines. *Micromedex Healthcare Series – Poisondex* 2004; 7.1.
20. Buckley NA, Whyte IM, Dawson AH. Cardiotoxicity more common in thioridazine overdose than with other neuroleptics. *J Clin Toxicol* 1995; 33: 199–204.
21. Haddad PM, Anderson IM. Antipsychotic-related QTc prolongation, torsade de pointes and sudden death. *Drugs* 2002; 62: 1649–1671.
22. Li C, Gefter WB. Acute pulmonary edema induced by overdosage of phenothiazines. *Chest* 1992; 101(1): 102–104.
23. Levine BS, Wu SC, Goldberger BA *et al*. Two fatalities involving haloperidol. *J Anal Toxicol* 1991; 15: 282–284.
24. Henderson RA, Lane S, Henry JA. Life-threatening ventricular arrhythmia (torsades de pointes) after haloperidol overdose. *Hum Exp Toxicol* 1991; 10: 59–62.
25. Trenton AJ, Currier GW, Zwemer FL. Fatalities associated with therapeutic use and overdose of atypical antipsychotics. *CNS Drugs* 2003; 17: 307–324.
26. Chue P, Singer P. A review of olanzapine-associated toxicity and fatality in overdose. *J Psychiatry Neurosci* 2003; 28: 253–261.
27. Smith RP, Puckett BN, Crawford J *et al*. Quetiapine overdose and severe rhabdomyolysis. *J Clin Psychopharm* 2004; 24: 343.
28. Tuohy K, Shemin D. Acute lithium intoxication. *Dialysis Transplant* 2003; 32: 478–481.
29. Spiller HA. Management of carbamazepine overdose. *Pediatr Emerg Care* 2001; 17: 452–456.
30. Schmidt S, Schmitz-Buhl M. Signs and symptoms of carbamazepine overdose. *J Neurol* 1995; 242: 169–173.
31. Isbister GK, Balit CR, Whyte IM *et al*. Valproate overdose: a comparative cohort study of self poisonings. *Br J Clin Pharmacol* 2003; 55: 398–404.
32. Spiller HA, Krenzelok EP, Klein-Schwartz W *et al*. Multicenter case series of valproic acid ingestion: serum concentrations and toxicity. *J Clin Toxicol* 2000; 38: 755–760.
33. Sztajnkrycer MD. Valproic acid toxicity: overview and management. *J Toxicol* 2002; 40: 789–801.
34. Reith DM, Fountain J, McDowell R *et al*. Comparison of the fatal toxicity index of zopiclone and benzodiazepines. *J Toxicol* 2003; 41: 975–980.
35. Isbister GK, O'Regan J, Sibbritt D *et al*. Alprazolam is relatively more toxic than other benzodiazepines in overdose. *Br J Clin Pharmacol* 2004; 58: 88–95.
36. Pounder D, Davies J. Zopiclone poisoning. *J Anal Toxicol* 1996; 20: 273.
37. Bramness JG, Arnestad M, Karinen R *et al*. Fatal overdose of zopiclone in an elderly woman with bronchogenic carcinoma. *J Forensic Sci* 2001; 46: 1247–1249.
38. Gock SB, Wong SH, Nuwayhid N *et al*. Acute zolpidem overdose – report of two cases. *J Anal Toxicol* 1999; 23: 559–562.
39. Garnier R, Guerault E, Muzard D *et al*. Acute zolpidem poisoning – analysis of 344 cases. *J Clin Toxicol* 1994; 32: 391–404.
40. Gable RS. Comparison of acute lethal toxicity of commonly abused psychoactive substances. *Addiction* 2004; 99: 686–696.
41. Caplehorn JRM, Drummer OH. Fatal methadone toxicity: signs and circumstances, and the role of benzodiazepines. *Aust NZ J Public Health* 2002; 26: 358–362.

Observations on the placebo effect in mental illness

The following considerations apply when interpreting the results of placebo-controlled studies. Although the references for each point are drawn from the depression literature, the same principles apply to the treatment of other disorders. The relative importance of each point will vary depending on the disorder that is being treated.

- Placebo is not the same as no care: patients who maintain contact with services have a better outcome than those who receive no care[1].
- The placebo response is greater in mild illness[2].
- The higher the placebo response rate, the more difficult it is to power studies to show treatment effects. Where the placebo response rate exceeds 40%, studies have to recruit very large numbers of patients to be adequately powered to show differences between treatments[3].
- It is difficult to separate placebo effects from spontaneous remission. The higher the spontaneous remission rate, the more difficult it is to power studies to show treatment effects[1].
- The placebo response rate in published studies is increasing over time[4]. This may be because of increasing numbers of mildly ill patients being recruited into trials because of clinicians' reluctance to risk severely ill patients being randomised into placebo arms.
- 'Breaking the blind' may influence outcome. The resultant 'expectancy effect' may explain why active placebos are more effective than inert placebos[5,6]. That is, if patients and observers note adverse effects, the placebo effect is enhanced.
- Most psychotropic drugs have side-effects such as sedation that may improve scores on rating scales without actually treating the target illness.
- Placebo response may be short-lived: studies are usually too short to pick up placebo relapsers[7].
- Statistical significance and clinical significance are not the same thing: a study may report on a highly statistically significant difference in efficacy between active drug and placebo, but the magnitude of the difference may be too small to be clinically meaningful.
- Publication bias remains a problem[8–10]. Many negative studies are never published. Underpowered positive studies often are.
- Placebo response increases according to expectancy. For example, placebo response is greater in studies randomising 2:1 active:placebo than in those randomising 1:1 (chance of receiving active is greater).
- Note that other effects may operate: 'wish bias' probably exaggerates the efficacy of new drugs compared with established agents[11].

References

1. Andrews G. Placebo response in depression: bane of research, boon to therapy. *Br J Psychiatry* 2001; **178**: 192–194.
2. Khan A, Leventhal R, Khan S *et al*. Severity of depression and response to antidepressants and placebo: an analysis of the FDA database. *J Clin Psychopharm* 2002; **22**: 40–45.
3. Thase M. Studying new antidepressants: if there was a light at the end of the tunnel, could we see it? *J Clin Psychiatry* 2002; **63**: 24–27.
4. Walsh BT, Seidman SN, Sysko R *et al*. Placebo response in studies of major depression: variable, substantial and growing. *JAMA* 2002; **287**: 1840–1847.
5. Kirsch I, Moore TM, Scoboria A *et al*. The Emperor's new drugs: an analysis of antidepressant medication data submitted to the U.S. Food and Drug Administration. *Prevention and Treatment* 2002; **5**: 10–23.
6. Moncrieff J, Wessely S, Hardy R. Active placebo versus antidepressants for depression. The Cochrane Library, 2001.
7. Ross DC, Quitkin FM, Klein DF. A typological model for estimation of drug and placebo effects in depression. *J Clin Psychopharm* 2002; **22**: 414–418.
8. Lexchin J, Bero LA, Djulbegovic B *et al*. Pharmaceutical industry sponsorship and research outcome and quality: systematic review. *BMJ* 2003; **326**: 1167–1170.
9. Melander H, Ahlqvist-Rastad J, Beerman B *et al*. Evidence based medicine selective reporting from studies sponsored by the pharmaceutical industry: review of studies in new drug applications. *BMJ* 2003; **326**: 1171–1173.
10. Werneke U, Horn O, Taylor D. How effective is St. John's wort? The evidence revisited. *J Clin Psychol* 2004; **65**: 611–617.
11. Barbui C, Cipriani A, Brambilla P *et al*. 'Wish bias' in antidepressant drug trials? *J Clin Psychopharm* 2004; **24**: 126–130.

Drug interactions with alcohol

Drug interactions with alcohol are complex. Many patient-related and drug-related factors need to be considered. It can be difficult to predict accurately outcomes as a number of processes may occur simultaneously.

Pharmacokinetic interactions[1,2]

Alcohol (ethanol) is absorbed from the GI tract and distributed in body water. The volume of distribution is smaller in women and the elderly where plasma levels of alcohol will be higher for a given 'dose' of alcohol than in males. Approximately 10% of ingested alcohol is subjected to first pass metabolism by alcohol dehydrogenase (ADH). The remainder is metabolised in the liver by ADH and CYP2E1. CYP2E1 plays a minor role in occasional drinkers but is an important metabolic route in chronic, heavy drinkers. CYP1A2 and CYP3A4 also play a minor role[3].

CYP2E1 and ADH convert alcohol to acetaldehyde which is the toxic substance responsible for the unpleasant symptoms of the 'antabuse reaction' (e.g. flushing, headache, nausea, malaise). Acetaldehyde is then further metabolised by aldehyde dehydrogenase to acetic acid and then to carbon dioxide and water.

All of the enzymes involved in the metabolism of alcohol exhibit genetic polymorphism. Forty percent of people of Asian origin are poor metabolisers via ADH. Chronic consumption of alcohol induces CYP2E1 and CYP3A4. The effects of alcohol on other hepatic metabolising enzymes have been poorly studied.

Metabolism of alcohol

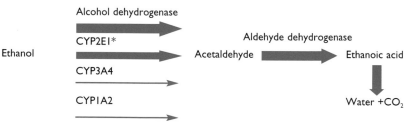

* Minor route in occasional drinkers; major route in misusers

Table Co-administration of alcohol and substrates for CYP2E1 and CYP3A4

	CYP2E1	CYP3A4
Substrates for enzyme (note: this is not an exhaustive list)	• Paracetamol • Isoniazid • Phenobarbitone	• Benzodiazepines • Carbamazepine • Clozapine • Donepezil • Galantamine • Mirtazapine • Risperidone • Tricyclics • Valproate • Venlafaxine • "Z" hypnotics
Effects in an intoxicated patient	Competition between alcohol and drug leading to reduced rates of metabolism of both Increased plasma levels may lead to toxicity	Competition between alcohol and drug leading to reduced rates of metabolism of both Increased plasma levels may lead to toxicity
Effects in a chronic, sober drinker	Activity of CYP2E1 is increased up to 10 fold Increased metabolism of drugs potentially leading to therapeutic failure	Increased rate of drug metabolism potentially leading to therapeutic failure

In chronic drinkers, particularly those who binge drink, serum levels of prescribed drugs may reach toxic levels during periods of intoxication with alcohol and then be sub-therapeutic when the patient is sober. This makes it very difficult to optimise treatment of physical or mental illness.

Table	Drugs that inhibit Alcohol Dehydrogenase and Aldehyde Dehydrogenase	
Enzyme	**Inhibited by:**	**Potential consequences:**
Alcohol dehydrogenase	• Aspirin • H₂ antagonists	Reduced metabolism of alcohol resulting in higher plasma levels for longer periods of time
Aldehyde dehydrogenase	• Disulfiram • Griseofulvin • Isoniazid • Metronidazole • Nitrofurantoin • Sulphamethoxazole • Isosorbide dinitrate • Chlorpropamide • Tolbutamide	Reduced ability to metabolise acetaldehyde leading to 'Antabuse' type reaction: facial flushing, headache, tachycardia, nausea & vomiting, arrhythmias and hypotension

Pharmacodynamic Interactions[1,2,4]

Alcohol enhances inhibitory neurotransmission at GABA$_a$ receptors and reduces excitatory neurotransmission at glutamate NMDA receptors. It also increases dopamine release in the mesolimbic pathway and may have some effects on serotonin and opiate pathways. Alcohol alone, would therefore be expected to cause sedation, amnesia, ataxia and give rise to feelings of pleasure (or worsen psychotic symptoms in vulnerable individuals).

Table		
Effect of alcohol	**Effect exacerbated by**	**Potential consequences**
Sedation	Other sedative drugs eg: • Benzodiazepines • Antipsychotics • Tricyclics • Z-hypnotics • Antihistamines • Opiates • Lofexidine • Baclofen • Tizanidine	Increased CNS depression ranging from increased propensity to be involved in accidents through to respiratory depression and death
Amnesia	Other amnesic drugs eg: • Benzodiazepines • Barbiturates • Z-hypnotics	Increased amnesic effects ranging from mild memory loss to total amnesia
Ataxia	• ACE inhibitors • B-blockers • Ca channel blockers • Nitrates Adrenergic alpha receptor antagonists eg • Clozapine • Risperidone • Tricyclics	Increased unsteadiness and falls

Alcohol can cause or worsen psychotic symptoms via increasing dopamine release in the mesolimbic pathways. The effect of antipsychotic drugs may be competitively antagonised, rendering them less effective.

Electrolyte disturbances secondary to alcohol-related dehydration can be exacerbated by other drugs that cause electrolyte disturbances such as diuretics.

Note that:
• **In the presence of pharmacokinetic interactions, pharmacodynamic interactions will be more marked.** For example, in a chronic heavy drinker who is sober, enzyme induction will increase the metabolism of diazepam which may lead to increased levels of anxiety (treatment failure). If the same patient becomes intoxicated with alcohol, the metabolism of diazepam will be greatly reduced as it will have to compete with alcohol for the metabolic capacity of CYP3A4. Plasma levels of alcohol and diazepam will rise (toxicity). As both alcohol and diazepam are sedative (via $GABA_a$ affinity), loss of consciousness and respiratory depression may occur.

Table   Psychotropic Drugs: choice in patients who continue to drink

	Safest choice	*Best avoided*
Antipsychotics	**Sulpiride & amisulpride** (non-sedative and renally excreted)	**Very sedative antipsychotics** such as chlorpromazine and clozapine
Antidepressants	**SSRI** Potent inhibitors of CYP3A4 may decrease alcohol metabolism in chronic drinkers (fluoxetine, paroxetine)	**TCAs**, because impairment of metabolism by alcohol (while intoxicated) can lead to profound hypotension, seizures, arrhythmias and coma Cardiac effects can be exacerbated by electrolyte disturbances Combinations of TCAs and alcohol profoundly impair psychomotor skills **MAOIs** as can cause profound hypotension Also potential interaction with tyramine-containing drinks which can lead to hypertensive crisis
Mood stabilisers	**Valproate** **Carbamazepine** Note: higher serum levels achieved during periods of alcohol intoxication may be poorly tolerated	**Lithium**, because it has a narrow therapeutic index and alcohol related dehydration and electrolyte disturbance can precipitate lithium toxicity

NB. Be aware of the possibility of hepatic failure or reduced hepatic function in chronic alcohol misusers. See page 293. Also note risk of hepatic toxicity with some recommended drugs (e.g. valproate).

References

1. Weathermon R & Crabb DW. Alcohol and medication interactions. *Alcohol Res Health* 1999; **23**: 40–51.
2. Tanaka E. Toxicological interactions involving psychiatric drugs and alcohol: an update. *J Clin Pharm Ther* 2003; **28**: 81–95.
3. Salmela KS, Kessova IG, Tsyrlov IB *et al*. Respective roles of human cytochrome P-4502E1, 1A2, and 3 in the hepatic microsomal ethanol oxidizing system. *Alcohol Clin Exp Res* 1998; **22**: 2125–2132.
4. Stahl S (1996). Essential Psychopharmacology: neuroscientific basis and practical applications. Cambridge University Press, UK.

Further reading

British National Formulary (2004). Appendix 1: drug interactions. British Medical association and Royal Pharmaceutical society of Great Britain.

ABPI Compendium of Summaries of Product Characteristics. Available at www.medicines.org.uk

Stockley I (1996). Alcohol Interactions in: Drug Interactions. The Pharmaceutical Press, London UK.

Miscellaneous

Nicotine

The most common method of consuming nicotine is by smoking cigarettes. One-third of the general population, 40–50% of those with depression and up to 90% of those with schizophrenia smoke[1]. Nicotine causes peripheral vasoconstriction, tachycardia and increased blood pressure[2]. Smokers are at increased risk of developing cardiovascular disease. As well as nicotine, cigarettes also contain tar (a complex mixture of organic molecules, many carcinogenic), a cause of cancers of the respiratory tract, chronic bronchitis and emphysema[3].

Nicotine is highly addictive. People with mental illness are 2–3 times more likely than the general population to develop and maintain a nicotine addiction[1]. Chronic smoking contributes to the increased morbidity and mortality from respiratory and cardiovascular disease that is seen in this patient group. Nicotine also has psychotropic effects. Smoking can affect the metabolism (and therefore the efficacy and toxicity) of drugs prescribed to treat psychiatric illness[4]. Nicotine use may be a gateway to experimenting with other psychoactive substances.

Psychotropic effects

Nicotine is highly lipid-soluble and rapidly enters the brain after inhalation. Nicotine receptors are found on dopaminergic cell bodies and stimulation of these receptors leads to dopamine release[1]. Dopamine release in the limbic system is associated with pleasure: dopamine is the brain's 'reward' neurotransmitter. Nicotine may be used by people with mental health problems as a form of 'self-medication' (e.g. to alleviate the negative symptoms of schizophrenia or antipsychotic-induced EPSEs or for its anxiolytic effect[5]). Drugs that increase the release of dopamine reduce the craving for nicotine. They may also worsen psychotic illness (see under smoking cessation below).

Nicotine improves concentration and vigilance[1]. It also enhances the effects of glutamate, acetylcholine and serotonin[5].

Schizophrenia

Up to 90% of people with schizophrenia regularly smoke cigarettes[1]. Possible explanations are as follows: smoking casues dopamine release, leading to feelings of well-being and a reduction in negative symptoms[5]; alleviation of some of the side-effects of antipsychotics such as drowsiness and EPSEs[1], and cognitive slowing[6], as a means of structuring the day (a behavioural filler) or as a means of alleviating the deficit in auditory gaiting that is found in schizophrenia[7]. Nicotine may also improve working memory[8]. It has been suggested that people with schizophrenia find it particularly difficult to tolerate nicotine withdrawal symptoms[4].

Depression and anxiety

In 'normal' individuals a moderate consumption of nicotine is associated with pleasure and a decrease in anxiety and feelings of anger[9]. The mechanism of this anxiolytic effect is not understood. People who suffer from anxiety and/or depression are more likely to smoke and find it more difficult to stop[9,10]. This is compounded by the fact that nicotine withdrawal can precipitate or exacerbate depression in those with a history of the illness[9]. Patients with depression are at increased risk of cardiovascular disease. By directly causing tachycardia and hypertension[2], nicotine may, in theory, exacerbate this problem.

Movement disorders and Parkinson's disease

By increasing dopaminergic neurotransmission, nicotine provides a protective effect against both drug-induced EPSEs and idiopathic Parkinson's disease. Smokers are less likely to suffer from antipsychotic-induced movement disorders than non-smokers[1] and use anticholinergics less often[4]. Parkinson's disease occurs less frequently in smokers than in non-smokers and the onset of clinical symptoms is delayed[1].

Drug interactions

Polycyclic hydrocarbons in cigarette smoke are known to stimulate the hepatic microsomal enzyme system, particularly P4501A2[5], the enzyme responsible for the metabolism of many psychotropic drugs. Smoking can lower the blood levels of some drugs by up to 50%[5]. This can affect both efficacy and side-effects and needs to be taken into account when making clinical decisions. The drugs most likely to be affected are: clozapine, fluphenazine, haloperidol, chlorpromazine, olanzapine, many tricyclic antidepressants, mirtazapine, fluvoxamine and propranolol.

Withdrawal symptoms[4]

Withdrawal symptoms occur within 12–14 hours of stopping smoking and include depressed mood, insomnia, anxiety, restlessness, irritability, difficulty in concentrating and increased appetite. Nicotine withdrawal can be confused with depression, anxiety, sleep disorders and mania. It can also exacerbate the symptoms of schizophrenia.

Smoking cessation

People with mental health problems generally have low motivation to stop smoking and may find withdrawal intolerable[8]. Although the efficacy of nicotine replacement treatments in people with enduring mental illness has not been evaluated in RCTs[11], the adverse effects of smoking on physical health are so great that patients should always be encouraged to stop. Nicotine replacement is available in the form of patches, microtabs, gum, lozenges and inhalers. Full details can be found in the *BNF*. Bupropion/amfebutamone (a noradrenaline and dopamine reuptake inhibitor) is also licensed for smoking cessation[12] and may be effective even in schizophrenia[13].

References

1. Goff DC, Henderson DC, Amico E. Cigarette smoking in schizophrenia: relationship to psychopathology and medication side-effects. *Am J Psychiatry* 1992; **149**: 1189–1194.
2. Benowitz NL, Hansson A, Jacob P. Cardiovascular effects of nasal and transdermal nicotine and cigarette smoking. *Hypertension* 2002; **39**: 1107–1112.
3. Anderson JE, Jorenby DE, Scott WJ *et al.* Treating tobacco use and dependence: an evidence based clinical practice guideline for tobacco cessation. *Chest* 2002; **121**: 932–941.
4. Douglas M, Ziedonis P, George TP. Schizophrenia and nicotine use: report of a pilot smoking cessation programme and review of neurobiological and clinical issues. *Schizophr Bull* 1997; **23**: 247–254.
5. Edward R, Lyon M. A review of the effects of nicotine and schizophrenia antipsychotic medication. *Psychiatr Serv* 1999; **50**: 1346–1350.
6. Harris JG, Kongs S, Allensworth D *et al.* Effects of nicotine on cognitive deficits in schizophrenia. *Neuropsychopharmacology* 2004; **29**: 1378–1385.
7. McEvoy JP, Freudenreich O, Wilson HW. Smoking and therapeutic response to clozapine in patients with schizophrenia. *Biol Psychiatry* 1999; **46**: 125–129.
8. Jacobsen LK, D'Souza DC, Mencl WE *et al.* Nicotine effects on brain function and functional connectivity in schizophrenia. *Biol Psychiatry* 2004; **55**: 850–858.
9. Alexander H, Glassman MD. Cigarette smoking: implications for psychiatric illness. *Am J Psychiatry* 1993; **150**: 546–552.
10. Wilhelm K, Richmond R, Wodak A. Clinical aspects of nicotine dependence and depression. *Medicine Today* 2004; **5**: 40–46.

11. Ziedonis DM, Williams JM. Management of smoking in people with psychiatric disorders. *Curr Opin Psychiatry* 2003; **16**: 305–315.
12. Electronic SPC. Zyban, 2002.
13. George TP, Vessicchio JC, Termine A *et al.* A placebo controlled trial of bupropion for smoking cessation in schizophrenia. *Biol Psychiatry* 2002; **52**: 53–61.

Further reading

De Leon J, Mahmood D, Canuso C *et al.* Schizophrenia and smoking: an epidemiological survey in a state hospital. *Am J Psychiatry* 1995; **152**: 453–455.
Desai HD, Seabolt J, Jann MW. Smoking in patients receiving psychotropic medications: a pharmacokinetic perspective. *CNS Drugs* 2001; **15**: 469–494
Zevin S, Benowitz N. Drug interactions with tobacco smoking. *Clin Pharmacokinet* 1999; **36**: 425–438.

Miscellaneous

Caffeine

Caffeine is probably the most popular psychoactive substance in the world. Mean daily consumption in the UK is 350–620 mg[1]. A quarter of the general population and half of those with psychiatric illness regularly consume over 500 mg caffeine/day[2]. Caffeine has *de novo* psychotropic effects and may also worsen existing psychiatric illness. It may also interact with psychotropic drugs.

Table Caffeine content of drinks	
Brewed coffee	100 mg/cup
Instant coffee	60 mg/cup
Tea	45 mg/cup
Soft drinks	25–50 mg/can

Chocolate also contains caffeine. Martindale lists over 600 medicines that contain caffeine[3]. Most are available without prescription and are marketed as analgesics or appetite suppressants.

Pharmacokinetics

Caffeine is rapidly absorbed after oral administration and has a half-life of 2.5–4.5 hours. It is metabolised by CYP1A2, a hepatic cytochrome enzyme that may exhibit genetic polymorphism. Metabolic pathways also become saturated at higher doses[4]. These factors may account for the large interindividual differences that are seen in the ability to tolerate caffeine[5].

Psychotropic effects

Caffeine is associated with CNS stimulation and increased catecholamine release[6]. Low-to-moderate doses are associated with favourable subjective effects such as elation and peacefulness[2]. Doses of >600 mg/day invariably produce anxiety, insomnia, psychomotor agitation, excitement, rambling speech (and sometimes delirium and psychosis)[7]. In sensitive people, these effects are produced by much lower doses. At high doses, caffeine can inhibit benzodiazepine-receptor binding[6,7]. Tolerance develops to the effects of caffeine and an established withdrawal syndrome exists (headache, depressed mood, anxiety, fatigue, irritability, nausea, dysphoria and craving)[8].

Caffeine intoxication (caffeinism)

The DSM-IV[9] defines caffeinism as the recent consumption of caffeine, usually in excess of 250 mg accompanied by five or more of restlessness, nervousness, excitement, insomnia, flushed face, diuresis, GI disturbance, muscle twitching, rambling flow of thought and speech, tachycardia or cardiac arrhythmia, periods of inexhaustibility and psychomotor agitation, when these symptoms cause significant distress or impairment in social, occupational or other important areas of functioning *and* are not due to a general medical condition or better accounted for by another mental disorder (e.g. an anxiety disorder).

Schizophrenia

Patients with schizophrenia often consume large amounts of caffeine-containing drinks[1]. This may be to relieve dry mouth (as a side-effect of antipsychotic drugs), for the stimulant effects of caffeine (to relieve dysphoria/sedation/negative symptoms) or simply because coffee/tea drinking structures the day or relieves boredom. Excessive caffeine consumption is of concern because caffeine increases the release of catecholamines and so may theoretically precipitate or worsen psychosis. Kruger[6] found that large doses of caffeine can worsen psychotic symptoms (in particular elation and conceptual disorganisation) and result in the prescription of larger doses of antipsychotic drugs. De Freitas and Schwartz[10] found that the removal of caffeine from the diets of chronically disturbed (challenging behaviour) patients, led to decreased levels of hostility, irritability and suspiciousness. These findings have not been replicated in less disturbed populations[11].

Caffeine can also interfere with the effectiveness of drug treatment. Clozapine serum levels can be raised by up to 60%[12], presumably through competitive inhibition of CYP1A2. Other drugs metabolised by this enzyme, such as olanzapine, imipramine and clomipramine, may be similarly affected. The potential effects of caffeine on the metabolism of other drugs, as well as the potential to induce a caffeine-withdrawal syndrome, should always be considered before substituting caffeine-free drinks.

Mood disorders

Caffeine may elevate mood through increasing noradrenaline release[13]. The practice of self-medication with caffeine to improve mood is common in the general population. Excessive consumption of caffeine may precipitate mania[14,15]. Depressed patients may be more sensitive to the anxiogenic effects of caffeine[16].

Caffeine can increase cortisol secretion (gives a false positive in the dexamethasone-suppression test)[17], increase seizure length during ECT[18] and increase the clearance of lithium by promoting diuresis[19]. Caffeine toxicity can be precipitated by drugs that inhibit CYP1A2. Fluvoxamine is an important example.

Anxiety disorders

Caffeine increases vigilance, decreases reaction times, increases sleep latency and worsens subjective estimates of sleep quality, effects that may be more marked in poor metabolisers. It can also precipitate or worsen generalised anxiety and panic attacks[20]. These effects are so marked that caffeine intoxication should always be considered when patients complain of anxiety symptoms or insomnia. Symptoms may diminish considerably or even abate completely if caffeine is avoided[21]. High doses of caffeine can reduce the efficacy of benzodiazepines (by reducing receptor binding[6,7]).

References

1. Rihs M, Muller C, Bauman P. Caffeine consumption in hospitalised psychiatric patients. *Eur Arch Psychiatry Clin Neurosci* 1996; **246**: 83–92.
2. Clementz G, Dailey JW. Psychotropic effects of caffeine. *Am Fam Physician* 1988; **37**: 167–172.
3. Martindale, *The Extra Pharmacopoeia*, 32nd edition. London: Pharmaceutical Press, 1999.
4. Kaplan GB, Greenblatt DJ, Ehrenberg BL *et al.* Dose-dependent pharmacokinetics and psychomotor effects of caffeine in humans. *Pharmacokinetics and Pharmacodynamics* 1997; **37**: 693–703.
5. Butler MA, Lang NP, Young JF *et al.* Determination of CYP1A2 and NAT2 phenotypes in human populations by analysis of caffeine urinary metabolites. *Pharmacogenetics* 1992; **2**: 1211–1214.
6. Kruger A. Chronic psychiatric patients use of caffeine: pharmacological effects and mechanisms. *Psychology Reports* 1996; **78**: 915–923.
7. Sawynok J. Pharmacological rationale for the clinical use of caffeine. *Drugs* 1995; **49**: 37–50.
8. Silverman K, Evans SM, Strain EC *et al.* Withdrawal syndrome after the double-blind cessation of caffeine consumption. *New Engl J Med* 1992; **327**: 1109–1114.
9. American Psychiatric Association. *Diagnostic and Statistical Manual of Mental Disorders*, 4th edition. Washington, DC: American Psychiatric Association, 1994.

Miscellaneous

10. De Freitas B, Schwartz G. Effects of caffeine in chronic psychiatric patients. *Am J Psychiatry* 1979; **136**: 1337–1338.
11. Roczapski A, Paredes J, Kogan C *et al*. Effects of caffeine on behaviour of schizophrenic inpatients. *Schizophr Bull* 1989; **15**: 339–344.
12. Carrillo JA, Herraiz AG, Ramos SL *et al*. Effects of caffeine withdrawal from the diet on the metabolism of clozapine in schizophrenic patients. *J Clin Psychopharm* 1998; **18**: 311–316.
13. Achor MB, Extein I. Diet aids, mania and affective illness. *Am J Psychiatry* 1981; **138**: 392.
14. Ogawa N, Oeki H. Secondary mania caused by caffeine. *Gen Hosp Psychiatry* 2003; **25**: 136–144.
15. Rauasia S. Mania associated with an energy drink: the possible role of caffeine, taurine and inositol. *Can J Psychiatry* 2001; **46**: 454–455.
16. Lee MA, Flegel P, Greden JF. Anxiogenic effects of caffeine on panic and depressed patients. *Am J Psychiatry* 1988; **145**: 632–635.
17. Uhde TW, Bierer LM, Post RM. Caffeine-induced escape from dexamethasone suppression. *Arch Gen Psychiatry* 1985; **42**: 737–738.
18. Cantu TG, Korek JS. Caffeine in electroconvulsive therapy. *DICP: Ann Pharmacother* 1991; **25**: 1079–1080.
19. Mester R, Toren P, Mizrachi I *et al*. Caffeine withdrawal increases lithium blood levels. *Biol Psychiatry* 1995; **37**: 348–350.
20. Bruce MS. The anxiogenic effects of caffeine. *Postgrad Med* 1990; **66**(Suppl. 2): 518–524.
21. Bruce MS, Lader M. Caffeine abstention in the management of anxiety disorders. *Psychol Med* 1989; **19**: 211–214.

Further reading

Drugdex Drug Evaluation. *Caffeine*. Micromedex Healthcare Series, Vol 109. Micromedex Inc. USA, 2002.
Paton C, Beer D. Caffeine: the forgotten variable. *Int J Psychiatry Clin Pract* 2002; **5**: 231–236.

Complementary therapies

A large proportion of the population currently use or have recently used complementary therapies (CTs)[1-4]. As health professionals are rarely consulted before purchase, a diagnosis is often not made and efficacy and side-effects are not monitored. The majority of those who use CTs are also taking conventional medicines[4] and many people use more than one CT simultaneously. Many do not tell their doctor[5]. The public associate natural products with safety and may be unwilling to report possible side-effects[6]. Herbal medicines, in particular, can be toxic as they contain pharmacologically active substances. Many conventional drugs prescribed today were originally derived from plants. These include medicines as diverse as aspirin, digoxin and the vinca alkaloids used in cancer chemotherapy. Herbal medicines such as St John's wort, *Gingko biloba* and valerian are increasingly used as self-medication for psychiatric and neurodegenerative illnesses[2,3,7]. Few CTs have been subject to randomised, controlled trials, so efficacy is largely unproven[2,8,9]. For a few complementary therapies, Cochrane Reviews exist. These include the use of kava to treat anxiety (some evidence of efficacy)[10], aromatherapy for behavioural problems in dementia (insufficient evidence, but worth further study)[11] and hypnosis for schizophrenia (insufficient evidence, but worth further study)[12]. There is little systematic monitoring of side-effects caused by CTs, so safety is largely unknown. Some herbs are known to be very toxic[13-17].

Whatever the perceived 'evidence base' for the use of complementary therapies, the feelings of autonomy engendered by taking control of one's own illness and treatment can result in important psychological benefits irrespective of any direct therapeutic benefits of the CT[4,18,19]. There are many different complementary therapies, the most popular being homeopathy and herbal medicine with its branches of Bach's flower remedies, and Chinese and Ayurvedic medicine. Non-drug therapies such as acupuncture and osteopathy are also popular. To master one can take years of study; therefore, to ensure safe and effective treatment, referral to a qualified practitioner is recommended. The majority of doctors and pharmacists have no qualifications or specific training in CTs. The following table gives a brief introduction. Further reading is strongly recommended.

References

1. Fisher P, Ward A. Complementary medicine in Europe. *BMJ* 2001; **309**: 107–111.
2. Barnes J, Anderson LA, Phillipson JD. *Herbal Medicines: A Guide for Health Care Professionals,* 2nd edition. London: Pharmaceutical Press, 2002.
3. Kessler RC, Soukup J, Davis RB. The use of complementary and alternative therapies to treat anxiety and depression in the United States. *Am J Psychiatry* 2001; **158**: 289–294.
4. Astin JA. Why patients use alternative medicine: results of a national study. *JAMA* 1998; **279**:1548–1553.
5. Berry MI, Tinorva E. The use of traditional Chinese medicine in Liverpool. *Pharm J* 1993; **251**: 12.
6. Barnes J, Mills SY, Abbot NC *et al.* Different standards for reporting ADRs to herbal remedies and conventional OTC medicines: face-to-face interviews with 515 users of herbal remedies. *Br J Clin Pharmacol* 1998; **45**: 496–500.
7. Pies R. Adverse neuropsychiatric reactions to herbal and over-the-counter 'antidepressants'. *J Clin Psychiatry* 2000; **61**: 815–820.
8. Kleijnen J, Knipschild P, Riet G. Clinical trials of homeopathy. *BMJ* 1991; 302: 316–323.
9. Reilly D, Taylor MA, Beattie NGM *et al.* Is evidence for homeopathy reproducible? *Lancet* 1994; **344**: 1601–1606.
10. Pittler MH, Ernst E. Kava extract for treating anxiety. The Cochrane Database of Systematic Reviews, 2003.
11. Thorgrimsen L, Spector A, Wiles A *et al.* Aroma therapy for dementia. Cochrane Database of Systematic Reviews, 2003.
12. Santiago I, Khan M. Hypnosis for schizophrenia. Cochrane Database of Systematic Reviews, 2004.
13. CSM. Kava Kava and hepatotoxicity. *Current Problems in Pharmacovigilance* 2002; **28**: 6.
14. CSM. Renal failure associated with traditional Chinese medicines. *Current Problems in Pharmacovigilance* 1999; **15**: 18.
15. CSM. Hypoglycaemia following the use of Chinese herbal medicine xiaoke wan. *Current Problems in Pharmacovigilance* 2001; **27**: 8.
16. Ernst E. Serious psychiatric and neurological adverse effects of herbal medicines – a systematic review. *Acta Psychiatr Scand* 2003; **108**: 83–91.
17. De Smet P. Health risks of herbal remedies: an update. *Clin Pharmacol Ther* 2004; **76**: 1–17.
18. Downer SM, Cody MM, McClusky P *et al.* Pursuit and practice of complementary therapies by cancer patients receiving conventional treatment. *BMJ* 1994; **309**: 86–89.
19. Oh VMS. The placebo effect: can we use it better? *BMJ* 1994; **309**: 67–70.
20. Fulder S. *The Handbook of Complementary Medicine,* 2nd edition. London: Hodder & Stoughton, 1989.
21 Mills SY. *The Essential Book of Herbal Medicine.* London: Penguin Arkana, 1991.
22. Pertiaric L, Shaw D, Murray V. Toxic effects of herbal medicines and food supplements. *Lancet* 1993; **342**: 180–181.
23. Wong AHC, Smith M, Boon HS. Herbal remedies in psychiatric practice. *Arch Gen Psychiatry* 1998; **55**: 1033–1044.
24. Aslam M, Davis SS. Heavy metal toxicity of some Asian medicines in the UK. *J Pharm Pharmacol* 1980; **32**: 83.
25. Homeopathy. *Effect Health Care Bull* 2002; 7: 1–12.

Further reading

Cooke B, Ernst E. Aromatherapy: a systematic review. *Br J Gen Pract* 2000; **455**: 444–445.
Ernst E, Rand JI, Stevinson C. Complementary therapies for depression. *Arch Gen Psychiatry* 1998; 55: 1026–1032.
Fugh-Berman A. Herb–drug interactions. *Lancet* 2000; **355**: 134–138.
Walter G, Rey JM. The relevance of herbal treatments for psychiatric practice. *Aust NZ J Psychiatry* 2000; **33**: 482–489.

Miscellaneous

Table An introduction to complementary therapies

	Homeopathy[11,12,20,25]	Herbal medicine (phytotherapy)[16,17,20-24]	Aromatherapy[20]
Health beliefs	• Treatment is selected according to the individual characteristics of the patient (hair colour and personality are as important as symptoms) • Treatment stimulates the body to restore health (there is no scientifically plausible theory to support this claim) • Like is treated with like (e.g. substances that cause a fever, treat a fever) • The more diluted the preparation, the more potent it is thought to be • Very potent preparations are unlikely to contain even one molecule of active substance	• Treatment is selected according to the individual characteristics of the patient (as with homeopathy) • Herbs are believed to stimulate the body's natural defences and enhance the elimination of toxins by increasing diuresis, defecation, bile flow and sweating • Attention to diet is important • The whole plant is used, not the specific active ingredient (this is believed to reduce side-effects) • Active ingredients vary with the source of the herb (standardisation is contrary to the philosophy of herbal medicine) • Herbalists believe that if the correct treatment is chosen, treatment will be completely free of side-effects	• Treatment is selected according to the individual characteristics of the patient (as with homeopathy and herbal medicine) • Illness is believed to be the result of imbalance in mental, emotional and physical processes, and aromatherapy is believed to promote balance • Purified oils are not used (the many natural constituents and believed to protect against adverse effects: similar to the beliefs held by herbalists) • There is no standard dose • Individual oils may be used for several unrelated indications
Used for	• A wide range of indications (except those outlined below) • May be taken with conventional treatments • Over 2000 remedies and many dilutions are available	• Everything except as outlined below • May be taken with conventional treatments but many significant interactions are possible (some have been reported) • Advertised in the lay press for a wide range of indications	• Everything except as outlined below • May be used as an adjunct to conventional treatments • Usually administered by massage onto the skin, which is known to relieve pain and tension, increase circulation and aid relaxation

	Homeopathy[11,12,20,25]	Herbal medicine (phytotherapy)[16,17,20-24]	Aromatherapy[20]
Not suitable for	• Infection • Organ failure • Vitamin/mineral/hormone deficiency	• Use in pregnancy and lactation (many herbs are abortifacient)[23] • Evening primrose oil should not be used in epilepsy[23]	• Use in pregnancy (jasmine, peppermint, rose and rosemary may stimulate uterine contractions) • Rosemary should be avoided in epilepsy and hypertension
Side-effects and other information	• None known or anticipated • Inactivated by aromatherapy and strong smells (e.g. coffee, peppermint, toothpaste) • Inactivated by handling • Healing follows the law of cure: symptoms disappear down the body in the reverse order to which they appeared, move from vital to less vital organs and ultimately appear as a rash (which is a sign of cure)	• Herbal remedies are occasionally adulterated (with conventional medicines such as steroids or toxic substances such as lead[24]) • Many side-effects can be anticipated (e.g. kelp and thyrotoxicosis, St John's wort and serotonin syndrome) • Overuse, adulteration, variation in plant constituents and misidentification of plants are common causes of toxicity Some Chinese herbs are toxic[13-15]	• Skin sensitivity • Significant systemic absorption can occur during massage • Ingestion can cause liver/kidney toxicity • All aromatherapy products should be stored in dark containers away from heat to avoid oxidation

Driving and psychotropic drugs

Many factors have been shown to affect driving performance. These include age, personality, physical and mental state and being under the influence of alcohol, prescribed medicines, street drugs or over-the-counter medicines[1]. Studying the effects of any of these factors in isolation is extremely difficult. Some studies have assessed the effect of medication on tests such as response-time and attention[2], but these tests do not directly measure ability or inability to drive.

It has been estimated that up to 10% of people killed or injured in road traffic accidents (RTAs) may be taking psychotropic medication[3]. Patients with personality disorders and alcoholism have the highest rates of motoring offences and are more likely to be involved in accidents[3]. Driving while unfit through taking prescribed or illicit drugs is an offence and may lead to prosecution. People whose driving ability may be impaired through their illness or prescribed medication should inform their insurance company. Failure to do so is considered to be 'witholding a material fact' and may render the insurance policy void.

Table Psychotropics and driving (see www.dvla.gov.uk)	
Drug	*Effect*
Hypnotics and anxiolytics	Benzodiazepines cause sedation and impaired attention, information processing, memory and motor co-ordination. The impairment is dose-related and greater with longer half-life drugs. When used as anxiolytics, benzodiazepines have been associated with an increased risk of RTAs[4]. One study found that zopiclone (despite having a short half-life) dramatically increased the risk of RTAs[4]. Another suggests middle-of-the-night administration of zolpidem can negatively affect driving ability[5].
Antipsychotics	Sedation and EPSEs can impair coordination and response time[1]. A high proportion of patients treated with antipsychotics may have an impaired ability to drive[6,7]. One study found patients with schizophrenia taking atypical antipsychotics or clozapine performed better in tests of skills related to car-driving ability than patients with schizophrenia taking typical antipsychotics[8]. Clinical assessment is required.
Antidepressants	TCAs have been associated with an increased risk of RTAs[9], although negative studies also exist[4]. SSRIs[10] and MAOIs may be safer long term but probably not during the acute phase of the illness[11] (where impairments may be illness- rather than medication-related[12]).
Anticonvulsants	Initial, dose-related side-effects may affect driving ability (e.g. blurred vision, ataxia and sedation). There are strict rules regarding epilepsy and driving.
Lithium	Lithium may impair visual adaptation to the dark[1] but the implications for driving safety are unknown. Elderly people who take lithium may be at increased risk of being involved in an injurious motor vehicle crash[13].
Alcohol	Alcohol causes sedation and impaired coordination, vision, attention and information-processing. Alcohol-dependent drivers are twice as likely to be involved in traffic accidents and offences than licensed drivers as a whole[3], and a third of all fatal RTAs involve alcohol-dependent drivers[3].

Miscellaneous

Effects of psychiatric medicines

Many psychotropics can impair alertness, concentration and driving performance. Drugs that block H_1, α_1-adrenergic or cholinergic receptors may be particularly problematic. Effects are particularly marked at the start of treatment and after increasing the dose. It is important to stop driving during this time if adversely affected. The use of alcohol will further increase any impairment.

Drug-induced sedation

Many psychotropic drugs are sedative. The more sedative a drug is, the more likely it is to impair driving ability. Other medicines, either prescribed or bought over the counter, may also be sedative and/or affect driving ability (e.g. antihistamines[3]). One study found that 89% of patients taking other psychotropic drugs in addition to antidepressants failed a battery of 'fitness to drive' tests[11]. Since the degree of sedation any individual will experience is very difficult to predict, patients prescribed sedative drugs should be advised not to drive if they feel sedated.

DVLA regulations

Although the DVLA give quite specific guidelines regarding illness and ability to hold a driving licence (see summary of DVLA regulations), the rules regarding taking medication and driving are rather more vague.

Note 6 of the 'At a Glance' guidelines for psychiatric disorders states that 'Driving while unfit through drugs ... is an offence', but what 'unfit through drugs' means appears to be at the discretion of the medical practitioner and individual concerned. The possible effects of various drugs are then listed, as in the table on the previous page.

DVLA – duty of the client
'If you have a medical condition which has become worse since your licence was issued, or you develop a new medical condition, you must write and inform the Drivers Medical Unit at the DVLA of the nature of your condition.' A list of the 'conditions' that interest the DVLA is provided, but medication used to treat these conditions is not mentioned specifically. Insurance companies should also be informed.

DVLA – duty of the prescriber
Doctors must advise patients on the effects that their illness and prescribed medication may have on their 'fitness to drive'. See also below.

The guidance also specified that patients under S17 of the MHA must be able to satisfy the standards of fitness for their respective conditions and be free from any effects of medication which would affect driving adversely, before resuming driving. Very few patients will fulfil these criteria.

GMC guidance on confidentiality[14]

If a patient lacks the capacity to understand the advice given by the doctor about "fitness to drive" or drives contrary to that advice, it is the duty of the doctor to inform the DVLA. This duty is absolute. There is no room for discretion.

In order to persuade a patient to desist from driving, their next of kin may be directly informed of the patient's lack of 'fitness to drive'.

Table Summary of DVLA regulations

Diagnosis	Group 1 Entitlement (cars and motorcycles)		Group 2 Entitlement (heavy goods or public service vehicles)	
	Notify DVLA?	Notes	Notify DVLA?	Notes
Uncomplicated anxiety or depression (without significant memory or concentration problems, agitation, behavioural disturbance or suicidal thoughts)	No	Consider effects of medication (see page 357).	No	Very minor short-lived illnesses need not be notified to DVLA. Consider effects of medication (see page 357).
Severe anxiety states or depressive illnesses (with significant memory or concentration problems, agitation, behavioural disturbance or suicidal thoughts)	Yes	Driving should cease pending the outcome of medical enquiry. A period of stability will be required before driving can be resumed.	Yes	Licence revoked for minimum of 6 months. Driving usually permitted if illness long-standing but controlled on medication that does not impair driving.
Acute psychotic disorders of any type	Yes	Driving must cease during the acute period. Relicensing can be considered (hypomania/mania following an isolated episode only) when all of the following conditions can be satisfied: a) has remained well and stable for at least 3 months b) is compliant with treatment c) has regained insight (hypomania/mania only) d) is free from adverse effects of medication which would impair driving e) subject to a favourable specialist report. Drivers with a history of instability or poor compliance will require a longer period off driving.	Yes	Licence revoked for at least 3 years. Driving will only be permitted again if medication is minimal and does not interfere with driving ability and there is no significant likelihood of relapse.
Hypomania/mania	Yes	See Acute psychotic disorders of any type. Repeated changes of mood: when there have been four or more episodes of mood swing in the last 12 months, at least 6 months' stability is required under condition (a) (above).	Yes	As above.
Chronic schizophrenia	Yes	See Acute psychotic disorders of any type. Continuing symptoms even with limited insight do not necessarily preclude driving. Symptoms should be unlikely to cause significant concentration problems, memory impairment or distraction while driving.	Yes	As above.

	Yes		Yes	
Dementia or any organic brain syndrome	Yes	Patient should inform DVLA (see guidance overleaf) Decision regarding fitness to drive based on medical reports. In early dementia, licence may be issued subject to annual review.	Yes	Licence revoked.
Learning disability	Yes	Severe LD – licence application will be refused. Mild LD – must be declared by patient on licence application form. Provisional licence may be issued: liaise with DVLA.	Yes	Only persons with minor degrees of learning disability will be considered for a licence.
Behaviour disorders (e.g. violent behaviour)	Yes	Court or patient should inform DVLA. Licence revoked. Licence reissued only after behaviour has been satisfactorily controlled. Medical report required.	Yes	Licence refused/revoked. Possibility of licence if person matures and psychiatric reports confirm stability.
Alcohol misuse 'Persistent misuse of alcohol confirmed by medical enquiry'	Yes	Licence refused/revoked for confirmed, persistent alcohol misuse until minimum of 6 months' controlled drinking or abstinence attained. Medical reports required.	Yes	Same as Group I except **I year's** controlled drinking or abstinence required.
Alcohol dependency	Yes	Licence refused/revoked until a 1-year period free from alcohol problems attained. Abstinence usually required. Medical reports required. Additional restrictions if seizures occur.	Yes	Licence not granted if there is a history of alcohol dependency in the past 3 years. Additional restrictions if seizures occur.
Alcohol-related disorders (e.g. psychosis)	Yes	Patient should inform DVLA. Medical reports required. Licence usually refused/revoked until satisfactory recovery.	Yes	Licence refused/revoked.
Drug misuse and dependency NB: Benzodiazepines prescribed above BNF limits for any reason constitute misuse/dependency for DVLA purposes	Yes	Licence revoked until drug-free period shown below is attained. Assessment and urine screen arranged by DVLA **may** be required. **6-month drug-free period** for cannabis, amphetamines, ecstasy and other psychoactive substances. **1-year drug-free period** for heroin, morphine, methadone (there are exceptions for those on a supervised maintenance programme), cocaine and benzodiazepines. Additional restrictions if seizures occur.	Yes	Licence revocation until drug-free period attained. Assessment and urine screen arranged by DVLA **will normally** be required. **1-year drug-free period** for cannabis, amphetamines, ecstasy and other psychoactive substances. **3-year drug-free period** for heroin, morphine, methadone, cocaine and benzodiazepines. Additional restrictions if seizures occur.
Full information can be found at: www.dvla.gov.uk.				

References

1. Metzner JL, Dentino AN, Goddard SL. Impairment in driving and psychiatric illness. *J Neuropsychiatry* 1993; **5**: 211–220.
2. Ray WA, Thapa PB, Shorr RI. Medications and the older driver. *Clin Geriatr Med* 1993; **9**: 413–438.
3. Noyes R. Motor vehicle accidents related to psychiatric impairment. *Psychosomatics* 1985; **26**: 569–580.
4. Barbone F, McMahon AD, Davey PG *et al.* Association of road-traffic accidents with benzodiazepine use. *Lancet* 1998; **352**: 1331–1336.
5. Verster JC, Volkerts ER, Schreuder AH *et al.* Residual effects of middle-of-the-night administration of zaleplon and zolpidem on driving ability, memory functions, and psychomotor performance. *J Clin Psychopharm* 2002; **22**: 576–583.
6. Grabe HJ, Wolf T, Gratz S *et al.* The influence of clozapine and typical neuroleptics on information processing of the central nervous system under clinical conditions in schizophrenic disorders: implications for fitness to drive. *Neuropsychobiology* 1999; **40**: 196–201.
7. Wylie KR, Thompson DJ, Wildgust HJ. Effect of depot neuroleptics on driving performance in chronic schizophrenic patients. *J Neurol Neurosur Psychiatry* 1993; **56**: 910–913.
8. Brunnauer A, Laux G, Geiger E *et al.* The impact of antipsychotics on psychomotor performance with regards to car driving skills. *J Clin Psychopharm* 2004; **24**: 155–160.
9. Currie D, Hashemi K, Fothergill J *et al.* The use of anti-depressants and benzodiazepines in the perpetrators and victims of accidents. *Occup Med* 1995; **45**: 323–325.
10. Hindmarsh I, Harrison C. The effects of paroxetine and other antidepressants in combination with alcohol on psychomotor activity related to car driving. *Acta Psychiatr Scand* 1989; **80**(Suppl. 350): 45.
11. Grabe HJ, Wolf T, Gratz S *et al.* The influence of polypharmacological antidepressive treatment on central nervous information processing of depressed patients: implications for fitness to drive. *Neuropsychobiology* 1998; **37**: 200–204.
12. Gerhard U, Hobi V. Cognitive-psychomotor functions with regard to fitness for driving of psychiatric patients treated with neuroleptics and antidepressants. *Neuropsychobiology* 1984; **12**: 39–47.
13. Etminan M, Hemmelgarn B, Delaney JAC *et al.* Use of lithium and the risk of injurious motor vehicle crash in elderly adults: case-control study nested within a cohort. *BMJ* 2004; **328**(7439): 558–559.
14. Morgan JF. DVLA and GMC guidelines on 'fitness to drive' and psychiatric disorders: knowledge following an educational campaign. *Med Sci Law* 1998; **38**: 28–31.

Further reading

Niveau G, Kelley-Puskas M. Psychiatric disorders and fitness to drive. *J Med Ethics* 2001; **27**: 36–39.

Miscellaneous

Communication with patients/service users

Follow the CAAT system.

Consultative

Those being prescribed medication should be consulted about their preferences with regard to adverse effects and likely outcomes with different medication. Patients' informed preferences should influence drug choice. Ideally, patients themselves should choose which medication they are prescribed. When patients are too ill to be consulted about drug choice, the opportunity for informative discussion should be provided as soon as appropriate.

Accurate

Patients have the right to factually accurate information about medicines and prescribing choices. Health-care workers should recognise the limits of their knowledge and refer for expert advice when necessary. Consider, also, the provision of written information and patient telephone helplines.

Appropriate

Information should be presented in such a way that it can be readily understood. It is more important to tell patients how medication affects symptoms than to try to explain complex theories of drug action. It is rarely necessary to discuss, for instance, receptor theory, but likely outcomes should certainly be discussed. Everyone should be afforded the opportunity to be given more information, having first reflected on the information initially provided or after having gained first-hand experience of medication prescribed.

True

Patients have the right to be told the truth about medicines. It is morally right to impart all *relevant* information to those prescribed medication. Being 'economical with the truth' is unethical and likely to damage relationships and perhaps lead to litigation. Clearly, it is impossible to tell patients everything that is known about a particular medication, but it is possible to direct patients to more comprehensive, well-grounded sources of information.

Use of antibiotics in psychiatry

Antibiotics are possibly the most frequently prescribed non-psychotropics in psychiatric institutions. Their use in psychiatry is often complicated by a number of factors: the absence of in-house specialist microbiologist advice; lack of experience or knowledge of modern antibiotic therapy; and restrictions on possible routes of administration because nursing staff are unlikely to hold necessary certification.

The following table sets out broad guidelines for the use of antibiotics in some commonly encountered conditions. In using this table, some general guidance should be noted:

- Take samples for microbiological examination before starting treatment.
- Start with oral therapy unless patient is very unwell or if condition requires a parenteral-only agent.
- Consult microbiology (where available) sooner rather than later – certainly if treatment has had no effect after 48 hours, ideally before starting treatment.
- Always check allergy status before giving any antibiotic. Check casenotes, the prescription chart and ask the patient.
- Be aware of the risk of antibiotic-associated colitis. Consult microbiology if this is suspected.

Infection/condition	1st line treatment	2nd line treatment
Ears, e.g. otitis externa, otitis media	• Consult microbiologist if otitis media suspected • Chloramphenicol 0.5% drops, four times daily	Neomycin or polymyxin drops
Fungal infections	Mouth/pharynx – Nystatin suspension (100 000 iu/ml), 1 ml four times daily Skin – Clotrimazole 1% cream three times daily Systemic or resistant skin infection – fluconazole 50 mg daily for 7–14 days Nail – terbinafine 250 mg daily (see *BNF* for duration)	Fluconazole Fluconazole Consult microbiology Consult microbiology
Gastroenteritis	Not usually indicated – consult microbiology	
Pelvic inflammatory disease	Collect high vaginal swab; if *Neisseria gonococcus* excluded: Metronidazole 400 mg three times daily for seven days plus doxycycline 100 mg twice daily for 2 weeks Give after food	Consult microbiology
Respiratory tract infections	Amoxycillin 250 mg three times daily or Erythromycin 500 mg three times daily	Co-amoxiclav 375 mg three times daily or Clarithromycin 250 mg twice daily
Throat infection	Usually has viral cause. Consult microbiology; if streptococcus confirmed: Phenoxymethylpenicillin 250 mg four times daily or cefadroxil 500 mg twice daily or erythromycin 500 mg three times daily	Consult microbiology
Tuberculosis	Consult microbiology	
Urinary tract infections	Trimethoprim 200 mg twice daily or amoxycillin 250 mg three times daily	Nalidixic acid 1 g four times daily or co-amoxiclav 375 mg three times daily or ciprofloxacin 250 mg twice daily
Vaginal candidiosis	Oral fluconazole 150 mg as a single dose or clotrimazole 500 mg vaginal pessary	Consult microbiology
Wounds, ulcers, pressure sores	Do not use topical agents If cellulitis present – consult microbiology	

Index

MAUDSLEY DISCUSSION PAPERS

There are currently eight discussion papers in print, as follows:

The titles above are priced at £4 each, including postage & packing.

Please make cheques payable to *King's College London* and send to:

Carole Dockett, Neuropsychiatry – P068, Institute of Psychiatry, De Crespigny Park, Denmark Hill, London SE5 8AF. Tel: 020 7848 0138. email: c.docket@iop.kcl.ac.uk